TELEPHONE TRIAGE:

Theory, Practice, and Protocol Development

Sheila Quilter Wheeler, RN, MA
with Judith H. Windt, PhD

Photographs by Richard Wheeler

NOTICE TO THE READER

The authors and publisher have made every effort to provide accurate information. However, they are not responsible for errors, omissions, or for any outcomes related to the use of the contents of this book and take no responsibility for the use of the products and procedures described.

Treatments described in this book are based on research and consultation with nursing, medical and legal authorities. To the best of our knowledge, the recommendations in this book reflect safe practice; nevertheless, they cannot be considered absolute and universal recommendations. The authors and publisher disclaim any responsibility for any adverse effects resulting from the suggested procedures, or from any undetected errors from the readers misunderstanding of the text.

TeleTriage Systems Publishers
44 Madrone Avenue
San Anselmo, CA 94960
415.453.8382
sw@teletriage.com

Printed in the United States of America

Library of Congress Cataloging in Publication Data

Wheeler, Sheila Q.
Telephone Triage: Theory Practice and Protocol Development
Includes bibliographical references and index

ISBN 978-0-9830769-3-3

1. Emergency Nursing 2. Triage (Medicine) 3. Telephone in medicine
4. Crisis Intervention (Psychiatry)

***** Note Regarding Telephone Triage Audio CD *****

The 60 minute Audio CD containing audio vignettes from 10 case studies is an integral part of the Audio Activities section at the end of the book. Due to publishing limitations this CD is not included with this book. However it will be sent to you upon purchase using the address information supplied when the book is purchased.

TABLE OF CONTENTS

CHAPTER 3 COMMUNICATION

SECTION 2

CHAPTER 4 TELEPHONE TRIAGE AND THE NURSING PROCESS

CHAPTER 6 HIGH-RISK POPULATIONS

SECTION 3

CHAPTER 7 CRISIS INTERVENTION

APPENDICES

FOREWORD

For 100 years, the telephone has given us unprecedented freedom in communication. The spectrum of uses for the phone has broadened considerably in just the past 20 years. Most of its expanded utility has resulted from technological innovations—facsimile machines, modems, satellites, answering machines. For the caller in crisis, however, advances in training for telephone triage have stood relatively still—that is, until now. A revolution has begun in this expanded nursing role. This book is about that revolution.

When I met Sheila Wheeler on a sunny Sunday morning in San Francisco, I was struck not only by her passionate interest in telephone triage, but by her vision of the field as an emerging subspecialty. Her pioneering work is a must for every student of nursing, and also has direct application to the work of the emergency medical dispatcher.

In 1979, the medical dispatcher was identified as the weak link in the delivery chain of emergency medical services. Since that time, an entire medical dispatch science has evolved to correct this sometimes lethal oversight. It took over 10 years for that evolution to result in a national standard of care for educating dispatchers. To date, such a revolution has not happened in the area of telephone triage by nurses.

The nurse has always acted as an advocate of the patient. But, as has been shown with paramedics and emergency medical technicians, physical expertise and understanding of bedside nursing principles do not necessarily add up to efficiency in history taking, evaluation, caregiving, and direction performed by phone. As a further limitation, telephone triage must be done without any visual clues whatever, and quite often, through a friend or relative. The potential for error when a patient is mistriaged is immense. As of the winter of 1992, I am aware of 13 current lawsuits in the United States involving the misadventures of ungoverned, untrained public safety dispatchers. As a rough estimate, these incidents will eventually cost municipalities and insurance companies between $50 million and $100 million.

Yet the state of telephone triage by both dispatchers and nurses remains largely at the "Dodge City" level—a state of lawlessness in which people can do whatever they want, whenever they want, to whomever they want. This doesn't sound like good risk management to me. In this excellent textbook, Sheila Wheeler has brought forward the first comprehensive work in the subject for the practicing nurse in the office, HMO, or hospital. Nurses and medical dispatchers alike can benefit from her clear and detailed presentation of a field of medical and nursing practice that until now has been either poorly defined or forgotten.

Anyone who believes that the way to avoid the ills of medical triage is simply not to do it fails to realize that every treatment and every decision in medicine has its consequences. Callers in crisis need rapid but careful evaluation, advice, and treatment. The work can be done right. Wheeler's excellent book has made that old phrase "hold the phone" safer and more effective than ever.

Jeff J. Clawson, M.D.
President, National Academy of Emergency Medical Dispatch

Dedication from the Author

To the vision, creativity, and resourcefulness of the expert nurse.

PREFACE

Access to health care is one of the most critical issues facing the industry in the 1990s. Access includes not only on-site appointments, diagnoses, and treatments, but also advice, information, counseling, and referral—often dispensed by telephone. Increased access to health care enhances cost effectiveness and empowers clients but must be safe, effective, and appropriate. Until recently, telephone triage was seen as unimportant. However, it promises to be a key vehicle for the delivery of health care services in the 21st century. It represents an expanded role for nurses with significant potential as a tool for client education and consumer advocacy.

However, as the "new kid on the block," telephone triage is still in an embryonic stage of development. As a novice telephone triage nurse, I was appalled by the lack of standards and became convinced that many mistakes could be prevented through formal training. Several years ago, I designed an orientation program that evolved into a series of seminars. These seminars led to the writing of a home study program and the original primer for telephone triage.

The material presented in this text is based on *The Fine Art of Telephone Triage*, published in the spring of 1988. I have since updated and adapted the material, incorporating new research, case histories, examples of model systems, and expert opinion to illustrate models of good practice. This new book reflects current practice and state-of-the-art information. It is based on 20 years of published research, personal experience, and interviews with experts. I have integrated the concepts of Benner, Marker, and Clawson, pioneers in the field of nursing expertise, quality assurance, and medical dispatch, respectively. Their writings and concepts form the foundation of this text.

HOW TO USE THIS BOOK

This text will enable telephone triage nurses to expand their roles and to practice with greater confidence, refinement, and sophistication. It provides guidelines for interview and documentation skills, protocol development, and applications for high-risk populations. It is a self-study course, designed to serve as a companion to a book of protocols as well as a text for improving practice and implementing new systems.

I wrote this book for all nurses who practice telephone triage, either formally or informally. Although the HMO "advice center" is most representative of current practice, the information applies to settings such as the office or clinic, and agencies such as hospice, public health, home health, occupational health, poison control, emergency departments, and student health. The content and concepts can be used to train physicians and emergency medical dispatchers (EMD).

One of the major difficulties in writing this book was to be authoritative about this newly developing and controversial field. In addition, most current studies focused on physicians' practice of "telephone medicine" rather than nurses. Thus, I have extrapolated from these studies to support my suggestions. Please bear in mind that the field is still fraught with controversy. At one end of the spectrum are those who maintain that no one should give advice over the phone. At the other are those who want technicians to perform the service with the aid of highly structured artificial intelligence computer systems. I agree with the experts who feel that nurses are best suited to perform telephone triage.

In the last decade, nurses have worked diligently to integrate nursing diagnoses into their existing nursing care plans and protocols. Although I believe that nursing will ultimately benefit from standardized diagnoses, it will take time before nurses successfully implement this step in every specialty. After much consideration, I decided not to use the current North American Nursing Diagnosis Association (NANDA) system. Instead I chose the "symptom-based" system now in current use in many telephone triage programs.

I had three reasons for this decision. First and most importantly, nursing diagnosis (and medical diagnosis, for that matter) presupposes empirical or firsthand knowledge or observations, which is impossible in telephone triage. Physicians appreciate these limitations and are reluctant to diagnose by phone, relying instead on a presumptive or "working diagnosis" approach, a safer, more effective and appropriate method which takes into consideration the limits of telephone triage practice. Secondly, most clients present symptoms in lay terms and prefer questions, answers, and explanations in nonmedical language. Finally, in telephone triage, timing is crucial. For nurses to switch their thinking from NANDA language to lay language many times each hour would be extremely burdensome.

Most of the examples cited, including those presented in the exercises, are based on actual case histories collected from nurses practicing in the field. Names of nurses and callers are fictional. The chapter exercises are based on Bloom's taxonomy of educational objectives, and are arranged in ascending order from knowledge and comprehension to application, analysis, and evaluation. The exercises can be used either for self-study or for group exercises.

Although most exercises can be performed by an individual, group learning offers additional benefits. Therefore, wherever possible, I encourage using preceptors to facilitate the mock call and protocol writing sections. I also encourage nurses to create their own mock call exercises and to audiotape their calls to further enhance self-evaluation and feedback. Finally, I recommend that all managers institute "phone rounds" (review of problematic calls) on a regular basis as a QA measure.

Standards, quality assurance, crisis intervention, and nursing expertise are covered in a general way only. I refer the reader to the texts by Marker (1988), Clawson and Dernocoeur (1988), and Benner (1984), which cover those subjects in greater detail. For additional information on psychological and medical crisis intervention, I refer the reader to Clawson and Dernocoeur's *Principles of Emergency Medical Dispatch* (1988), which presents the approach in more detail as well as a set of "pre-arrival instructions" or protocols.

Chapter five covers protocol and form design and development extensively and is intended to present models of excellence and design flaws. A task force of six expert nurses can create a customized set of protocols (using this book and the suggested resources) in about three to four months. This text is a cost-effective alternative to expensive and inflexible turnkey telephone triage programs. When protocols and a standards manual are combined with this book, they form the basis for a comprehensive system that can be customized to the needs of the sponsoring institution.

The Audiotape Activities section will help to further refine your analytical and critical skills. The Activities are designed to work with the *Telephone Triage Audiotape* containing reenactments of calls to suicide prevention, poison control, medical advice and the like. To order your *Telephone Triage Audiotape* simply complete the order form in the back of this book and return it to Delmar Publishers, Inc.

ACKNOWLEDGEMENTS

Writing this book has been an adventure, a test of faith and friendship, full of ups and downs. Four years ago, it took eight rejected proposals before finding a publisher who believed in the project. This was not surprising, since at that time telephone triage was a relatively unknown subject, and the market for a book like this was small. I thank Delmar Publishers and Beth Williams, my editor, for their support and encouragement. After 2 years of going it alone, I found a co-author and collaborator, Judith Windt, who shared the load with me, offering support, conscientious attention to detail, excellent insights, and feedback. My children Joe and Kate, and my husband Richard, have endured a distracted mother and wife as I wrestled with the book month after month.

I owe a special thanks to friends and my extended family—Jane Kennedy, Chree Quilter, Deborah Quilter, and Zida Borcich for their moral support, insight, encouragement, and especially their humor; my mentor/colleagues—Jeff Clawson, M.D., Carolyn Smith-Marker, M.S.N., and Jean Shepherd Ph.D., provided inspiration and encouragement.

Finally, the quality of certain sections was the result of collaboration with several key people. Barbara Siebelt R.N., B.A., gave enthusiastic support and timely contribution to the chapter on medicolegal aspects. Nancy Okamoto, R.N., M.S. gave a timely, expert appraisal and thoughtful suggestions for the audiotape exercise. Charles Clark did a meticulous and brilliant copy edit/review—resulting in a stronger and more lucid text. Thanks to all nurses who have shared their expertise and experiences, and offered criticism—all of which served to enhance and give credibility to this book. Finally, many thanks to Debra Norris, who helped with the preparation of the final manuscript—a painstaking and labor-intensive task.

ABOUT THE AUTHORS:

Since 1984, Sheila Quilter Wheeler has pioneered in the field of telephone triage through practice, research, writing, teaching, consulting, and media production. She assisted in the production of "Anonymous Heroes," an award-winning training videotape for medical dispatchers who work on 911. Ms. Wheeler has written for the *Journal of Emergency Nursing,* lectured nationally, and has been a guest lecturer at the Emergency Nurses Association Scientific Assembly and the Ambulatory Ob/Gyn conferences. She holds a diploma in nursing from St. Vincent's College of Nursing in Los Angeles, California, an MA in Film from San Francisco State University, and is currently pursuing a masters degree in community health nursing at the University of California, San Francisco. Ms. Wheeler is a member of the College of Fellows of the National Academy of Emergency Medical Dispatch (NAEMD).

Judith H. Windt, Ph.D., is a freelance health and medical writer living in Menlo Park, California. She has written about AIDS, blood banking, and pharmaceutical research, and has edited newsletters and published articles in medical journals. She is an active member of the American Medical Writers Association and is also the author of over a half-dozen published short stories and two novels.

Barbara Siebelt, B.A., R.N. is Assistant Vice President, Risk Management Consultant at Willis Corroon Corporation of Maryland. She was the first president of the American Association of Critical Care Nurses. Ms. Siebelt is also a staff nurse in the emergency department in Silver Springs, Maryland.

Richard Wheeler is a photographer based in San Rafael, California. Uses for his style of human interest photography span the commercial spectrum from annual reports to editorial illustration.

SECTION 1

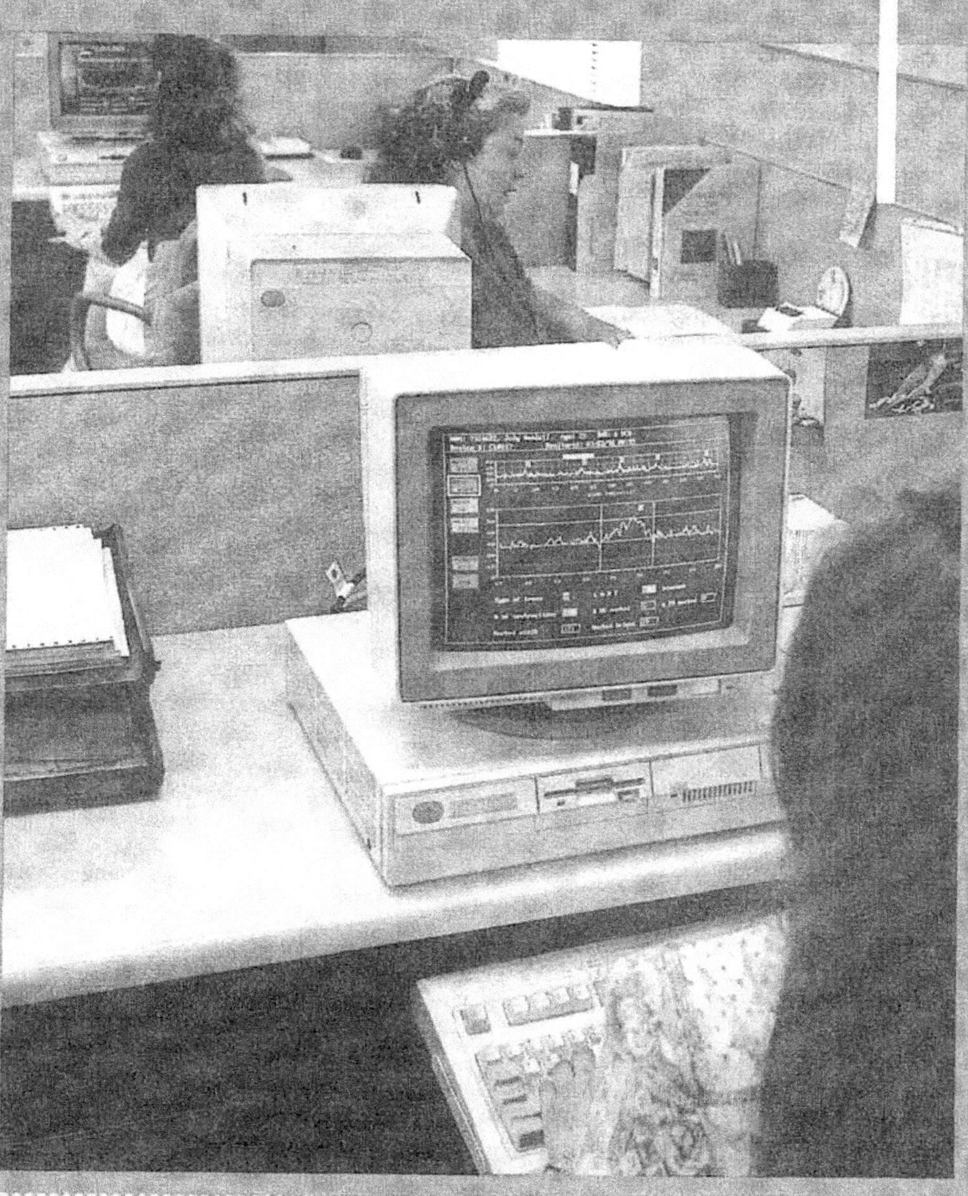

(Photo on previous page) *Nurses monitor and manage high-risk mothers at home using telemetry and the telephone. Advanced communication technology make is possible to visualize and document the caller's uterine activity. (Courtesy Kaiser Permanente, Northern California Regional Center for Preterm Birth Prevention. Santa Clara, California. Russ Lee, photographer.)*

CHAPTER 1
Telephone Triage: An Overview

Sometimes when I consider what tremendous consequences come from little things . . . I am tempted to think . . . there are no little things.
–Bruce Barton

TELEPHONE TRIAGE DEFINED

In one 8-hour shift, a telephone triage nurse may field up to 80 telephone calls—one every 6 minutes—painstakingly assessing headaches, newborn rashes, chest pain, possible allergic reactions, medication questions, and seasonal flu and fevers. Nurses may direct clients to obtain a second medical opinion or advise them where to find relevant, current information. They might counsel someone threatening suicide. Many traditional functions of emergency rooms, clinics, and physicians' offices have evolved into a new specialty called telephone triage.

Triage means a sorting out. Telephone triage involves ranking clients' health problems according to their urgency, educating and advising clients, and making safe, effective, and appropriate dispositions—all by telephone. It may include everything from AIDS counseling and child abuse hot lines to 911 and telemetry monitoring, and takes place in settings as diverse as emergency rooms and hospices.

HISTORY AND BACKGROUND

The concept of triage began during World War I in France. It was designed to salvage the "walking wounded" and not waste valuable resources on victims with fatal injuries. Informal telephone triage is as old as the telephone itself. In fact, one of the first calls made by Alexander Graham Bell was for assistance following a battery acid burn (Grumet, 1979). In the early days, physicians were quick to install telephones in their offices, seeing that this new technology could help their practices. Currently, telephone management accounts for a large percentage of physicians' practices.

Health maintenance organizations (HMOs) were the first to institute advice (gatekeeper) services in the 1970s. In 1984 a small hospital emergency department (ED) in the Northwest developed a "24-Hour Nurse Advice" program. This later evolved into the first marketing (welcome mat) system complete with computerized protocols, a sophisticated advertising campaign, and tracking systems for future marketing ventures. A wide variety of similar systems have sprung up over the last decade. In 1990, the term "telephone triage" appeared on Medline® indexes, a formal acknowledgement of this new subspecialty.

Studies of Telephone Triage

As soon as telephone medicine emerged as a part of health care systems, researchers began to study the phenomenon. They found it sorely lacking. Studies in the past 20 years have uncovered serious faults in practice. Most research has focused on the quality of physicians' task performance in the office setting. Several authors have suggested that physicians and other health care providers show deficiencies in taking histories and identifying problems, frequently jumping to conclusions and discounting clients' previous history (Johnson & Johnson, 1990; Margolis et al, 1987; Sloane et al, 1985; Wood et al, 1989; Yanovski et al, 1992). Physicians especially spend more time giving treatment instructions than listening to the client. Overall, researchers judge assessments to be inadequate due to insufficient "talk time."

In a study of emergency department nurses' performances, Verdile, Paris, Stewart, and Verdile (1989) found that nurses also failed to collect adequate data and histories, provided erratic and faulty advice, had poor interviewing skills, and failed to use protocols or to document calls. The authors recommend that the ED adopt training programs modeled after the training program for emergency medical dispatchers set forth by Jeff Clawson, M.D. (Clawson & Dernocoeur, 1988).

Another study (Levy et al., 1980) found that emergency room staff often failed to obtain necessary baseline information and that treatment of clients was frequently "cavalier" (p. 327) and potentially dangerous. The researchers point out the need to develop ways to obtain more accurate information from clients. They suggest that the wide variation in advice given for similar complaints evidences a need for training.

A few studies (Fosarelli & Schmitt, 1987; Pitts & Whitby, 1990) have focused on physicians' dissatisfaction with what they feel is an extra burden on them. The large volume of calls during regular hours and frequent or inappropriate after-hours calls can contribute to fatigue, mistakes, stress, and frustration. One of these studies (Caplan & Straus, 1988) recommends a potentially risky practice for reducing after-hours calls: having a recording refer the client to a second number. Others offer a more reasonable solution: delegating telephone work to someone other than the physician. For example, Strain and Miller (1971) described how a nurse in a pediatric office was trained to assume a large part of the telephone workload. But this success story represents only a single individual trained to fill the needs of a particular office.

Not surprisingly, those studies critical of the current state of affairs call for development of *formal* training programs in telephone management. They suggest that *experience and observation are inadequate training methods.* They call for additional research focusing on protocols and specialized training. Fischer and Smith (1979) assessed the use of the telephone in a family practice setting. They note that in an earlier study (Katz, Pozen, & Mushlin, 1978), training of pediatric health assistants specifically to handle calls reduced the number of office visits and reduced home management of 30% of clients, a greater percentage than in their own study (6%), in which no training was done. Kelley and Mashburn (1990) surveyed telephone calls handled by nurse-midwives in a practice that included both certified nurse-midwives and physicians practicing obstetrics and gynecology (ob/gyn). Large percentages of nonpregnant (53.1%) and pregnant (46.6%) clients wanted counseling or information about medications or tests. The authors recommend more training in telephone technique, interviewing, and counseling methods, as well as physiologic principals and technical subject matter.

Clearly, nurses can learn to do telephone triage effectively and safely—if they are well trained, have access to high-quality protocols, and have frequent performance evaluations. A good rule of thumb (see Schmitt, 1980) is to delegate this important task to medical personnel *at a lower rank than physicians* (for economic reasons), but *with enough medical expertise* to perform the work safely and effectively. Because physicians have severe time constraints, nurses can offer much that physicians do not: listening to, communicating with, and teaching patients, and serving as advocates for better care.

Caller Population and Call Content

Studies have found predictable patterns of caller types, peak call periods, and call content. Armed with this knowledge, staff in offices, clinics, and emergency departments (EDs) can prepare for these calls by writing protocols for the most likely problems and establishing orderly procedures.

Who Calls? Women, children, and the elderly make up a large proportion of callers and clients in certain settings. In internal medicine, women called twice as often as men (Johnson & Johnson, 1990). In family and internal medicine practices analyzed by Radecki, Neville, and Girard (1989), a similar ratio was discovered. Knowles and Cummins (1984) found that while twice as many women as men called an ED, 27% of the calls were about someone else. In other studies in which more women called than men, the proportion of women callers was similar to that of the practice population (Curtis & Talbot, 1979; Spencer & Daugird, 1988).

Spencer and Daugird (1988) observed that the number of calls made about children under 2 years of age was disproportionately large compared to the number of children of that age in the family practice studied. In another study of a family practice, 17% of the calls were about children aged 1 to 4 years (Curtis & Talbot, 1979).

In two studies of family practice, researchers found that the elderly tend to be relatively frequent callers (Daugird & Spencer, 1989; Spencer & Daugird, 1988). Radecki, Neville, and Girard (1989) analyzed internal medicine practices and found that clients over 65 constituted 29.3% of those receiving telephone care, the largest proportion compared to other age categories.

When Do Clients Call? When considering all calls in a family practice, Spencer and Daugird (1988) found that while most occurred during office hours, 14.6% came on weekends. Of those coming in during the week, 13.5% occurred from 5:30 P.M. to 11:30 P.M. but only 8.3% came between 11:30 P.M. and 7:30 A.M.. In general practice offices, peak calling time was between 10 A.M. and noon (Johnson & Johnson, 1990). Knowles and Cummins (1984) report that peak calling time in an ED occurred during the same hours (10 A.M. to noon).

Half of all after-hours calls in a family practice occurred on weekends (Curtis & Talbot, 1979). Of those occurring on weekdays, most came between 5:30 P.M. and 11:30 P.M., with few calls coming during the middle of the night. Evens, Curtis, Talbot, Baer, and Smart (1985) report a similar pattern of late afternoon calls during the week in a family practice setting. The authors theorize that clients become aware of their own problems or symptoms after the demands of work are finished; or, if calling about their children in the late afternoon, they notice that the children are not well when they are reunited with them after work.

What Do Clients Call About? A few complaints make up the bulk of calls, although the chief complaint categories differ by specialty. For example, Fischer and Smith (1979) report that 25 common complaints made up 80% of calls in several family practice settings surveyed. Most common were upper respiratory infections (URI) (24.2%) and fever (15.9%), with all other categories representing less than 5% of the total each.

In other studies of family practices (Curtis & Talbot, 1979; Curtis & Talbot, 1980; Evens, Curtis, Talbot, Baer, & Smart, 1985; Spencer & Daugird, 1988), top diagnoses included gastrointestinal (GI) problems, URI, viral infections, minor trauma, back pain, anxiety, otitis, and urinary infection. Spencer and Daugird noted that almost twice as many of the calls were follow-ups to previously existing problems as opposed to new problems.

The specific types of complaints reported in a pediatric practice were similar to those in family practice settings. Levy et al. (1980) found that 85% of the calls were about respiratory problems, fever, GI problems, skin and infectious diseases, and trauma.

Johnson and Johnson (1990) surveyed seven internists and found that 39% of the calls were about acute concerns and 69% were about chronic problems. The top diagnoses, in rank order, were in the following categories: cardiology, gastroenterology, endocrinology, ear/nose/throat, pulmonary, and rheumatology.

In the ED investigated by Knowles and Cummins (1984), the top presenting problem categories (44% of the total) were GI, respiratory, ob/gyn, and trauma. Calls to an ob/gyn office show that not all clients are calling about symptoms. Aside from gynecological problems, which constituted the most frequent category among nonpregnant women, the top categories for calls were medication, counseling, test results or requests, and pain. Among pregnant women (excluding inquiries about pregnancy), the major categories were body systems complaints, counseling, test results or requests, pain, and medication (Kelley & Mashburn, 1990).

Thus, telephone triage nurses should expect calls about administrative issues, lab results, and prescriptions as well as about symptoms. Administrative calls comprised 13% and 12% of the total, respectively, in the practices investigated by Knowles and Cummins (1984) and Johnson and Johnson (1990). In these studies, 2% and 16%, respectively, of the calls were requests for laboratory results.

Until recently, little research has been done on medications prescribed over the phone. Johnson and Johnson (1990) found that the most frequently prescribed drug categories in rank order were antibiotic, cardiovascular, anti-inflammatory, analgesic, antihistamine/decongestant, GI, and psychotropic. Another 1990 study (Spencer & Daugird) found that 31.0% of calls to a rural two-person private family practice involved filling a prescription. The most frequently prescribed new prescription types in rank order were "upper respiratory (URI) drug treatment... (antihistamines, decongestants, and antitussives)." Next were "antibiotics, pain medications, psychotropics, steroid creams" and medications for musculoskeletal disorders (p. 206). The most frequently prescribed drugs that were refills, in rank order, were psychotropics, antihypertensives, pain medications, cardiac medications, drugs for upper respiratory infections, and antibiotics. Most of these drug classes suggest chronic conditions, for which clients would be likely to request refills.

Daugird and Spencer (1989), in their study of clients who are frequent users of telephone medicine, give a useful insight into the needs of frequent callers. They found that these clients were older, tended to call about chronic complaints rather than acute symptoms, and were more likely to be taking long-term or psychotropic drugs.

Practitioner and Client Satisfaction. Traditionally, physicians have found after-hours calls stressful and exhausting, while clients have eagerly sought this service. An early study shows that although family practice residents felt satisfaction with 70% of after-hours calls, they also felt angry and frustrated 13% of the time, and indifferent 17% of the time (Curtis & Talbot, 1979). This study raises some issues worth considering. Physicians judged that 40% of the calls were prompted by anxiety about a problem. These physicians were more likely to feel angry and frustrated about calls they felt had a psychosocial rather than an organic source. On the other hand, 49% of clients surveyed felt that *reassurance was more important than relief of symptoms.*

Johnson and Johnson (1990) corroborate these findings. They note that "two thirds of the phone calls resulted in 'discussion/reassurance' only" (p. 238) without need for an appointment. And 27% of the clients in the study by Evens, Curtis, Talbot, Baer, and Smart (1985) called because of worry or concern about a problem rather than because of physical discomfort from the problem itself. Sixty-six percent of the callers were satisfied with reassurance, advice, and explanation, as opposed to a specific action such as being seen. In an ambulatory care clinic, clients who had access to a telephone service for referrals, appointments, prescription refills, questions about insurance, or even "simply the need to talk to someone" (p. 741) showed significantly greater satisfaction with their care than did controls without access to the service (Stirewalt, Linn, Godoy, Knopka, & Linn, 1981).

Clearly, reassurance and thoughtful attention to client concerns, whether medical, informational, or even administrative, usually fills clients' needs and satisfies them. Out of the apparent conflict between practitioners' and clients' needs, a solution may emerge. Telephone encounters, if handled sensitively, can help eliminate unnecessary appointments (thus, in the long run, relieving physicians of some of their work load), can educate clients, and can improve the relationship between physician and client. Curtis and Talbot (1979) suggest a need for reorientation of medical practice "since the traditional organic approach frequently does not coincide with patients' needs or expectations" (p. 909).

CURRENT PRACTICE

Rising costs have changed the face of health care in the United States. Health care providers try to cope by decentralizing or limiting services. Clients try to cope by turning to the ED as their primary care provider.

Trends in Health Care

A mother delivers her firstborn and is discharged within 24 hours to go home.

An elderly woman returns home with tubes and dressings after a brief hospital stay for a hysterectomy.

A person with AIDS, unable to work, has lost his health insurance. He is at home, dying of cancer.

A stressed-out mother tries to cope at home with a premature infant who requires complicated care.

Following major elective surgery, a man from a distant part of the state stays in a "recovery care" hotel until he can manage riding home in the car several days later with his family.

A woman who has had exploratory surgery for infertility remains in the recovery room at the surgicenter for an hour before her husband takes her home.

What do the people in these scenarios have in common? They are caught in a major shift to a decentralized health care system. Spiralling costs have resulted in strategies to shorten hospital stays and ration health care. This shift has resulted in a proliferation of home health services and the diversion of health care to decentralized facilities. Unfortunately, rationing often makes health care unavailable to many who need it.

As a result, people are increasingly filling the gap by using hospitals, clinics, medical offices, EDs, and other facilities for telephone advice and support. While call volume is growing in all such facilities, EDs especially are experiencing an upsurge, as people use the ED as the primary provider. Because many clients, particularly the medically indigent, have no physician, calls which formerly

FIGURE 1.1 Telephone Triage: A Partial Solution to the Health Care Gap

INCREASED NEEDS	DIMINISHED RESOURCES
Growing uninsured population	Decreasing number of hospital beds
Growing AIDS population	Decreasing number of EDs
Growing elderly population	Rising health care costs→inaccessibility
Rising crack/AIDS infant population	Diagnosis related groups
Rising violence	Decreased health benefits
Rising maternal/child population	
Early hospital discharges	

WHERE TELEPHONE TRIAGE CAN HELP

Increasing telephone support for:
- Home health and ambulatory care
- Home deaths and hospices
- Home births, postpartum stays of 24 hours or less
- Hot lines (AIDS, suicide prevention, etc.)
- Home treatment via monitoring and telemetry

went to the physician's office now come to the ED. Staff and client perceptions of the services of the ED are widely divergent. Clients may think of the ED as everything from an advice hot line to a drop-in clinic to a trauma center. Clients rely on the free, professional, accessible, instantaneous medical advice available by telephone 24 hours a day. In fact, a 1984 study found that the community expected telephone triage as an expanded role of the ED (Knowles & Cummins).

Health care has become more complex, expensive, and specialized, thus making triage necessary to meet the needs of the high number of clients who require immediate attention. Telephone triage allows for a quick assessment to discern who takes priority. (See Figure 1.1.)

Within the current crisis in health care are the seeds of opportunity. Forces such as decentralization, rationing, specialization, and the growing use of EDs can produce new technology, new services, and new methods to deliver care. Telephone triage will be a major vehicle for health care in the 21st century, easing some of the stress and confusion engendered by the health care crisis.

Telephone Triage Today

Telephone triage practice has three dimensions: acuity, spectrum, and volume. *Acuity* refers to the urgency and the severity of the problem—whether, for example, it presents an immediate threat to life, limb, or a major organ. Calls may thus be classified as high, moderate or low acuity. Systems which triage problems of high acuity include 911 and EDs. Moderate-level problems are usually triaged by HMOs, clinics, and offices. Informational, referral, and AIDS hotlines handle problems of low-level acuity. *Spectrum* refers to the *range* of problems presented. For example, if presenting symptoms at a facility range from chest pain to chickenpox, it is a wide-spectrum system. On the other hand, if all the calls related strictly to AIDS information or ob/gyn problems, it is a narrow spectrum system. *Volume* refers to average number of calls per hour. Ten or more per

FIGURE 1.2 Acuity, Spectrum, and Volume of Calls in Different Systems

SYSTEM	ACUITY	SPECTRUM	VOLUME
Telephone triage (ED, clinic, advice)	High to Low	Wide	High
911 calls	High	Wide	Moderate
Crisis intervention hot line	High	Narrow	Moderate
Ob/gyn physician's office	High to Low	Narrow	Low

hour are considered high volume, five to ten are considered moderate volume, fewer than five are considered low volume.

Thus, as illustrated in Figure 1.2, dispatch centers are high-acuity, wide-spectrum facilities, whereas AIDS hotlines are low-acuity, narrow-spectrum systems. ED nurses may have the greatest challenge of all: their calls range from low to high acuity and include a wide spectrum of problems.

Currently, telephone triage is practiced in three major settings: EDs, HMOs, and marketing systems. It is also practiced in a number of minor settings, such as crisis and support lines. Of the major practitioners of telephone triage, EDs are the least organized and fail to confront the reality that they do now and will continue to receive an increasing volume of wide-spectrum, high-acuity calls. HMOs are better organized but often fail to live up to their own standards. Marketing systems are costly, well staffed, and well equipped, but standards may be inadequate and triage policies too restrictive or conservative. One attempt to set standards is Clawson's emergency medical dispatch program (Clawson & Dernocoeur, 1988), the most highly-developed model system to date.

The Emergency Department. EDs, though nominally high-acuity facilities, in reality receive calls and visits that encompass all levels of acuity and the full spectrum of problems. One study of the calls to an ED (Knowles & Cummins, 1984) illustrates this point well. Administrative calls (including lab test results) comprised 15% of the phone contacts, and 36% of the calls concerned routine ob/gyn, respiratory, and GI symptoms. Forty-eight percent dealt with minor problems, 32% were strictly informational, and 17% were urgent (requiring medical attention within a few hours). One-fourth of the callers described acute problems which required either first aid information or over-the-counter medications. Forty-four percent sought advice regarding problem disposition (whether they should come to the ED). Eight percent of the calls involved trauma, and only 1% were true emergencies.

Knowles and Cummins (1984) conclude that the use of EDs for telephone advice does bring benefits: ED medical advice reflects a true community need; it fills an important public relations need; and many callers (50%) view the ED as an extension of hospital services. On the other hand, such calls also create problems. Staff spent about 90 minutes per day on calls. The volume of calls increased during the late morning and early afternoon—periods of high ED activity. The staff viewed the calls as an interruption of more important work. Finally, advice was based on informal, on-the-job training and experience only, without the use of protocols. The authors make three recommendations: (1) that the ED make a single person responsible for performing telephone triage, spending 5 minutes per call, (2) that protocols be implemented, and (3) that documentation be required.

EDs sorely need to implement such advice. Even when taking calls about high-acuity problems (their traditional sphere of activity), the average ED lacks standards and training programs. Telephone triage performance has been found to be inadequate, with clerks or orderlies often making decisions regarding client disposition and advice. Two examples from a 1980 study point out shortcomings of such a system (Levy et al.):

> *A mother calling for her two-month-old infant gave a previous diagnosis of pneumonia. The infant had a high fever and trouble breathing. The nurse advised nose drops.*
>
> *Another parent reported that an 8-month-old infant, who had been previously diagnosed with otitis media and was on antibiotics, was acting confused and delirious. The nurse gave no further advice and failed to recommend that the child be brought in for observation.*

The ED staff (1) **failed to obtain baseline information,** (2) in 46% of the calls, **failed to obtain the age of the child,** and (3) frequently **gave advice without obtaining adequate histories**—thus violating three cardinal rules of telephone triage (Levy et al., 1980).

Two recent studies also found serious flaws (Verdile, 1989; Isaacman et al., 1992). In the 1989 study, for example, a research assistant posed as a caller. She reported that her father was having "bad indigestion and heartburn," a scenario that could reasonably be interpreted as myocardial ischemia. If additional questions were asked, she described the client as a "56-year-old man who smoked cigarettes, did not drink alcohol, and had no previous cardiac history" (p. 278). If additional questions were asked about the heartburn, the caller described it as "a squeezing sensation, in the chest, associated with nausea and sweating" (p. 279).

The data from the calls were analyzed and showed that:

- Three out of 46 nurses refused to give any advice or information over the phone, with two of those stating this was a hospital policy.
- Clerical employees answered and managed 9% of the calls.
- Over half (56%) of the nurses failed to ask the caller any questions about the client or the chief complaint.
- Thirty-two percent instructed the caller to give the client antacids, several giving this advice *after* receiving information which pointed to myocardial ischemia.
- One nurse advised the caller to give "sublingual nitroglycerin to the patient every five minutes" (p. 279). When the caller asked what nitroglycerin was and how to obtain it, the respondent told the caller to "ask any cardiac patient, they all have nitroglycerin" (p. 279).
- Only four nurses advised the caller to call 911 and have the client brought to the ED.

Thus, as demonstrated by these current studies, EDs often have inadequate resources to manage calls. Nurses may field calls without protocols, training, documentation, adequate staffing, or standards. Two recent policy statements (see Chapter 2, Figures 2.1 and 2.2) illustrate renewed concern about standards for telephone advice in the ED setting.

EDs are designed for on-site treatment of serious medical, trauma, drug, and emotional problems. In fact, as the uninsured population grows, EDs—even as their numbers diminish (Will, 1990)—are the only resource for the poor and uninsured, many of them acutely ill. If EDs do not use telephone triage more effectively, they will suffer increasing system dysfunction, inappropriate use, and waste of scarce resources.

Few emergency nurses openly acknowledge telephone triage as an expanded emergency nursing role. When surveyed informally, however, they admit to giving telephone advice despite administration directives forbidding it (Wheeler, 1989). Most are torn between providing what they consider reasonable and expected care by phone and suffering the legal consequences, and not providing care by phone at all.

Health Maintenance Organizations. In the early 1970s, several HMOs began to use nurses rather than physicians to screen calls. This "gatekeeper" approach is designed to cut costs by using less expensive staff (nurses rather than physicians) to eliminate unnecessary office visits and to encourage self-care at home when possible. When high standards are maintained, telephone triage in HMOs is a successful, highly appreciated, and integral part of the larger system. Although HMOs have the largest pool of nurses practicing telephone triage, few have developed the role. Some systems are actually understaffed, offer little training, have few standards, and rely heavily on protocols some of which are sketchy.

In addition, the gatekeeping function gives rise to an unanticipated danger (Kerr, 1989). Some HMOs specify that unless the problem is life-threatening, clients experiencing an emergency must use the HMO's own ED unless they obtain permission to go elsewhere, a practice that may result in delays. Clients or callers—already under stress—must decide for themselves whether to call the paramedics or the HMO, or whether to choose another, possibly closer, facility. They then risk a retroactive ruling against coverage if the HMO later decides they made the wrong decision.

Nonetheless, HMOs are often better organized than ED systems. Protocols are provided, although they may vary in quality and spectrum. Orientation is usually limited to several weeks of on-the-job training that consists of observing, emulating, and being monitored by a preceptor. Because gatekeeping is the major function of these systems, call volume is extremely high. Such intense, unrelenting workloads lead to burnout and lower standards. Nurses have computers to quickly access information such as the caller's name, medical record on numbers of calls answered and minutes elapsed before management of the problem. Many nurses resent this use of computers and feel demeaned and harassed by such a bottom-line mentality—leading to lower morale.

Although HMO advice systems were the first to recognize telephone triage as a separate subspecialty, training and standards in these systems have failed to keep pace with technological advances. For example, some HMOs are developing computerized protocols but have failed to develop training programs for protocol design, in a sense, putting the cart before the horse. The resulting protocols are often flawed and ill conceived. The computerized version is essentially an electronic book of poorly written protocols, weak in content while *appearing* very sophisticated in form. Because of this high-tech equipment (telephone systems and computers), many systems look impressive at first. Upon closer inspection, however, the nurses who staff them may be undertrained and overworked. Such programs may not be user-friendly and fail to provide safe, effective, and appropriate dispositions.

Hospital Marketing Systems. Community relations are a major marketing force in today's competitive health care market. In the mid-1980s one group of health care marketers saw the potential of telephone triage to simultaneously increase hospital revenue and to provide a community service. They created a telemarketing tool that enhances the hospital image while encouraging increased ED visits and use of in-house programs, services, and physicians. Like other marketing systems, it started out as a physician referral system, later adding the advice component.

Marketing systems tend to be high-tech and marketing-intensive. Nurses are referred to as "telemarketers," who track client populations and later develop other marketing strategies based on the statistics they collect. These marketing systems come with generic advertising packages (radio, television, billboard, and newspaper ads), a direct mail campaign, and promotional items including phone stickers, refrigerator magnets, mugs, and T-shirts. Marketing systems are very costly (in 1988, $42,000 for a turnkey package, and between $160,000 and $360,000 annually for expenses) and by one estimate can garner over $300,000 in increased hospital revenue per year (Health Care Advisory Board, 1988). Most systems are sold with an exclusive geographic marketing area, giving the hospital a competitive advantage against other local hospitals. A survey of marketing systems showed an increase in ED visits and new hospital admissions (Health Care Advisory Board, 1988).

Although marketing systems are models of high-tech sophistication, they discourage nursing autonomy by using extremely conservative protocols. On the plus side, marketing systems often are staffed better than HMOs and many have higher "talk time" standards (10 calls per hour or 6 minutes per call).

One "anti-marketing" system (Smith, 1990) targets the medically indigent. Among its goals is to "save . . . tax dollars currently being wasted due to ignorance and inappropriate use of the health care system" (p. 21). The assumption is that many problems are safely manageable at home if callers receive sound advice and if they are warned about possibly life-threatening developments. Such a program could, for example, ease the ED burden. It offers recommendations on the level of health care needed, referral to a specific health care provider, and education. Because it has been proposed that this program be mandatory for clients on Medicaid and Medicare, the author acknowledges the need for the highest medical standards. Driven as they are by the bottom line, however, such programs risk being overly strict gatekeepers and limiting needed health care.

Hot Lines and Support Lines. With the continued breakdown in the health care system and the rise of consumerism in health care, it is not surprising that hot lines have proliferated over the last 20 years (Figure 1.3). The telephone, that most accessible and democratic of all communications tools, is the vehicle for everything from AIDS information to cocaine abuse counseling to parental stress counseling. Most of these "mini-systems" are staffed by lay counselors and may provide companionship, information, referral, or may act as a safety net for the medically indigent. One support line links bored, lonely, frightened, or troubled latchkey children with older adults who have been trained to talk and listen to children. All the calls are reviewed; potential problems, such as reports of teachers hitting children, are followed up; and volunteers are instructed to use 911 in emergencies (Marshall, 1977).

FIGURE 1.3 Telephone Triage Offshoots: Minisystems and Hot Lines

This list is a small sample of the hundreds of hot lines and other programs operating nationwide.

GRANDMA, PLEASE: intergenerational support hot line for latchkey kids

HELPLINE: counseling and crisis intervention hot line located at the site of potential suicide (bridge phone)

DOCTORS BY PHONE: 900 hot line medical advice for $3 per minute

TELECARE: emotional support for the elderly

CHEST PAIN HOTLINE: information and triage for all chest pain

LIFELINE: emergency monitoring for the elderly

PHYSICIAN FINDER: physician referral

COPELINE: parental stress support line

PHARMACY DRUG INFORMATION SERVICE: 24-hour drug information hot line

DIAL-A-DIETICIAN: hot line to disseminate nutrition information

800-4-CANCER: cancer information, referral, and support group

800-222-LINK: self-help clearinghouse in California for statewide support group referral

TEL MED: taped medical information

TEL HOSPITAL: reassurance and informational tapes for clients anticipating surgery or diagnostic tests

AIDS and HERPES hotlines: information, support group referral

COCAINE HOTLINE: chemical abuse counseling, information and referral

SUICIDE PREVENTION: counseling, referral, psychological crisis intervention

RAPE HOTLINE: counseling, support groups, informational referral

HEALTHCALL: medical information by telephone for 300 health topics 24 hours a day for $1.50

HEALTHLINK: health information, physician referral and community resource referral

LUNGLINE: nurses answer questions on respiratory disease, allergies and immune disorders

---

Other mini-systems include more specialized versions of marketing systems and target populations such as the elderly, children, and women. Some hospitals have library-based information hot lines that are marketing vehicles for in-house programs.

Crisis Lines. Obvious examples of crisis intervention lines are poison control centers, suicide prevention lines, and 911. When demand drove hundreds of hospital EDs to became poison control centers, they failed to train staff adequately or to expand facilities or personnel. As a result, ED staff were ill prepared for crisis calls about poisonings. A 1983 study (Thompson, Trammel, Robertson & Reigart) concluded that incorrect treatment recommendations were nine times greater in EDs than in regional poison control centers. Another study showed that regional centers had continuous availability, comprehensive information, written protocols, and qualified staff. They surpassed ED poison control centers in populations served, call volume, staffing, medical direction, staff orientation and follow-up protocols (Geller, Fischer, Leeper, & Ranganathan, 1988). By the mid-1980s, most of the ED poison control hot lines shut down and regional poison control centers took their place. Even among regional centers, however, standards vary from community to community. For example, some poison control staff require that victims always come to the ED, while others often treat clients over the phone.

Callback Systems. An unanticipated development of telephone triage is the rising number of hospital callback programs. Nurses or social workers called back selected clients who had been discharged from the ED (Jones, Bradford, & Dougherty, 1987) or from regular hospital stays (Cave, 1989; Riley, 1989). Of the ED clients, 95% felt the calls were useful and felt they should be continued. Health care workers were able to provide useful follow-up care in the form of additional advice about treatment or medications, clinic or physician visits, home health assistance, or rehospitalization. In addition, because of feedback provided by clients, one hospital altered procedures to decrease the discomfort of clients (Riley). With a simple phone call, these facilities were able to provide increased quality assurance and enhance their image with the public.

Another program encouraged post-myocardial infarction (MI) or cardiac surgery clients to call a nursing coordinator at any time of the day or night with questions and concerns (Nicklin, 1986). This program is part of an educational program that includes preoperative, postoperative, and predischarge teaching. While 43.6% of the calls required that clients go to the ED or contact their doctor, other callers were given information and home treatment advice. The author notes that some client concerns provide clues to needed predischarge education. She recommends a follow-up class for clients and families two weeks after discharge, based on call content.

Whether health professionals call clients or clients call the health facility, callback programs become a vehicle for increasing the hospitals' responsiveness to clients' needs. Both in direct health care and in education, callback systems are becoming a health management tool. A study by Wasson et al. (1992) showed phone calls could be successfully substituted for clinic appointments.

Other Uses of Telephone Triage. The telephone is being used as a health management tool in a number of new and creative ways. Tel-Med® offers communities all over the United States free recorded advice on over 200 health topics (Harsham, 1982). Many hospitals have physician referral services (Anon., *Hospitals,* May 20, 1987). One hospital uses regular phone calls from the coronary care unit nurse to post-MI clients to assess their conditions and to review the procedures for emergency health care. Then, if clients experience new MI symptoms, they call a hot line, transmit an electrocardiogram (EKG) as previously instructed, using a pocket-sized heart monitor, and may receive instructions to self-inject with lidocaine. Meanwhile, the nurse dispatches paramedics (Van Every & Curwen, 1985).

Emergency Medical Dispatch: A Model Program. Medical dispatchers are nonmedical personnel or paramedics who respond to calls for ambulance, fire, or police on 911. They assess by phone the need for emergency service and are responsible for dispatching medical rescue vehicles to victims. Fifty-percent of medical dispatchers are at least high school graduates, two thirds are female, and most have no previous medical training. (McMurray, *Personnel Communication,* June 15, 1992). Until recently, medical dispatchers were considered the weak link in the emergency response system.

In the late 1970s, Jeff Clawson, a Salt Lake City physician developed a system for emergency medical dispatch (EMD). Clawson's training program (Clawson & Dernocoeur, 1988) is the most complete and effective in the nation. The 40-hour program includes training and coaching techniques for CPR, the Heimlich maneuver, childbirth, and some 30 other medical problems. Such programs raise questions for ED physicians and nurses: if medical dispatchers are trained to coach by telephone, why are not physicians and nurses equally well trained?

Coordination of resources and equipment is a specialty of EMDs. With a knowledge of medical principles, they can ask the right questions and coordinate an intelligent system response. For example, they must have the judgment to reserve hazardous red-light-and-siren paramedic trips for true emergencies. They must be able to contact other resources such as poison control centers, child abuse agencies, and power companies at a moment's notice. They must be able to dispatch emergency vehicles efficiently, taking into consideration traffic, physical barriers, distance from the emergency, and other emergency locations from which vehicles may be returning. But the training Clawson and Dernocoeur (1988) urge also includes communications skills. For example, they mention the need for "training in hysteria control" (p. 4); for making a good impression by using a "warm, caring, polite, interested, nonjudgmental" voice (p. 11); and for avoiding an angry response to anger. While acknowledging the importance of experience, they also suggest that dispatchers learn to "wipe the emotional slate clean" (p. 11) between calls and avoid letting past experience influence present responses. Telephone triage nurses or physicians in EDs, clinics, or offices could also use these techniques.

Looking Into the Future. Currently, physicians can install highly efficient systems that enable them to practice office telephone triage as an integral part of client care (Ghitelman, 1988). A system with multiple lines, for example, allows calls to be automatically routed to the next higher number so that clients do not experience annoying and potentially dangerous busy signals. One-button dialing is available for emergency and frequently used numbers. Headsets free the hands to document calls. Simple expedients such as using an internal communication system can speed communication from room to room and maintain confidentiality.

More exotic technological developments in computers and telecommunications are also driving telephone triage to the frontiers of health care. In more formal systems, computers, for example, are used in marketing, quality assurance (QA) and advice. As marketing tools, they are used to track and compile demographic information; as QA tools, to compile statistics on staff productivity, call acuity, and staffing needs. In the future computerized protocols will expedite the advice as well as document the process. Computerized protocols will go beyond the "electronic book" stage, using artificial intelligence to make telephone triage more efficient and effective.

Telemetry is also expanding the horizons of telephone health care. Several recent studies have established the feasibility of monitoring clients at home via telemetry. Echocardiography transmitted by telephone has been used for children with heart disease (Finley et al., 1989). In a rural area, adults with heart disease can transmit their EKGs by placing the telephone mouthpiece on a transmitter positioned over their sternum (Zelus & Hughes, 1988). Computerized home telemetry has been used to monitor blood pressures of hypertensive pregnant women from their homes (Dalton, Manning, Roberts, Dripps, & Currie, 1987). Women at risk for preterm labor have been successfully monitored by tocodynamometry (Lindsay et al., 1990; Gonen, Braithwaite, & Milligan, 1990; Acker, Corwin, Sachs, & Schulman, 1989). Currently, nurses with one California company monitor uterine activity of high-risk obstetrical clients as far away as Alaska. Through telemetry and the tocodynamometer, nurses monitor clients 24 hours a day. This advanced technology eliminates the need for bed rest and makes lengthy and expensive preterm hospitalizations obsolete.

Integrated systems of computers and telecommunications may soon make it possible for medical personnel to see and hear clients while monitoring the client's heart and temperature by telephone. Telephone advances with fiberoptic technology and "video windows" will make such services possible ("Glass Cable," 1990). According to Clawson and Dernocoeur (1988), by the year 2025, callers to 911 will be able to defibrillate victims by using the earpiece and receiver of the telephone! As the 21st century approaches, telephone triage looks to an exciting future and expanding potential.

Meanwhile, a recent article in *The Wall Street Journal* ("Nurses on Call," 1991) yields some provocative statistics. An on-call nurse program established in an HMO in Detroit generated 10,000 calls in its first year. While research findings are not yet complete, the coordinator of the program found that 2,951 emergency room and clinic visits were prevented, savings totaled $48,000, physicians agreed with 99% of nurses' decisions, and clients were satisfied more than 92% of the time. Public enthusiasm is helping to make telephone triage an established part of the health care system.

CHAPTER 1

EXERCISE: TRUE/FALSE

Note to the reader: This is a pretest.

OBJECTIVE: To test current knowledge of telephone triage.

METHOD: Mark each statement true or false.

______ 1. A recent study found that nurse practitioners manage common pediatric problems by phone better than pediatricians.

______ 2. Pediatricians spend about 27% of their total practice time on the phone.

______ 3. When practiced effectively, telephone triage increases cost effectiveness.

______ 4. A severe language barrier is a "red flag."

______ 5. Children and frail elderly need not be given special consideration when doing telephone triage.

______ 6. Second-party information can sometimes be adequate for collecting data.

______ 7. Poor client triage results in missed diagnoses, increased client anxiety, office confusion, and legal liabilities.

______ 8. Benner's domains of nursing expertise have little relevance to telephone triage practice.

______ 9. Nurses must elicit information rather than solicit responses.

______ 10. In Perrin and Goodman's study, nurses spent less time per call than physicians.

______ 11. A study of medical students' telephone advice technique showed that as efficiency increased proficiency increased as well.

______ 12. A nurse recommending a self-help or support group should add a disclaimer statement.

______ 13. Most telephone triage nurses are taught to recommend libraries and bookstores as resources for health information to callers.

______ 14. There are hot lines for information and referral for herpes, AIDS, and parental support.

______ 15. Person-centered speech focuses on the nurse/client roles rather than an encounter between individuals.

______ 16. Self-help groups are voluntary, small groups structured for mutual aid, formed by peers, under a professional's direction and supervision, to help satisfy a common need, overcome a common handicap or life-disrupting problem, and bring about personal change.

______ 17. Mothers of twins have found the experience so stressful that they have formed Mothers of Twins Clubs.

______ 18. Women are at higher risk than men for AIDS, for completed suicide, and as victims of violent crime.

______ 19. Infants, especially those under 6 months of age, are considered to be at risk for complications of illness.

______ 20. Activities of daily living are not useful in assessing a child's state of health.

______ 21. La Leche League is a support group devoted to promoting natural childbirth and home deliveries.

______ 22. Parental stress hot lines can provide an outlet for negative emotions, help clients to define and solve problems, and instill confidence and self-esteem.

______ 23. Childbearing years are the ages of 20-50.

______ 24. Professional women are not considered by marketing firms to be a viable target for marketing of health care services.

______ 25. Common complaints presented by women of childbearing age include minor birth control complications, vaginal infections, abdominal pain, bleeding, and breast lumps.

______ 26. There are no support groups for women with endometriosis, women who've undergone mastectomies, new mothers, or women who have undergone cesarean sections.

______ 27. If no rape hot line is available in the community, the nurse must never offer any kind of advice because she might be considered legally liable.

______ 28. Old age is a low-risk period of life.

______ 29. The elderly are more susceptible to completed suicide than teenagers.

______ 30. Elderly persons often react to loss with anger, depression, or hypochondria.

______ 31. Threats or serious neglect are not considered child abuse.

______ 32. When faced with calls needing advanced or basic life support, the nurse should document name, address, phone number, age, complaint, level of consciousness, breathing, and heart status.

______ 33. When interviewing the client in a crisis situation, it is useful and permissible to use leading questions.

______ 34. Three possible transportation interventions for emergent or urgent calls are advanced life support transport, basic life support transport, or private car.

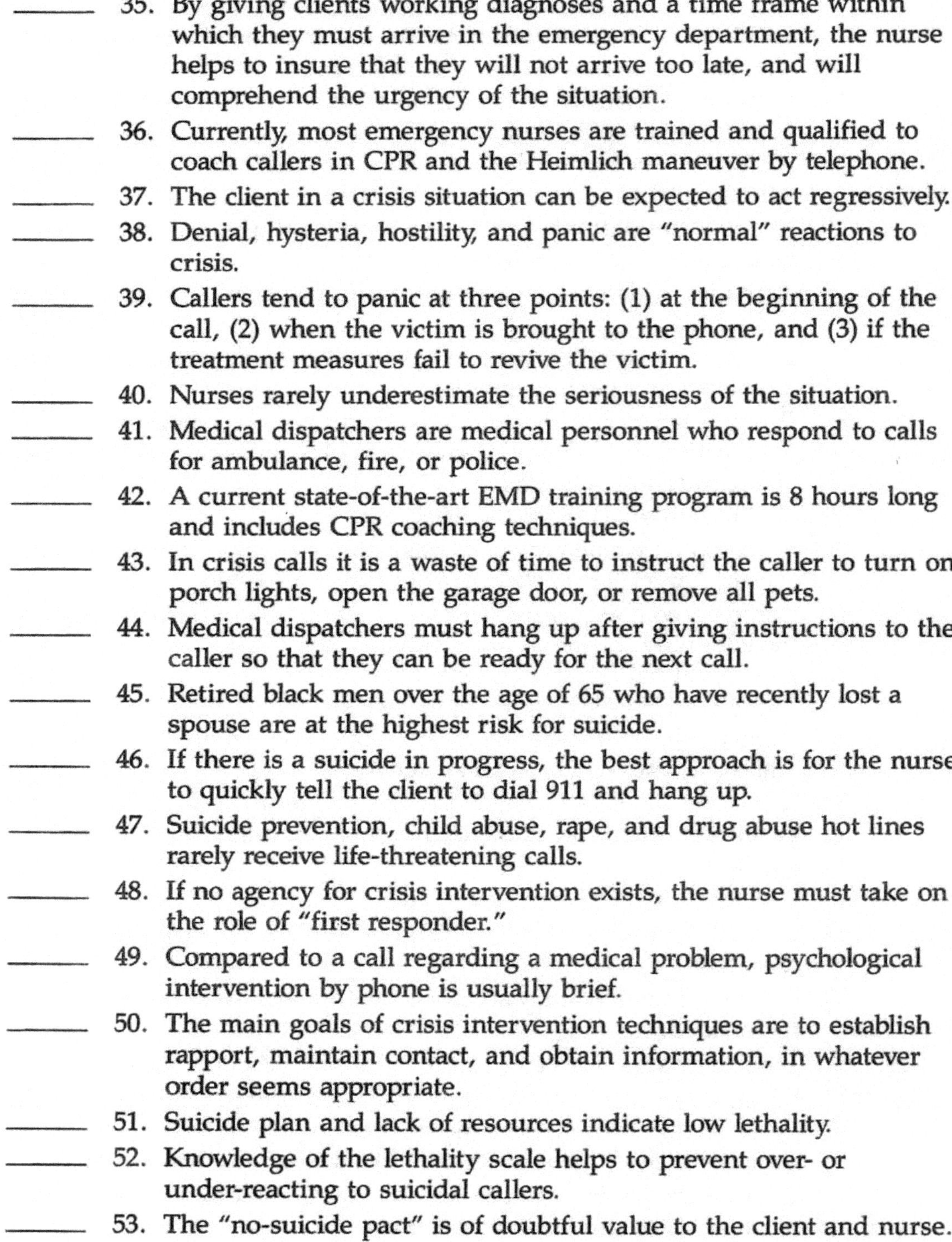

______ 35. By giving clients working diagnoses and a time frame within which they must arrive in the emergency department, the nurse helps to insure that they will not arrive too late, and will comprehend the urgency of the situation.

______ 36. Currently, most emergency nurses are trained and qualified to coach callers in CPR and the Heimlich maneuver by telephone.

______ 37. The client in a crisis situation can be expected to act regressively.

______ 38. Denial, hysteria, hostility, and panic are "normal" reactions to crisis.

______ 39. Callers tend to panic at three points: (1) at the beginning of the call, (2) when the victim is brought to the phone, and (3) if the treatment measures fail to revive the victim.

______ 40. Nurses rarely underestimate the seriousness of the situation.

______ 41. Medical dispatchers are medical personnel who respond to calls for ambulance, fire, or police.

______ 42. A current state-of-the-art EMD training program is 8 hours long and includes CPR coaching techniques.

______ 43. In crisis calls it is a waste of time to instruct the caller to turn on porch lights, open the garage door, or remove all pets.

______ 44. Medical dispatchers must hang up after giving instructions to the caller so that they can be ready for the next call.

______ 45. Retired black men over the age of 65 who have recently lost a spouse are at the highest risk for suicide.

______ 46. If there is a suicide in progress, the best approach is for the nurse to quickly tell the client to dial 911 and hang up.

______ 47. Suicide prevention, child abuse, rape, and drug abuse hot lines rarely receive life-threatening calls.

______ 48. If no agency for crisis intervention exists, the nurse must take on the role of "first responder."

______ 49. Compared to a call regarding a medical problem, psychological intervention by phone is usually brief.

______ 50. The main goals of crisis intervention techniques are to establish rapport, maintain contact, and obtain information, in whatever order seems appropriate.

______ 51. Suicide plan and lack of resources indicate low lethality.

______ 52. Knowledge of the lethality scale helps to prevent over- or under-reacting to suicidal callers.

______ 53. The "no-suicide pact" is of doubtful value to the client and nurse.

ANSWER KEY

EXERCISE: TRUE/FALSE

Numbers in parentheses indicate chapter in which correct answer may be found.

1. T (1)
2. T (6)
3. T (1)
4. T (4)
5. F (4)
6. T (4)
7. T (1)
8. F (3)
9. T (3)
10. F (3)
11. F (1)
12. T (4)
13. F (4)
14. T (1)
15. F (3)
16. F (4)
17. T (6)
18. F (6)
19. T (6)
20. F (4)
21. F (6)
22. T (6)
23. F (4)
24. F (6)
25. T (6)
26. F (6)
27. F (6)
28. F (6)
29. T (6)
30. T (6)
31. F (6)
32. F (7)
33. T (7)
34. T (7)
35. T (4)
36. F (7)
37. T (7)
38. T (7)
39. T (7)
40. F (7)
41. F (7)
42. F (1, 7)
43. F (7)
44. F (7)
45. F (7)
46. F (7)
47. F (7)
48. T (7)
49. F (7)
50. T (7)
51. F (7)
52. T (7)
53. F (7)

CHAPTER 2
Medicolegal Aspects of Telephone Triage

"Things which matter most must never be at the mercy of things which matter least."
–Goethe

The legal principles and practices discussed in this chapter may not be the same in all jurisdictions. Also, the issue of negligence, its scope and relationship to policies, and the relationship of employer policies to nursing standards as well as licensure are not covered in this chapter. However, the master-servant relationship between employer and employee has several implications, one being that the employer can be responsible for the actions of the employee (B. Siebelt, Personal communication, June 15, 1992). For a more complete discussion of these issues, please refer to Ford, 1985. While this chapter sets forth some general guidelines, it cannot completely answer all questions regarding the legalities of telephone triage.

THE DILEMMA OF TELEPHONE TRIAGE

From a legal standpoint, many telephone triage nurses consider the telephone more foe than friend. Because it is a fledgling specialty, telephone triage is controversial, and experts are still struggling to determine its legal parameters. There are few precedent-setting cases relating directly to telephone triage as practiced by nurses. However, it is possible to apply the legal principles derived from cases involving nursing in general to telephone triage. Many experts cautiously recommend practicing only with standards, training, protocols, and adequate staff (Katz, 1990; Scott & Packard, 1990; McGear & Simms, 1988; Politis, 1988; Dunn, 1985; Halberstam, 1977; Willett, 1977). On the other hand, hospital administrators almost unanimously forbid emergency department nurses to give advice by phone. Both the American College of Emergency Physicians (ACEP) and the Emergency Nurses Association (ENA) have issued statements regarding telephone advice (Figures 2.1 and 2.2), two of the few available guidelines.

FIGURE 2.1 American College of Emergency Physicians (ACEP) Statement on Emergency Telephone Advice

Telephone advice is often used to provide immediate information to a caller who is concerned that an emergency exists. The goal is to provide a public service while controlling costs by reducing unnecessary hospital visits. Although there is a recognized need to be responsive to the public, the College recommends against any substantial diagnosis or treatment recommendation by telephone. When any doubt exists, a recommendation should be made for the caller to come to the emergency department.

While telephone diagnosis is never recommended, the American College of Emergency Physicians endorses the following principles for dealing with the public's expectation for telephone advice:

- Clients who have recently been discharged from the emergency department may call for additional explanation of medical services already rendered to them, including response to questions about their medication, discharge instructions, or referral.
- Telephone advice should provide first aid information and recommendation on how to access medical care.
- Telephone advice should be given only by qualified medical professionals who know the limitations and ramifications of providing this service. The quality of telephone advice should be assured through the use of policies, protocols, documentation and quality assurance programs to monitor outcomes.

Statement approved by the ACEP Board of Directors, September 8, 1989

FIGURE 2.2 Emergency Nurses Association (ENA) Position Statement

Statement of Problem: Many consumers perceive the emergency department as a resource for free health care advice and guidance over the telephone. Rising health care costs as well as decreased or absent insurance coverage have contributed to an increase in the number of emergency department telephone calls for assistance and advice. Emergency nurses are often the emergency department personnel who answer these calls.

The caller may or may not accurately perceive or evaluate the urgency of the situation or condition that prompted the call. Often times the nurse may be asked to provide an opinion regarding potential medical or nursing diagnoses. When addressing medical diagnosis, the nurse may be in violation of state nurse practice acts and may be practicing beyond the scope of nursing practice. Whether addressing medical or nursing diagnoses, the emergency nurse providing advice over the telephone can be liable for that advice.

Emergency department telephone advice has been an integral component of emergency nursing practice in some institutions. However, in places that utilize this system, there are limited resources for nurses answering these calls.

Association Position: ENA believes that in the best interest of the patient, the nurse should not render opinions regarding diagnoses or treatment over the telephone. The emergency nurse should inform the person calling that the problem cannot be diagnosed over the telephone and that they should either come to the emergency department for examination and treatment or see their private physician or health care provider. In some cases, it may be necessary for the nurse to assess the urgency of the situation to determine if it is life threatening. In life-threatening situations, it may be appropriate for the nurse to teach CPR or other life saving measures over the phone. In these situations, Emergency Medical Services (EMS) should be accessed. The nurse should carefully document each conversation.

ENA recognizes that some institutions have developed sophisticated telephone triage programs. These programs should be predicated on clearly defined protocols with medical direction by experienced, professional emergency staff members. Staff members should have specialized education in triage, telephone assessment, legal aspects and limits and capabilities of the service. A quality assurance program is essential to assure quality control of the telephone triage program.

Rationale: With the best patient outcome in mind, emergency nurses should assess and evaluate each situation independently to determine actions that would result in the best patient outcome. The emergency nurse should also practice within the scope of their state nurse practice act while being aware of his/her own legal liability for advice given over the telephone.

Statement approved by the ENA Board of Directors, April 27, 1991

Herein lies a dilemma. Clearly, the recommendation of no advice is unfeasible. The telephone is a fact of life, and callers will continue to seek medical advice by phone. Nurses will risk liability by continuing to offer telephone advice because they feel a professional and personal obligation to do so. One study (Trautlien, Lambert, & Miller, 1984) notes an "irreducible minimum, a so-called 'white noise' of error in human activity" (p. 771). Even if one cannot eliminate all risk, one can reduce it by following what Trautien et al. describe as "one of the . . . operational definitions of excellence," that is, "doing ordinary things extraordinarily well" (p. 771). Because telephone triage is an extension of nursing practice, the best way to manage risk, to find a route out of the dilemma, is by doing the best and most professional job of which one is capable. This includes obtaining the highest degree of training and specialization possible under the circumstances (Tennenhouse, 1991). *At the same time, nurses must take care to do no more than what they are licensed to do in the first place.*

It is difficult to apply principles from other nursing specialties to telephone triage. For example, what is the nature of the nurse/client relationship on the phone? What exactly is the telephone triage nurse's responsibility? Is diagnosis by phone feasible? Do protocols and documentation provide risk management? While there are few definitive answers, existing nursing standards help address these questions and serve as a guide upon which to base telephone triage practice.

Telephone Triage as a Nursing Function

Telephone triage is a nursing function based on the nursing process (Scott & Packard, 1990; McGear & Simms, 1988). This process involves assessment, diagnosis, formulating a plan, intervention, and evaluation. Thus, standards applicable to nursing practice in general apply to telephone triage in particular. Nursing care must be "safe, effective and appropriate" (Marker, 1988).

Experts stress three procedures to help protect telephone triage nurses from legal liability: use of protocols, documentation of calls, and quality assurance checks (Dunn, 1985; McGear & Simms, 1988; Scott & Packard, 1990; Tennenhouse, 1991; Wood, 1986).

Mindlessly following a protocol will not protect a nurse from legal liability. As professionals, nurses must be accountable and autonomous. Accountability means the nurse makes conscientious use of protocols, complete documentation and adherence to standards and quality assurance guidelines. Autonomy means the nurse must use independent judgment and occasionally override protocols when the situation warrants it. Adhering to these principles helps defend against allegations of malpractice.

Although there is always the possibility of human error, protocols help maintain a high standard of consistent, thorough care over a wide variety of conditions (e.g., when the nurse becomes "burned out" during high-volume periods, or when the caller is emotionally overwrought). Protocols can be presented in court as examples of the advice habitually offered for a given problem in a particular institution. They are the standard of care for that institution.

Documentation is another safeguard. Thorough, accurate documentation of calls increases defensibility in a court of law, as it augments memory (Scott &

Packard, 1990; Daugird & Spencer, 1988; Dunn, 1985; McGear & Simms, 1988) and offers proof of advice given (Willett, 1977; Wood, 1986). Protocols have a role in documentation as well, by expediting the collection and recording of information (Tennenhouse, 1991). Several authors (Katz, 1990; McGear & Simms, 1988; Schmitt, 1980; Scott & Packard, 1990) have developed documentation forms which can help in the efficient and accurate recording of information. Tennenhouse (1991) suggests using logbooks or triplicate forms which are later added to the client's record, and Daugird and Spencer (1988) suggest space-saving forms taped shingle-style to charts. McMahon (1986) notes that documenting client dissatisfaction is a useful risk management measure.

Finally, documentation enhances quality assurance. Records can be used to compile statistics so that the agencies can have a better idea of the kinds of services needed (Dunn, 1985) and to help determine nurses' workload (McMahon, 1986). Daugird and Spencer (1988) point out that forms may prompt physicians to record information they otherwise might have neglected and contend that documentation of telephone calls should become a standard of care. Other quality assurance measures include daily audits of records and consumer satisfaction surveys (McMahon, 1986). In addition, ongoing in-service training programs, courses, and conferences help nurses hone their skills.

Nursing Standards

Standard I of the American Nurses Association Standards of Nursing Practice states: "The *collection of data about client health status is systematic and continuous.* The data are *accessible, communicated and recorded*" (p. 183). The rationale for this standard is that complete and ongoing data collection determines the client's nursing needs (Ford, 1985).

Each state has its own nurse practice act. In California and some others states, nursing is considered a profession. This means that a nurse's conduct is measured by a professional standard of care rather than a general standard. In California, nursing practice calls for:

> *Observation of signs and symptoms of illness, reaction to treatment or general behavior, or general physical condition, and (1) determination of whether such signs, symptoms, reactions, behavior, or general appearance exhibit abnormal characteristics; and (2) implementation, based on abnormalities, or appropriate reporting, or referral, . . . or the initiation of emergency procedures ("Nursing Practice in California," 1989, p. 26).*

Two other sources include standards adhered to in specialty areas and policies and procedures or standards of the nurses' employers.

The nurse must *listen, elicit, assess, and communicate significant information* (American Nurses Association, 1980). Nursing and statutory standards apply to the communications function—essentially all that is available to the telephone triage nurse by which nurses' actions can be measured.

Telephone triage is an extension of the nursing function. Thus, nurses are accountable for the advice and care recommended to clients. In telephone triage, there is limited contact between nurse and client. The nurse's role is limited to communicating—accurately and effectively—through receiving, recording, and conveying information. So failure to communicate may prove to be negligent. In order to bring a successful lawsuit, the plaintiff must demonstrate the four elements of negligence.

THE ELEMENTS OF NEGLIGENCE

The section on Elements of Negligence was written by Barbara Siebelt, RN, BA, Assistant Vice President, Willis Corroon Corporation of Maryland. All the case studies described are based on actual court cases.

Dramatic increases in health care costs have necessitated the widespread use of telephone triage, not only as a screening device for high volumes of calls, but also as a vehicle for advice, crisis intervention, and management. One problem inherent in telephone triage practice is the absence of the client. The nurse must rely either on a client's description of a problem or, worse yet, another party's secondhand description.

The nurse performing telephone triage is, first and foremost, a communicator and has a charge to "do the ordinary extraordinarily well." In addition to communicating well, the nurse must have effective public relations skills in order to develop a rapport with the caller, so that the information the nurse provides will be accepted by the caller. The nurse can lessen liability exposure by communicating effectively.

Documented protocols are essential to telephone triage. They usually contain key questions, phrases, or words to trigger the most accurate response from the caller. Another essential element is the need for almost instantaneous rapport between caller and nurse to facilitate effective and accurate data collection. The nurse should use protocols, technical knowledge, communication skills, and common sense to identify problems, assess acuity, and determine a course of appropriate action.

Telephone triage nurses increase their defensibility and enhance their quality of care by using documentation which is designed to correlate with established protocols. No matter which mode of documentation is used (written, taped, typed, etc.) one must be able to prove that there were no alterations, deletions, or corrections that cannot be defended as the truth and verified by the person who wrote, dictated, or taped them.

Everyone has a duty to behave reasonably. A failure to act reasonably that results in injury to another constitutes negligence, and each person is responsible for his or her own negligence. Any individual who alleges negligence must provide proof that the person accused of negligence failed to act reasonably when they had a duty to do so and that the failure to act reasonably caused an injury that can be related to the breach of duty. Malpractice is negligence committed by a professional in the performance of professional duties. When negligence is alleged, the plaintiff (the party alleging negligence) must prove negligence on the part of the defendant (the party accused of negligence). The plaintiff must prove that the defendant had a duty to perform an act, that he or she was negligent, and that the negligence caused injury or harm. Four elements must be established in order to prove negligence.

Duty to Meet the Standard of Care

The standard of care is the level of care that would be given by a reasonably prudent nurse under the same or similar circumstances. The standard is determined by expert witnesses. An expert is a person who may express an opinion regarding the standard of care and whether it was met, and may testify for either the plaintiff or the defendant. Theoretically, only nurses should be able to testify to the standard of care of other nurses because they have the same background. In reality though, physicians frequently testify to the standard of nursing care.

Verification of the standard of care can be supported by various types of documented information such as published nursing standards, policies and procedures, nurse practice act interpretation, published articles, job descriptions and any information specific to the alleged malpractice. The following case study illustrates the question of standard of care.

> *Mrs. Jones called the advice line of HMO Y about her husband, who was complaining of neck and jaw pain that radiated to the left shoulder. She was greeted by the advice nurse for the shift, who asked Mrs. Jones her reason for calling. Mrs. Jones explained that her husband was having pain in this neck and jaw. The nurse asked if there was pain in any other part of the body. Mrs. Jones stated that her husband also had shoulder pain, but that it had gone away. The nurse then asked if the pain was always present in Mr. Jones' neck and jaw and if the shoulder pain was present during the call. The patient's response was, "yes." She also asked if the pain was accompanied by sweating, nausea, or vomiting. The nurse asked to speak to Mr. Jones directly, but his wife stated that he did not wish to come to the phone. The nurse asked then if Mr. Jones had a history of problems related to his circulation, heart, or lungs, or had ever been treated for a problem like this. Mrs. Jones replied "not to her knowledge." When the nurse asked if Mr. Jones' pain was*

related to movement Mrs. Jones answered "no." Mrs. Jones then stated that she had some Tylenol #3 left from a tooth extraction that she could give to her husband. The advice nurse said that was a good idea and Mr. Jones should take two pills and call back if the pain was not relieved. Five hours later, Mrs. Jones called the nurse back to relate that her husband's "pain was somewhat relieved." Without hesitation, the nurse told Mrs. Jones to observe her husband and bring him to the center in the morning. The nurse asked the above questions after referring to a protocol that was used to rule out the presence or absence of cardiac related pain.

Breach of the Duty to Meet the Standard of Care

When a nurse fails to do what a reasonably prudent nurse would do under the same or similar circumstances, the standard of care could be considered breached. Issues to be addressed regarding an established standard are:

- Does the HMO Y have an established protocol for possible cardiac-related pain?
- What would a response be if Mrs. Jones called the second time stating that her husband's pain was not relieved by the suggested treatment?
- What alternative to observation at home should the nurse have offered to Mrs. Jones?
- What supportive documentation was readily available on file to review the first response to Mrs. Jones when she stated she had called earlier?

The Breach of Duty Causes Foreseeable Harm

The third element of liability is that of foreseeable harm that can be attributed to the breach of duty. This may also be referred to as proximate cause. In the case of Mr. Jones, it was foreseeable that Mr. Jones might have had a problem which warranted physical examination and observation because the location, duration, and severity of his pain was significant. Mr. Jones' pain was only "somewhat relieved" as related by Mrs. Jones. Therefore, the unrelieved symptoms warranted additional evaluation, since this type of pain could have been cardiac related and had potentially serious implications.

Actual Harm or Injury

As a result of the breach of duty, some actual harm or injury must occur. The morning following his initial episode of pain, Mr. Jones began vomiting, perspiring, and complaining of shortness of breath. His wife called the rescue squad. He had a cardiac arrest en route to the hospital and died shortly after arrival.

The following case studies illustrate additional situations that present legal implications for telephone triage practice:

Mrs. Smith, a 29-year-old woman, was the mother of one child and had no previous prenatal problems. Five-months pregnant with her second child, she called the advice nurse at HMO X complaining of back pain that was not localized to any particular area. She also complained of a "slight brownish red discharge" accompanied by an "occasional cramp." The nurse asked Mrs. Smith if she had any bright bleeding and if the cramps were ever constant. Mrs. Smith answered all of the questions in the negative. The nurse told Mrs. Smith to watch for bright bleeding and that if this did occur she should call back. Did the nurse meet the standard of care requiring that the nurse refer to the established protocol for vaginal bleeding in pregnancy? (standard of care.) In this case, the nurse failed to use the protocol.

Several hours later, Mrs. Smith made a second call with the same complaint of back pain, bleeding, and cramping with no relief and was instructed to remain at home, stay in bed, and see her primary care physician in the morning. Was there a protocol which offered alternatives suggesting that the patient be evaluated by a physician and did the nurse follow it? (breach of the standard.) The protocol offered alternatives, but the nurse failed to use them. At that point, Mrs. Smith said that she was "worried." The nurse asked what concerned her, and told her that many times the bleeding stops spontaneously. Was the patient at risk when she stated that she was "worried." (foreseeability of harm.) The patient was at risk.

The next morning Mrs. Smith was transported by the rescue squad to the HMO's Urgent Care Center. She had profuse vaginal bleeding and was pale and diaphoretic. Her blood pressure was 82/50 and an intravenous of lactated Ringer's solution was started. She was transferred to a local hospital where it was discovered that she was spontaneously aborting. A nonliving female child was delivered. Was there actual harm or injury? Yes, Mrs. Smith went into shock and delivered a nonliving child. (actual harm or injury.)

Mr. Green, a 69-year-old widower, called HMO Z complaining of pain in the middle of his back that sometimes hurt in his "stomach." The nurse asked if he had nausea, vomiting, or diarrhea, all of which he denied. He stated that he had been working outside earlier in the day. Without further questions, the nurse told Mr. Green to take an extra strength Tylenol, go to bed with a heating pad, and call in the morning.

Was there an established protocol for abdominal or back pain and was it referred to by the nurse? (standard of care.) There was a protocol, but the nurse failed to refer to it.

Mr. Green did as he was told but awakened during the night with "worsening" pain. He then called the HMO to ask for additional advice, adding that it felt worse on movement. He was told that back pain can get worse before it gets better, and to continue the prescribed treatment. Did the established protocol give alternatives to suggest that the patient be seen by a physician? The protocol offered alternatives, but the nurse failed to use it. (breach of the standard.)

Mr. Green got no relief from anything, so he called 911 early in the morning and was transported to the nearest hospital. He was diagnosed with a bleeding abdominal aneurysm and became a surgical emergency. The diagnosis of bleeding abdominal aneurysm indicates that a rupture could occur at any time and that internal bleeding could occur that would be irreversible. (foreseeability of harm.) His aneurysm ruptured in the operating room and he suffered a cardiac arrest and died during surgery. Perhaps if Mr. Green's diagnosis had been made sooner, surgery would have been performed under less urgent circumstances and his life would have been saved. (actual harm or injury.)

To be defended adequately when negligence is alleged, it is important that at least the following be available to be used as defense evidence:

- Dated policies and procedures
- Telephone triage protocol designed specifically for the facility
- Job description for the nurses who perform telephone triage
- Information relative to the procedures for telephone triage education
- Call documentation

Policies and procedures should be kept on file for at least as long as the statute of limitations in your jurisdiction.

AREAS OF CONTROVERSY

Implied Relationship

Is there an implied relationship between caller and nurse? This is an area of much controversy and there is no case law specific to this area at this time.

Tennenhouse (1988) compares nurses to medical dispatchers, stating that nurses in the HMO, physician's office, and emergency settings have an implicit relationship with callers. On the other hand, Dunn (1985) suggests that the nurse/client relationship begins when the nurse begins to give advice. However, even if no relationship is implied, to assume that advice need not be given may be risky as well.

Arguments can be made to support that giving advice can provide reasonable alternatives to a patient when a problem is identified that warrants some form of attention as determined by the caller/patient. Ultimately, that advice can be to seek care in an acute care facility using an emergency transport system. On the other hand, giving advice to the caller/patient is subject to interpretation and could cause the patient to choose an alternative not appropriate for the problem that was described. In any event, when the ultimate alternative advice given is to seek care in a hospital or similar acute care environment, using the emergency medical tranport system, the acceptable standard of care can be met.

Assessment and Working Diagnosis

Nurses cannot diagnose by phone, nor should they lead the caller to believe that they are getting a diagnosis. Strictly speaking, diagnosis involves identifying and determining the nature of a disease or condition through examination. Neither physician nor nurse can make a diagnosis without examining the client. Even at the bedside, making a diagnosis is a painstaking process requiring time, careful examination, and often laboratory tests. At the bedside as well as by phone, however, it is an accepted practice to form *initial* impressions or a working diagnosis. In both instances, the working diagnosis forms the basis for subsequent treatment and further diagnostic tests. Telephone assessment, however, is limited because hearing is the main tool of evaluation and because the work must be done quickly—often within six to eight minutes. Therefore, unlike face-to-face assessment and diagnosis, telephone triage dictates limited assessment and working diagnosis. Rather than *seeking to determine specific causes of symptoms,* the telephone triage nurse aims *to identify symptoms and classify them by acuity.* "Ruptured aortic aneurysm; impaired tissue perfusion" is a diagnosis which specifies a cause for symptoms. "Severe abdominal pain, etiology unknown," on the other hand, is a *working diagnosis,* which names the symptom and classifies it according to potential seriousness. The disposition is based upon this assessment.

On the telephone, the only diagnosis which can be made by a physician or nurse is a presumptive or working diagnosis. The nurse or doctor must always inform the client of the presumptive status of this evaluation. The nurse must use discretion in the choice of words used to transmit this information, taking care not to leave the caller with the impression that a firm diagnosis has been made by telephone.

The working diagnosis is best stated simply, both for the record and to the caller. Using approved nursing diagnostic terms as some authorities (Scott & Packard, 1990) suggest may create unwarranted assumptions among health care providers. It seems risky to state that abdominal pain is related to tissue perfusion when one cannot see the client and there are other possible sources of pain, bowel obstruction and gastroenteritis, for example. In addition, "abdominal pain related to tissue perfusion, alteration in gastrointestinal" is circuitous and time-consuming to write, while "severe abdominal pain, etiology unknown" is clearer and more direct. If anything, telephone assessment needs to be more streamlined and simplified, not more complicated.

Using medical diagnostic terms can also confuse the client. Instead, use lay language: "Based on your description of the symptoms, this sounds like a severe nosebleed." Most published protocols use diagnostic titles based on lay terms (Clawson & Dernocoeur, 1988; Schmitt, 1992). Abdominal pain, rash, and headache are universally recognized and accepted as protocol titles. This approach is direct and expeditious.

Once the problem has been named, the next step of the process is to classify it according to its acuity. *Acute* problems require visits to a physician or ED. *Nonacute* symptoms can be managed by clients for short periods with home treatment. In such cases, however, clients should be directed to monitor treatments and report back if symptoms worsen, fail to progress, or change markedly (McGear & Simms, 1988; McMahon, 1986). In addition, to meet *informed consent* requirements, verbalize to all callers that this assessment or working diagnosis, is not "written in stone" and is subject to change. Failure to communicate the limitations of telephone diagnosis may mislead callers into thinking that the diagnosis is definitive and liabilities may result.

Crisis Intervention

Nowhere are system flaws more relentlessly revealed than in crisis intervention. Attorney Jeanne Dunn (1985), one of the most conservative of experts on telephone triage liability, recommends not giving advice over the phone except in life-threatening emergencies. Yet, if nurses are forbidden to give advice for routine calls, they will be less prepared for crisis-level calls. Because such callers are often severely distraught or have impaired judgment, they are ill-equipped to manage the situation without professional assistance. Rigorous crisis intervention training helps insure high standards and that the call will be safely managed.

Even so, crisis calls inevitably tax a system, and under such stress, mistakes are more likely to happen. Clawson and Dernocoeur (1988) cite "the emergency rule," (p. 211–212) which offers some protection to emergency medical dispatchers. Even though telephone triage nurses, like medical dispatchers, should be trained to handle emergencies, extremely high volumes of emergency calls may come in at once, overwhelming available personnel and equipment. The courts then recognize that the system is laboring under its own emergency, and the person on the phone cannot be reasonably held to the same level of conduct as in periods of normal call volume.

Reasonably Safe Disposition

As in any situation involving nursing practice, clients receiving telephone advice should be able to expect recommendations for a reasonably safe disposition. Considering both the volume of care provided by phone (some HMOs average 10,000 to 20,000 calls per day) and the litigiousness of our times, relatively few malpractice actions have occurred (Dunn, 1985; McGear & Simms, 1988; Willett, 1977).

Part of the communications function which is unique to telephone triage is the "duty to terrify." Tennenhouse (1988) states that the "duty to terrify is a duty based on the liability from an injury to the noncompliant patient who claims that his or her noncompliance was due to an inadequate understanding of the urgency of the situation." The nurse must always err on the side of caution, but especially with certain clients. For example, depending upon additional information presented, a woman of childbearing age who presents with severe abdominal pain (possible ectopic pregnancy) could be told, "These symptoms could be life-threatening. Go to the emergency department within the next 15 minutes." Directives should be specific enough to convey the concept of urgency, yet not so specific that the nurse seems to be making a diagnosis or prognosis. Nurses must err on the side of caution when in doubt.

Misrepresentation

A recent study of urgent care centers showed that out of 100 calls made for advice, receptionists gave advice 45 times (O'Brien & Miller, 1990). Receptionists must not give advice, represent themselves as nurses, or let callers believe they are speaking with a nurse. Likewise, nurses must never hold themselves out as physicians nor let the caller believe they are talking with a physician. Tell the caller immediately, either by introductory tape or in person, to whom they are speaking. For example, a statement such as "this is the advice nurse (secretary), how can I help you?" is probably sufficient. Failure to clarify a role in this way may result in legal liabilities.

Documentation by Exception and Documentation by Inclusion

When it comes to documentation at the bedside, some maintain "if you don't document it, it wasn't done." Can the same be said for telephone triage questions asked and information received? Since all the telephone triage nurse has to work with are the communications transmitted and received, does that become equivalent to bedside observations and treatments? Many experts agree that documentation of telephone interactions is important (Clawson & Dernocoeur, 1988; Scott & Packard, 1990; McGear & Simms, 1988; Wood, 1986). However, at least one study of family medicine residents found that, even when documentation was required, compliance was variable (Hamedeh, 1989). What constitutes safe, effective and appropriate documentation is an area of considerable controversy, and there are at least two schools of thought on the issue: documentation by exception and documentation by inclusion. Each has certain advantages and risks.

Documentation by exception means standardized questions are asked but negative responses need not be documented. For example, if the client has chest pain, it would not be necessary to document "denies sweating, shortness of breath" because the policy is that questions must be asked but the answers not necessarily documented. The advantage is that this approach reduces charting to a minimum and is less time-consuming. The nurse is not made to look negligent for anything not documented. The risks are that no one can prove that standardized questions were indeed asked or what the response was.

By contrast, documentation by inclusion maintains that negative responses to certain standardized protocol questions (and any other intuitive questions) must be documented. If they are not, it may appear that the nurse failed to ask certain questions. It places a greater burden on the nurse to perform additional charting and is more time-consuming. However, it presents a more comprehensive picture of what happened during the call. *In either case, there should be written policies stating the approved approach to documentation.*

Then there is the problem of the documentation form. By their very format (blank or detailed), forms often lean in the direction of one of the above approaches. For example, blank forms are simple, lined sheets which require little more than demographic information. Thus, such data categories as "Assessment, Diagnosis, Plan, Evaluation" or "symptoms, characteristics, location, onset, pregnancy, allergies, medications" are not printed on the form to cue the nurse as to key questions. This format places few documentation demands on nurses but makes heavy assumptions about the quality of memory, expertise, competence, reliability, and conscientiousness of the nurse using it.

On the other hand, detailed forms require charting by inclusion because standard required data are printed on them. (See Figures 5.15, 5.16, and 5.17) This forces the nurse to address each item in writing or run the risk of being considered negligent for not having completed required documentation.

There are several ways to overcome the drawbacks of each of these approaches. One possible solution is to use the detailed form with written policies which direct nurses to leave no blanks and to write "not applicable" next to items which do not apply. For example, if the caller is a male, pregnancy would not apply. A second approach is to use a blank form but to place the list of required data items by the phone as a quick reference. A third approach is to use the detailed version of the form as an interim training tool. It would then only be used during a period of orientation or as a remedial measure for QA.

Taping of Calls and Written Documentation

Should calls be taped or written? Wood (1986) states that though tapes are the most complete and direct record of telephone encounters, they are costly and time-consuming to review. According to her study, medical records made by residents corresponded reasonably well with transcripts of audiotapes. One may therefore conclude that in a facility where personnel keep scrupulous telephone records while using effective, comprehensive protocols and documentation forms, the written record will provide a reasonably accurate account of what transpired and tapes would not be necessary.

Finally, telephone triage must be practiced as carefully and professionally as other nursing functions. Ultimately, "good patient care is your best defense against being sued for malpractice" (Ford, 1985 p. 180).

CHAPTER 2

EXERCISE: MULTIPLE CHOICE

OBJECTIVE: To understand basic legal aspects of telephone triage.

METHOD: Choose the best answer or answers.

______ 1. Telephone triage:
- a. is not a nursing function.
- b. is a nursing function.
- c. must only be practiced by physicians.

______ 2. The duty of due care is:
- a. care which a physician would have given under the circumstances.
- b. care which an experienced nurse would have given under the circumstances.
- c. care which a reasonably prudent nurse would have given under the circumstances.

______ 3. Breach of duty means:
- a. The nurse was late on duty or was absent without prior notification.
- b. The nurse was under the influence of drugs or alcohol on duty.
- c. The nurse failed to render the level of care which a reasonably prudent nurse would have rendered under the same circumstances.

______ 4. The "duty to terrify" means:
- a. "A duty based on the liability from an injury to a compliant patient who claims that his or her compliance was due to an inadequate understanding of the urgency of the situation."
- b. "A duty based on the liability from an injury to the noncompliant patient who claims that his or her noncompliance was due to an inadequate understanding of the urgency of the situation."
- c. Nurses and clients have a duty to terrify one another whenever possible.

______ 5. Causation means:
- a. the injury was caused by a failure to meet the standard of care.
- b. failures to meet the standard of care can cause client injuries.
- c. the root of the problem can usually be traced to the nurse.

_____ 6. Actual harm means:
   a. that the nurse's license will be suspended if he or she is caught.
   b. that the client is never told that actual harm occurred.
   c. that actual harm or injury to the client has occurred.

_____ 7. Calls received in an ED:
   a. should be documented under all circumstances.
   b. need only be documented if they did not result in an appointment.
   c. need only be documented if they involve potential liability.

_____ 8. The best defense against a malpractice suit is:
   a. a nurse attorney with experience in telephone triage.
   b. malpractice insurance.
   c. high standards of nursing practice.

_____ 9. ENA and ACEP are two organizations which:
   a. regulate governmental guidelines for telephone triage practice.
   b. have formulated policy statements regarding the practice of telephone triage in emergency departments.
   c. have sponsored several joint conferences for telephone triage nurses.

_____ 10. ANA Standards of Nursing Practice require:
   a. that data collection be systematic and continuous.
   b. that data be written in English only.
   c. that data be accessible, communicated, and recorded.

_____ 11. Nurses must:
   a. listen, elicit, assess, and communicate significant information.
   b. listen and solicit information which is contained in the protocol questions.
   c. listen for at least 1 minute and before instructing clients in self-care treatment.

_____ 12. Nurses must:
   a. formulate a nursing diagnosis using only NANDA approved terms.
   b. formulate a working diagnosis using terminology approved by his or her facility.
   c. formulate a medical diagnosis which is later approved by a physician.

_____ 13. Liability can be limited by:
   a. malpractice insurance and knowledge of the Nursing Practice Act.
   b. taping of calls, quality assurance, and thoughtful advice.
   c. conscientious use of protocols, documentation, and quality assurance.

______ 14. Receptionists:
   a. may give advice as authorized by their employers.
   b. must only take information and never make recommendations.
   c. may act in place of a nurse when the nurse is out of the office.

______ 15. It is essential that:
   a. the nurse remain open to new information from the client.
   b. that the nurse know self-relaxation techniques.
   c. that the nurse speak several languages.

ANSWER KEY

EXERCISE: MULTIPLE CHOICE

1. b
2. c
3. c
4. b
5. a
6. c
7. a
8. c
9. b
10. a, c
11. a
12. b
13. c
14. b
15. a

CHAPTER 3
Communication

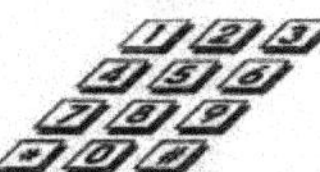

> *"We are what we repeatedly do. Excellence, then, is not an act, but a habit."*
> *–Aristotle*

COMMUNICATION THEORY

Successful communication involves the exchange of information between one person and another. The message must not only be sent via some medium such as words, pictures, or signals, but received and understood. Thus, a successful communication requires a sender, a message, a medium, and a receiver. For the message to be complete, information usually has to flow in both directions (Figure 3.1). In the interview situations a telephone triage nurse is likely to encounter, completing the loop is essential.

FIGURE 3.1 The Communication Loop

COMMUNICATOR → MESSAGE → MEDIUM → RECEIVER

(Who) (What) (How) (To Whom)

FEEDBACK

(With what effect)

(Reproduced by permission from Lancaster, Jeanette and Lancaster, Wade, editors: *Concepts for Advanced Nursing Practice: The Nurse as a Change Agent,* St. Louis, 1982, The C.V. Mosby Co.)

If too little or too much information is transmitted, the chances of the message being received and understood diminish. Most communications have the luxury of a broad scope. For example, painting uses form, color, texture, and symbolism. Face-to-face conversation embraces spoken and body language, facial expression, touch, and even smell. By contrast, in telephone triage, the scope of communication is narrow and therefore subject to misinterpretation. Verbal messages are restricted to words and to the tone, quality, and inflection of the voice. Telephone triage suffers from lack of visual input. Thus, because the "signal" is incomplete, barriers which in person are not very formidable can become nearly insurmountable in telephone triage (see Figure 3.2).

FIGURE 3.2 Telephone Triage Communication Barriers

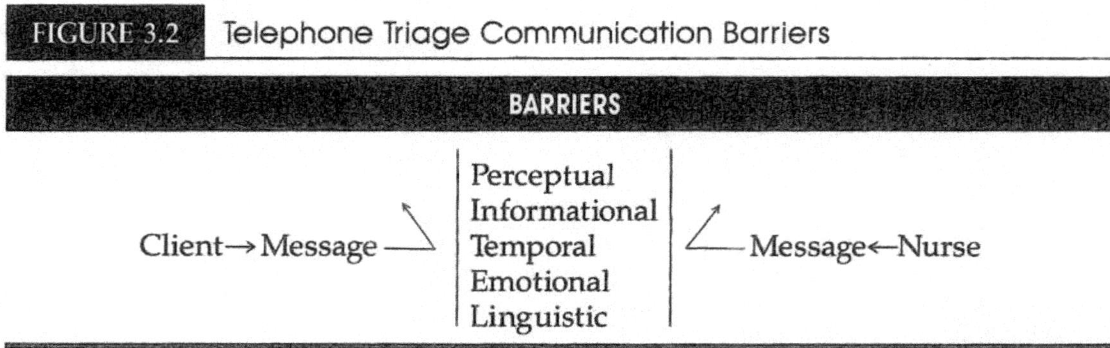

Messages are impaired by poor relationships and by feelings, needs, and biases. Clients' and nurses' beliefs, attitudes, and perceptions of symptoms become obstacles in themselves. Therefore, nurses must do everything they can to prevent this from happening (see Figure 3.3).

FIGURE 3.3 Barriers and Facilitators to Communication

	BARRIERS	FACILITATORS
1. Perceptual	Misperception of the problem, biases or stereotyping	Being concrete, openminded
2. Emotional	Lack of trust, emotional overload, denial	Trusting relationship
3. Informational	Not listening, leading questions	Active listening, open-ended questions
4. Temporal	Insufficient talk time	Sufficient talk time
5. Linguistic	Language barrier Medical jargon	Bilingual capabilities Lay language

As agents of change, nurses must understand the communication process, including the characteristics of verbal and nonverbal interactions, obstacles to communication, and means to facilitate the process.

Like all communications, the goals of telephone triage include giving and receiving information, understanding the information, release of anxiety, and problem solving. In telephone triage practice, nurses can facilitate communication by attending to and receiving messages, clarifying or asking for examples, reflecting and paraphrasing to check the accuracy of the message, speaking in lay language when instructing, and validating and summarizing messages in closing. *Finally, communication depends on receiving information as much as on sending it.*

Telephone Charisma

To a large degree, all nursing care hinges upon communication. At the bedside, speech, smell, touch, sight, and emotional cues paint a rich picture of the client's condition, while on the phone, communications are limited to verbal and emotional cues. In telephone triage, as suggested above, the risk of miscommunication is great. Although it is possible to gain limited tactile and visual information conveyed indirectly by callers, nurses receive information, analyze, solve problems, and instruct without observing the client. Despite limited sensory input, telephone interactions are multidimensional and multifunctional and can include counseling, coaching, monitoring, teaching, and crisis intervention. The challenge is to push the limits of what is possible and unique to this specialty.

Even with these limitations, many nurses demonstrate resourcefulness, expertise and imagination. From the first words of greeting, and from the way they listen, respond, and question, they demonstrate the warmth, caring, and trustworthiness that is charisma. Their voices seem to smile.

More, their success depends on their ability to gather information about each case and to communicate. Nurses not only intervene in emergencies and instruct and direct clients in self-monitoring procedures, they also plan and coordinate health care. To do this well, they must be expert information brokers.

Information is a tangible product. It is the precursor of expert care. But, as the following scenario demonstrates, the information conveyed in telephone triage work can be as "bare bones" or as sophisticated as the nurse makes it:

> *Wanda, a new mother, calls with what she describes as breastfeeding problems. She complains of sore, cracked nipples and says the child is nursing incessantly. She is weepy and exhausted, feeling beleaguered by the demanding newborn. She is recovering from a C-section. Her questions revolve around her "sore, cracked nipples."*

Anna, the nurse, responds: "How can I help you?" but her voice is tired and flat. Her manner lacks congruence. She refers to the "Breastfeeding Problems" protocol, listlessly reading the standard advice. To expedite the call, she discourages additional client self-disclosure or exposure of a possible hidden agenda. She offers no options, explanations, or referral. Her manner is "time-driven" and she makes little attempt to build rapport. The call is over within 3 minutes. The caller, dissatisfied with the brevity of the call and lack of emotional support, fails to follow the advice. She grows increasingly depressed. She calls back two days later with worsening symptoms.

Sophia, another nurse, addresses the problem holistically. She visualizes a new breastfeeding mother, post-C-section, deprived of sleep, and exhibiting possible symptoms of postpartum depression. She elicits concrete information from the client about ineffective nursing techniques and, using self-disclosure (the appropriate sharing of personal experience), briefly alludes to her own difficulties as a new nursing mother. She acts as a catalyst, tactfully refraining from making decisions but encouraging the client to "own" the problem and the solution. She tailors the standard advice to fit the client's needs, and then documents deviations from standard advice. Her recommendations are concrete. In addition to breastfeeding and post-C-section support group referrals, she offers book titles and the name of a lactation consultant. Finally, she elicits hidden agendas from the client, who, it turns out, feels guilty for feeling unexpected anger at her situation. The call lasts 7 minutes.

In the second case, the caller leaves the interaction feeling empowered and self-confident. Although Sophia used over twice the time as Anna, her resourcefulness, creativity, and warmth made her more proficient, and the system more effective.

The foregoing example illustrates the entire thesis of this chapter: that the manner of communication is almost as important as what is communicated. Effective telephone technique inspires, persuades, and engenders trust. "Telephone charisma" is the personal magic characterized by self-disclosure, empathy, respect, warmth, and authenticity.

A Communication Model

As currently practiced, telephone communication between clients and health care providers is often one-sided and unbalanced. Providers do most of the talking. Clients receive treatment advice and little support or encouragement. Thus, the information flow between caller and provider never becomes integrated, resulting in ineffective communication and inappropriate dispositions. For example, one study (Sloane, Egelhoff, Curtis, McGaghie, & Evens, 1985) shows that some physicians gather information for as little as 1 minute before formulating a working diagnosis and giving instructions. This is not enough time to hear the patient out.

Telephone triage nurses should spend at least 2–3 minutes gathering data and collaborating with the client on a working diagnosis. They should spend the remaining time reiterating the history, answering questions, explaining the diagnosis and the treatment plan, and eliciting hidden agendas—areas which are usually neglected. Figure 3.4 illustrates approximate time allotments for various functions in an average 6-minute call.

FIGURE 3.4 Telephone Triage Interaction: Information Flow and Approximate Time Allotments

PROCESS OBJECTIVE	NURSE	INFO FLOW	CLIENT	# MIN
1. Data Collection Phase				2–3
	Gathers data, listens	⟵	States problem	
Generic protocol	Writes, clarifies	⟵	Explains, emotes	
Specific protocol	Asks questions	⟵	Describes, explains	
2. Confirmation Phase				1–2
Implement protocol	Reiterates	⟶	Confirms, redefines	
Formulate working diagnosis	States diagnosis in lay language	⟵	Corrects working diagnosis	
3. Disposition Phase				2–3
	States solution	⟶	Listens	
Make disposition Give advice	Explains, elaborates	⟶	Writes	
	Educates, reiterates plan	⟶ ⟵	Agrees to plan	

*Based on an average talk time of 6 minutes. Some calls will be longer and others shorter than this average and should be proportioned as appropriate.

Figure 3.4 also illustrates a communication model. This information flow and time allotment chart shows the interaction in three phases. (For more information about therapeutic communication, see Bernstein and Bernstein, 1985.)

In the early data collection phase, nurses should remain receptive and encourage clients to present problems or symptoms through *active listening* and *open-ended,* as opposed to leading, questions. Open-ended questions do not limit the scope of the answer to yes or no. (Active listeners demonstrate through verbal and nonverbal cues, such as a simple "uh-huh," that they are paying attention to, but not judging, what the client is saying. By contrast, a passive listener remains silent and unresponsive, simply allowing the client speak into a void.)

Ideally, the client does most of the talking. Warmth, empathy, and respect characterize this stage (Hornsby & Payne, 1979). At the bedside, voice, gestures, touch, and facial expression communicate warmth. But on the phone, only the voice—well modulated, of moderate speed, congruent—is available to convey warmth and engender trust. (Congruence means that the speaker's words and nonverbal behavior match. To say "I understand how you must feel" with irritation in one's voice is incongruent and communicates only impatience and boredom.) Empathy, active listening, and showing confidence in the client's ability to manage problems all bolster trust. Thus, as the nurse gathers data, she or he is also building a relationship.

The second stage, confirmation, is collaborative. The nurse reiterates what the client has said, refines it, and confirms the problem history. Information flows back and forth. This transitional stage may involve risk-taking. (Hornsby & Payne, 1979). The trusting relationship established in the first stage enables the nurse to elicit from the client a clear, concrete picture of the symptoms. The client must feel that the nurse cares. Self-disclosure, sharing of feelings and experiences, and authenticity—simply being oneself—facilitate this stage (Hornsby & Payne, 1979).

Finally, in the disposition phase, the nurse becomes the more active one, classifying the problem and providing protocol advice. Now the client is more receptive, asking questions and clarifying instructions. Confrontation, immediacy, and empowerment of the client are the key elements of this phase (Hornsby & Payne, 1979). Without trust, confrontation can backfire. Clients can become defensive or hostile. Trust is the foundation upon which confrontation becomes a building block toward empowering clients to modify their own behavior.

In real life, of course, telephone interactions seldom flow as smoothly as described above. The client and nurse, for example, may have to repeatedly backtrack to earlier stages to obtain information or clarification missed the first time.

While the brevity of telephone encounters makes long-term behavior modification unlikely, *helping clients to alter behavior for the moment or for brief periods is a realistic goal.* For example, when clients agree to follow advice or contact a support group, they are modifying behavior. Presenting options and forming verbal contracts will develop, strengthen, and maintain new behaviors or discourage unhealthy behaviors.

Some argue that with only 6 to 8 minutes in which to work, achieving quality interactions is impossible. In fact, quality interactions can develop in small but genuine measure. Even brief, anonymous encounters can save lives. Trained dispatchers build trust by giving concrete directives, explaining necessary absences from the phone, staying with the clients, and discouraging ineffectual behavior while helping to develop new behavior. They empower panic-stricken clients to initiate lifesaving activities. Within seconds, client and practitioner forge a relationship and begin a problem-solving collaboration.

The goal of telephone triage communication is not to change people's behavior or attitudes forever (although in some cases this may happen) but to change clients' immediate behavior and attitudes as these relate to the presenting problem.

A Functional Model

The model described above focuses on the *form* of interpersonal communications in telephone triage. It is a method for enhancing the personal relationship between nurse and client to facilitate information exchange and action. Nurses must never forget, however, that the nursing function is at the heart of assessing a client's needs, whether in person or by telephone.

Patricia Benner (1984) argues that nursing expertise falls into seven domains or functions: helping, coaching/teaching, diagnosing/monitoring, crisis intervention, monitoring therapeutic interventions, quality assurance, and organizational skills monitoring. These functions apply to telephone triage as well. In telephone triage, however, communication necessarily becomes the major *vehicle* for the entire nursing process. This section elaborates Benner's concepts in terms of telephone communication. Each function is illustrated by an example, showing its application to telephone triage practice.

The Helping Function. In telephone triage, the key aspects of the helping role are *creating a healing relationship, 'presencing' (i.e., being present), maximizing clients' control, and providing comfort* through voice (rather than touch) (Benner, 1984). The following example illustrates how a nurse's expertise turned a near-disaster into a successful outcome:

> *Mrs. Chapman called, insisting on talking with her child's pediatrician. Noting her abrupt manner, Barbara, the nurse, calmly probed for additional information. After several minutes, Mrs. Chapman revealed that her husband (a drug abuser) was physically abusing both*

the caller and her infant. He demanded that she wean her child and was threatening both of them. She wanted a physician to talk to her husband. Barbara scheduled an appointment with a social worker immediately. Later on, Barbara learned that the woman left her spouse and moved to a distant community to begin anew. Barbara later revealed that had she reacted with hostility to the caller's abrupt behavior, she never would have had the opportunity to intervene at all. (Case history, Wheeler, 1989)

Benner calls the "act of just *being* with the clients" *presencing*. The nurse's receptive presence enabled the client to disclose her painful, frightening situation. This nurse created a healing relationship by presencing and by helping the client obtain the information she needed.

The Coaching/Teaching Function. Even within the constraints of the 6-minute talk time, a surprising amount of teaching and health promotion is possible. *Timing, eliciting interpretations of illness, and providing rationales for home treatment* are key teaching and coaching functions (Benner, 1984). Expert nurses identify "client readiness" and they seize opportunities to help clients learn to change behaviors and attitudes. Informing clients about their rights, informed consent, and second medical opinions constitute teaching, and are acts of empowerment.

John, a college student, calls regarding AIDS symptoms. He says that he recently attended a wild fraternity party where he engaged in group sex without using condoms. He can barely remember the night, having used cocaine and alcohol. He denies IV drug use, but acknowledges that some friends have dabbled with IV drugs. He sounds worried and remorseful. He is well educated regarding AIDS and safe sex practices. Nonetheless, this knowledge has not resulted in a change in sexual behavior. Prior to this incident, John felt invincible, but suddenly he feels vulnerable and fearful.

The nurse's response requires much more expertise than simply providing treatment information. David, the nurse, seizes the moment to correct the client's misperceptions and provide rationales for new behavior, using a sophisticated approach which requires risk-taking and resourcefulness. He uses the client's rational fear as leverage to elicit a verbal commitment to safe sex and avoidance of IV drug use. He confronts behavioral discrepancies and risky sexual practices in a nonjudgmental way, while maintaining the trusting relationship with the caller. David credits the client's awareness of safe sex: "You are well informed about the need to use condoms." He then points out, "But what many people don't know is that using drugs and alcohol is also a high-risk activity when it comes to AIDS. It can make you lose control, even forget what you know. Do you think maybe drugs caused you to get into a dangerous situation without intending to?"

The Diagnostic Function. Strictly speaking, telephone triage is not designed to diagnose. However, within limits, nurses can *detect and document significant changes in the client's condition, anticipate problems, and formulate treatment strategies* (Benner, 1984). Protocols help to detect, identify, and classify significant changes in clients' conditions. (The diagnosis function is discussed in detail in Chapter 4.)

> *Mrs. Green called about her 3-year-old child who had fallen with a stick in his mouth. Although there was no visible bleeding, the nurse, Suzanna, recommended that she bring him in for an examination. The physician discovered a 6 cm jagged laceration in back of the throat about 1 cm away from the carotid. (Adapted from case history, Wheeler, 1989)*

In this case, Suzanna intuitively *anticipated possible complications and formulated a strategy* (Benner, 1984) to eliminate problems by recommending that the client be brought to the ED.

The Crisis Intervention Function. Nowhere else is the instant *grasp of rapidly changing situations* more vital than in crisis intervention by phone (Benner, 1984). At the bedside the crash cart provides lifesaving drugs and equipment. By phone, lifesaving instructions and coaching techniques (*"crash cards"* or protocols) are a client's lifeline. Crash cards are directives read verbatim to callers over the phone to coach them in CPR, the Heimlich maneuver, childbirth techniques, and first aid for some 30 other problems.

> *Gina, a young mother, called in a panic saying, "My baby isn't breathing." Kathy, the nurse, dispatched an ambulance. The mother said that the child was getting blue. Kathy gave CPR instructions and the mother dropped the phone and ran to administer CPR to the child until the ambulance arrived. Resuscitation attempts were unsuccessful, and the child eventually died. (Adapted from case history of sudden infant death syndrome, Wheeler, 1989)*

Even though the outcome was death, the nurse gave the mother a chance to do all that was possible via telephone CPR coaching. Currently most nurses, with the exception of medical dispatchers, have no protocols or specialized training for coaching in CPR. Some are able to "wing it" while others feel frustrated and helpless in managing these calls. It is likely that crash card training will be required in the future. (Specific crisis intervention techniques are discussed in detail in Chapter 7.)

The Monitoring Function. Currently, monitoring is not a major function of telephone triage nurses. As technology and the field of ambulatory care continue to grow and expand, however, the demand for nurses with skills in *minimizing the risks and complications of intravenous therapy and in the administration of medication* will rise (Benner, 1984). The hazards of immobility resulting from an illness will become greater as more clients are treated at home. Currently, some nurses monitor simple interventions and home treatment and instruct clients in administering nonprescription medication. In addition, several pioneering home telemetry systems have been instituted (see Chapter 1). A possible model for the sophisticated telemetry practices of the future is the high-risk obstetric monitoring of the Tokos Company. Tokos nurses monitor their high-risk obstetric clients 24 hours a day via telemetry and telephone contact. Lifeline is another telemetry-based system which offers support to frail elderly in the home. (Both of these systems are described in Chapter 6.) In the future, technology such as telemetry and home monitoring will expand and develop to meet the needs for more decentralized health care.

FIGURE 3.5 Telephone Triage Nurse as Coordinator of Resources

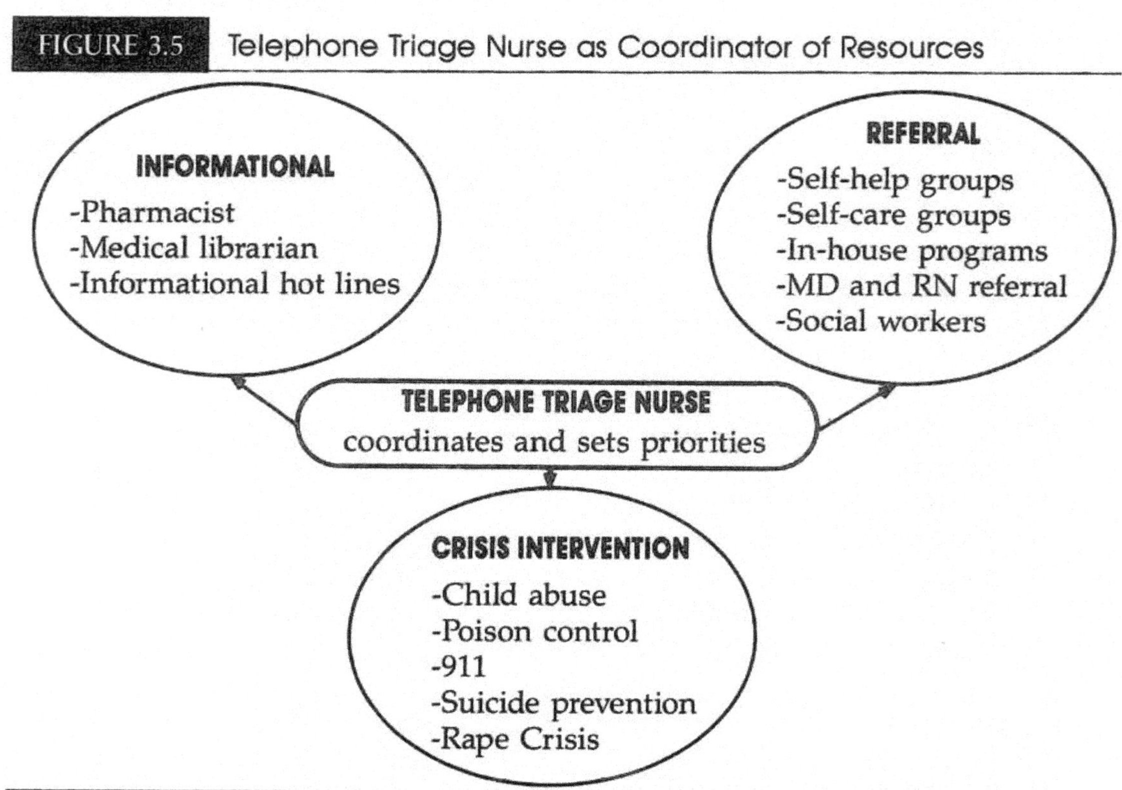

The Coordinating and Quality Assurance Function. Telephone triage, like other nursing activities, involves *building and coordinating resource teams to meet the various needs of clients* (Benner 1984). Currently, most systems have not developed extensive coordinating capabilities or quality assurance activities. (See Chapter 4 for more details on quality assurance standards.) In the future, telephone triage nurses may be called on to coordinate activities for informational, referral, and crisis intervention agencies (see Figure 3.5), and will refer callers to one or many resources.

DEVELOPING COMMUNICATION SKILLS

Good communication depends on respecting the client. The nurse should allow enough time for a complete picture to emerge, formulate questions that allow clients to describe their symptoms fully, and create a safe, understanding atmosphere that neither patronizes the client nor belittles the problem.

Allow Enough Time

There are no short cuts in telephone triage. Ineffective communication leads to increased legal liability, substandard client care, and possible legal complications (Thayer, 1984). With some specialists spending up to 28.5% of their time on the phone (Radecki, Neville, & Girard, 1989), it is understandable that many physicians feel oppressed by their telephones, as Fosarelli and Schmitt (1987) showed in a survey of pediatricians. As a result, overburdened physicians may stint on time spent per call. In one study of a private practice, average length of time for phone calls was approximately $1\frac{1}{2}$ minutes long (Spencer & Daugird, 1988), while in another study of seven internists, mean call lengths were 3.4 minutes, with 41% of calls lasting only 1 to 2 minutes (Johnson & Johnson, 1990). The amount of time spent gathering data must inevitably suffer if total call length is this short. In a 1987 study (Margolis et al.), a woman posing as a mother whose child had diarrhea made calls to 31 participating family practice residents who were not aware that the call was part of the study. According to the results, residents spent three times as much time talking as the caller, completeness of history-taking was directly related to time spent talking by the caller, and important diagnostic questions were often omitted. Furthermore, as physicians gain experience, they spend progressively less time on the phone asking questions and gathering diagnostic data and more time giving treatment advice (Sloane, Egelhoff, Curtis, McGaghie, & Evens, 1985). Smith and Fischer (1980) evaluated the effectiveness of telephone management instruction for medical students. This study shows that high efficiency (speed with which call was handled) was often associated with poor proficiency (competence, effectiveness, and safety). The authors conclude that trainees should strive for an acceptable level of proficiency first and then refine techniques for efficiency.

A key study in the *The New England Journal of Medicine* compared the performance of pediatric nurse practitioners with pediatricians (Perrin & Goodman, 1978). The authors discovered that pediatric nurse practitioners performed as well as or better than physicians in telephone triage of common pediatric problems. The nurse practitioners were judged to be warmer and more open to questions, and they left callers feeling more satisfied. They spent *significantly more time per call* than physicians (MDs spent 3 to 5 minutes; RNs spent 5 to 7 minutes). Perrin and Goodman consider that this additional time was invested in client education. The study finds, however, that both groups lacked skills in explaining the working diagnosis and the home care treatment.

Sloane, Egelhoff, Curtis, McGaghie, and Evens (1985), argue that problem solving among experienced physicians may rely as much on intuition as on empirical data gathering. Relying solely on experience and intuition, however, is risky. Nurses, too, can bring their experience and intuition to bear, but to promote high standards, they should allow enough time for clients to speak. This practice is safer in the long run. Failing to listen to the caller jeopardizes the trust between nurse and client. A client who feels rushed may be reluctant to open up with unforeseen but crucial information, and a disposition based on sketchy information may be inaccurate.

Fosarelli and Schmitt (1987) suggest that clients or parents of pediatric clients can be trained to use the phone appropriately, thus reducing some of the phone burden for physicians. According to another study (Katz, Pozen, & Mushlin, 1978), trained pediatric health assistants helped to reduce the number of phone encounters for physicians from 25 to 3 a day by educating parents so that they became less dependent on the pediatric office for their children's mild, self-limiting conditions. They also increased parental satisfaction by acting friendly and supportive on the phone rather than businesslike and laconic. Client satisfaction can help build client independence and foster additional learning. The director of a telephone communications program suggests that client satisfaction and compliance with proposed treatment can be adversely affected by workers who fail to convey important information because of poor communication skills (Zylke, 1990). Thus, although the telephone has proved to be a burden for some, it can be turned into an advantage by training staff in telephone communication techniques and the appropriate delivery of medical information. The goal is to educate clients about their own medical problems, to empower them to understand the treatment advice, and to motivate them to comply with it fully. The process used to achieve this goal is to train nurses in proper telephone communication techniques and in the proper use of protocols. More time spent initially saves time later (Egger, 1986). The result is better client care.

An average phone call should last 6 to 8 minutes (see Figure 3.4). Once nurses are willing to spend enough time on the phone for clients to relate symptoms, the way is clear to practice effective communication skills. In addition to *listening*, nurses must *elicit, assess,* and *communicate* significant information. Eliciting requires using open-ended questions in the interview process. Assessment is enhanced by using a client-centered communication style in which the nurse and the client feel free to talk back and forth to confirm, correct, and appraise the problem. In addition to client-nurse communications, telephone triage nurses must give written and verbal communications to other health care providers as appropriate. They must document to certain standards to insure continuity of care from all who subsequently encounter clients. These topics are discussed more fully in Chapter 4.

Ask Open-Ended Questions

History taking is the main method of data collection. The successful interviewer asks open-ended questions. (This process corresponds to the data-gathering phase in the model of information flow, in which the nurse is receptive and noncontrolling.) Asking leading questions—a flawed technique in which the interviewer solicits specific responses—yields faulty data. Margolis et al. (1987) found notable deficiencies in history taking among the residents they studied, and noted that four out of five questions asked were leading questions. It is important to resist the urge to control the conversation in this way. Leading questions cloud the picture by providing the answer in the question: "Is the pain *severe?*" "Are you having *bloody* stools?" "Are you having *difficulty* breathing?" Leading questions usually elicit yes or no answers. Open-ended questions or directives such as "Describe the pain," "What are the stools like?" or "Tell me about your breathing" eliminate yes or no responses. Always start data collection with open-ended questions. Prompt clients to describe symptoms fully.

Open-ended questioning is also effective when appointments are in short supply. Manipulative clients know that by giving affirmative responses, they will get appointments. If not given the chance to respond with an automatic affirmative answer, they are less likely to abuse the system by obtaining unnecessary appointments.

Feeding the answers to clients when interviewing is a common pitfall of time-driven systems. It may also be the result of improper training or faulty technique. Often clients unconsciously supply the answers that they sense the nurse wants to hear. One study points out the "tendency to alter communications in the direction of reciprocal exchange, so that any inherent mechanism of denial operating within the physician may be intensified in his communications with a disavowing patient" (Spitz & Bloch, 1981, p. 91). Leading questions can result in *mutual denial* and inappropriate or unsafe dispositions. With rare exceptions, it is better to use leading questions only as a last resort.

The exceptions to this rule are calls from children, frail elderly, and clients confused because of drug abuse or psychological or neurological impairment. In these cases, facilitative questions are a compromise between open-ended and leading approaches. For example: "Is the pain better, worse, or the same as it was yesterday?" "Is the bleeding dark red or light red?"

Another exception is the crisis intervention call, where assessments must be made within seconds. In a crisis, leading questions are compulsory: "Is the victim conscious? Breathing? Is there a heartbeat?" When an immediate disposition is imperative, open-ended questions are too time-consuming and diagnostic.

Develop Client-Centered Communication Styles

One theory postulates that communication styles are either "person-centered" or "position-centered" (Kasch & Knutson, 1985). Person-centered communications appeal to clients' logic and reasoning. Nurses give reasons for treatments and treat clients as intelligent adults. On the other hand, position-centered approaches favor an authoritarian stance based on one's role, and seek to coerce clients into a certain action.

An especially pernicious variation on the authoritarian approach is to treat all callers as potential customers. Some revenue-conscious marketing systems encourage this attitude. Nurses see themselves as "telemarketers" first and nurses second, and erode client trust by resorting to aggressive marketing tactics. Programs advertised as "community services" lose credibility when the bottom line is revenue rather than service.

On the other end of the scale, Bernstein and Bernstein (1985) developed a person-centered approach to interviewing—essential for obtaining an accurate history—which posits the *understanding response* as most likely to encourage a trusting relationship, elicit needed information, and foster client satisfaction. The authors contrast this ideal with response types that they characterize as *hostile*, *evaluative*, *reassuring*, or *probing*. As they describe them, these responses are almost guaranteed to dishearten and frustrate clients and make them withdraw.

For instance, in the example given at the beginning of this chapter, the telephone nurse might have responded with *hostility* to the discouraged postpartum nursing mother: "C'mon, it's not all that bad! Grow up!" The nurse implies that the mother's feelings are wrong and humiliates her. A response like this can only result in negative interaction and possible termination of communication. Less astringent approaches, however, while appearing to lay the groundwork for a trusting relationship, actually squelch it at the outset. In an example of an *evaluative* response, the nurse might say, "You shouldn't feel so negative about nursing. Millions of mothers have nursed their babies and put up with a little discomfort." In making a judgment about the woman's feelings, the nurse only prevents her from expressing other concerns. Even if the nurse gives what seems to be a *reassuring* response such as, "I hear that from most new mothers. Don't worry. The sore nipples clear up eventually," she denies the client's problems and feelings, making her feel they are not problems at all. Though the mother may feel temporarily mollified, her depression soon returns because its source has not been addressed. The client would be similarly left with guilt and depression if the nurse made a *probing* response, asking for more information: "Have you tried cocoa butter? Does the baby tend to keep the nipple in his mouth after he falls asleep?" She implies that if the client supplies an answer, she can supply a solution—an unlikely event. Probing questions may help to uncover problems, but if used simply to confer an air of authority upon the nurse, they will not help the client develop autonomy. If, however, the nurse *understandingly* says, "You sound exhausted. I'll bet you're surprised—maybe even a little angry—at how much a baby can disrupt your life," the mother is likely to feel safe. She will be more willing to explore her sense of inadequacy and take action to solve the problem. The empathic response respects the client and puts the nurse and the client on the same level, where they can work out a solution together.

Sometimes, even impeccable techniques are insufficient to prevent roadblocks to communication. The next section deals with developing the expertise to break through these barriers.

OVERCOMING COMMUNICATION ROADBLOCKS

Clients may call and then deny or evade the problem. They may fail to follow instructions through misunderstanding or fear. A skilled nurse recognizes and breaks through these failures of communication, opening the way to excellent care.

Denial

Denial is a normal human defense mechanism for handling unpleasant experiences. It exists in nurses as well as clients. In clients, it takes several forms: minimizing symptoms, noncompliance, the "good patient syndrome," and circumlocution. The following examples show how minimizing symptoms and noncompliance are related:

Ralph, a 35-year-old man called from his office complaining of "chest pain while jogging that morning." He wanted to know if it was "serious." Greta, the nurse, spent considerable time and effort to convince him to come to the emergency department, but was unable to achieve compliance. She finally hand carried the message to the physician.

Manuel, an elderly Hispanic man, called complaining of severe chest pain, sweating, and difficulty breathing. He refused to come to the emergency department as advised. Lola, the nurse, suspected that, like other elderly callers, he was afraid that he might die if he came to the hospital.

Callers who minimize symptoms to the point of noncompliance put nurses in a bind. If clients refuse to come in after continued urging, use the chain of command and physician leverage as appropriate. Always document client noncompliance.

A nurse can also fall into the trap of concurring with the client's minimizing for reasons unknown to herself. Spitz and Bloch (1981) describe a case of a resident who received a call 15 minutes before midnight on New Year's Eve from a woman whose mother was suffering gastrointestinal symptoms and low back pain. Because the caller seemed calm and in control, the resident felt the symptoms were not serious, and prescribed flu medication. When he expressed concern about the availability of the medication late on New Year's Eve, the caller again acted confident that she would be able to find an open pharmacy. Because of her calm demeanor, the resident failed to realize the seriousness of the situation. The woman died the next morning (diagnosis not given).

The "good patient syndrome" is another facet of denial: overly compliant, suggestible clients who lack self-confidence. A case history depicted on television's "60 Minutes" illustrates the syndrome well:

A son made three separate calls to 911 regarding his mother's severe back and abdominal pain. Untrained medical dispatchers first told the family she had food poisoning, and on the second call diagnosed the condition as hyperventilation. The dispatcher then instructed the son to have her blow into a paper bag. While the son was attempting to bring her to the car, she had a seizure. At that point the family again called 911 and the dispatcher sent the paramedics, but by that time the woman was in cardiac arrest and eventually died. ("60 Minutes," December 25, 1988)

In this case, the dispatcher's authoritarian, position-centered, "you're not sick until I say you are" stance compounded the family's self-doubt. Dispatchers minimized the caller's fears and the client's symptoms. Because dispatchers failed to collect adequate data, they jumped to conclusions and misdiagnosed the problem twice. Both father and son relied too heavily on the dispatchers' authority, lacking the self-confidence to demand the paramedics. The need to be "good patients" led them to deny what clearly was a serious situation.

A seven-year study of 249 deaths of young children both at home and in the hospital graphically demonstrates the prevalence of the good patient syndrome. The researchers found a tendency for deaths to occur at home over the weekend when family physicians were unavailable. Apparently, parents felt the children were ill, but "not ill enough" to bother the doctor on the weekend (Emery, 1959).

Distortion of clinical facts, abnormal emotional responses, and circumlocution are other forms of denial (Spitz & Bloch, 1981). Circumlocution is the use of an unnecessarily large number of words to express an idea. It may stem from efforts to give a coherent history while experiencing severe emotional distress (Spitz & Bloch, 1981). The following example illustrates how emotional overload creates a very disorganized history:

> *Tom, a middle-aged man, called Jonathan, the ED nurse. Going into minute detail, Tom said that he had come to town to visit his brother. The caller reported that he and his brother had been sitting and talking, and rambled on in this vein for approximately 3 minutes. He then said that while they were talking, his brother had grabbed his chest, gasped, and slumped to the floor. The brother was now lying on the floor, not breathing, and was blue. When he was finally brought in, they were unable to resuscitate him.*

The nurse, unaware of the circumlocution, failed to confront the situation in a timely way. Circumlocution may be difficult to assess. Expert questioning, direct confrontation, and interpretation of hidden agendas are methods to short-circuit circumlocution. Expert questioning involves asking direct, leading questions or making confrontational observations. For example: "Is she breathing?" or "You're talking in circles!" The effective use of confrontation is illustrated in this scenario:

> *A resident became suspicious when a husband kept emphasizing insignificant details surrounding his wife's acute illness. The resident finally said emphatically to the husband: "Now something is going on there. What is it?" The husband then became tearful, and proceeded to describe very accurately "an acute abdomen." (Adapted from Spitz & Bloch, 1981)*

In such cases, nurses must act quickly and within the first 30 seconds, direct callers to come to the point—especially in the ED, where calls are more likely to be urgent.

Clients are not the only ones guilty of denial. Nurses often fall victim to this pitfall. For example, novice nurses may overlook symptoms that seem irrelevant. Or as in the case of the resident who received a call on New Year's Eve, physicians receiving calls at intrusive times may feel conflicted about their need to serve clients and their need not to be disturbed. Denial can occur because of inexperience, a resistant mind-set, lack of confidence, a previous "misdiagnosis," or previous telephone abuse. Nurses should be aware of their own hidden agendas. To avoid this pitfall, they should consult with colleagues in questionable cases, acknowledge and remedy their own knowledge deficits, and refine and develop protocols. Finally, they should obtain training and use extra vigilance with chronic callers.

Noncompliance

Despite advances in diagnosis and treatment, noncompliance continues to plague providers. In telephone triage, nurses are likely to encounter clients who refuse to make and keep verbal contracts. In extreme cases, noncompliance can lead to medical complications.

Noncompliance stems from several sources. Clients may have health beliefs or hold spiritual or other values incompatible with the advice given. Cultural influences may intervene. Clients may be inadequately informed.

An often overlooked reason clients fail to come in for appointments is that they cannot afford treatment. Indigent and low-income families and even middle-class clients often wait until the symptoms have reached crisis proportions. Socioeconomic status is always a possible factor in noncompliance, especially as health care becomes more expensive and less accessible. To be most effective, explore reasons for noncompliance before proceeding with further advice.

Facilitating Compliance. To facilitate client compliance, first understand the client's perception of the problem. The understanding nurse who acknowledges the postpartum mother's anger without judging exemplifies an empathic response. She further reduces the mother's sense of alienation and isolation by pointing out that her emotions are common in new mothers—she is not the only one. In the case of the elderly Hispanic man with cardiac symptoms who refused to go to the emergency room, the nurse might voice her suspicion and gently ask, "Are you afraid you might die if you go?" This acknowledgement might have helped the man realize that he could die at home, too, if he does not seek help.

Empathy includes not only tuning in to possible hidden agendas and different value systems, but discerning that the client might have a different level of knowledge. The client is most likely not a health professional. Therefore, give concrete instructions. For example, if a child has gotten a foreign substance in her eye, don't simply say, "Wash her eye with water." Rather, instruct the parent, "Wrap her in a beach towel to keep her from wiggling around, lay her on her back on the drainboard. Trickle a *slow* stream of *cool* water from the faucet into her eye for *five minutes* by the clock. Then call me back." Keep sentences short. Use lay language. Do not say, "My diagnosis is that it's a viral infection which is causing a flu-like syndrome. Better use acetaminophen instead of aspirin." Say instead, "Your child may have flu. Aspirin can be dangerous for children under 16 years of age. Use Tylenol® instead." Directives can be kept to a minimum and yet be safe and effective.

When you have shown an empathetic understanding of the client's perception of the problem, congruence, authenticity, and self-disclosure will improve the quality of the nurse/client relationship. The nurse can say to the fearful man, "I had to go to the hospital last year because of appendicitis. I was frightened, too." The client may then be prompted to say, "You're better now?" A route has been opened to problem solving. The client might now be willing to make a verbal contract: "I'll ask my son to drive me to the emergency room if they will let him stay with me." Appropriate self-disclosure makes nurses more effective and credible. For example, parenthood is a rich resource of life experience from which to draw when counseling clients.

Verbal contracts or plans of action bolster compliance. Clients who repeat a mutually agreeable course of action are more likely to carry it out. Verbal contracts foster ownership of problems and solutions, whether to administer Tylenol® and call back or to come to ED within 20 minutes. The more collaborative the interaction, the better. Facilitate decision making and problem solving by presenting ideas, information, or options to callers. Resist the impulse to "fix" problems and take control—it increases clients' feelings of dependency and powerlessness.

As an added benefit, increasing compliance has value in risk management. Clients who are informed *and* involved in decision making are less likely to bring suit against the provider because of their collaborative role (Thayer, 1984).

Knowledge Deficits

Lack of adequate knowledge can cause problems in compliance. Knowledge deficits stem from several sources: lack of exposure, lack of recall, misinterpretation, cognitive limitations, or lack of motivation to learn. Clues to knowledge deficits appear when clients describe problems, fail to follow through on instructions, state misconceptions, or ask questions. Sometimes clients call in a state of heightened awareness, anxious to stop old behaviors or learn new ones. Some refer to this as the "teachable moment," a time when a person is ready to make a change. Timing is important in identifying and seizing teachable moments. Telephone nurses can be change agents if they know when to confront problems and do so without alienating clients.

But the nurse's role as educator goes beyond the solution of immediate problems. The bulk of the work in telephone triage falls into the teaching and coaching function, and this function is part of preventive medicine and consumer advocacy. Thus, a mother who learns over the phone that a serious complication of diarrhea in infants is dehydration can also learn the simple measures for rehydration. The next time the baby has diarrhea, she can prevent serious complications—and can teach others. A teenager who learns to treat a first-degree burn by running cool water over it until the pain stops feels empowered—and can teach others.

Traditionally, client teaching has been undervalued and neglected. As an area of independent nursing, however, it presents unlimited opportunities to develop an autonomous, creative practice.

CHAPTER 3

EXERCISE 1: DIFFERENTIATING BETWEEN OPEN-ENDED AND LEADING QUESTIONS

OBJECTIVE: To practice distinguishing between open-ended and leading questions.

METHOD: Mark "O" for open-ended or "L" for leading. Generally, leading questions can be answered with a simple yes or no. By providing the answers in the questions, leading questions may cause the client to give misleading information. Open-ended questions allow the client to respond in a more creative, spontaneous, and accurate way.

EXAMPLE: O Describe your symptoms.
L Is your urine cloudy?

EXERCISE

______ How are you feeling?

______ Is it getting worse?

______ Have you ever had a bladder infection before?

______ Have you ever had anything like this before?

______ Did the pain begin suddenly?

______ How did the pain begin?

______ Where exactly is the pain located?

______ Is the pain above your pubic bone?

______ How are you feeling in general?

______ Do you feel run down, fatigued?

______ Tell me about the pain.

______ Is your pain sharp?

______ Are you having difficulty breathing?

______ How is your breathing right now?

______ Do you have any other symptoms going along with this?

______ Are you having shortness of breath, sweating, dizziness?

______ Give me a rating on a scale of 1 to 10, if 10 is the worst pain you've ever had.

______ Is this the worst pain you've ever had?

______ How many loose stools have you had today?

______ Have you had severe diarrhea?

EXERCISE 2: FORMULATING OPEN-ENDED QUESTIONS

OBJECTIVE: To formulate open-ended questions.

METHOD: In teams or individually, formulate open-ended alternatives to the following leading questions.

EXAMPLE: L: Are your stools black or bloody?
O: Describe your stools.

EXERCISE

L Is this pain in your lower abdomen?

______ ______________________________

L Does it look like chicken pox?

______ ______________________________

L Do you have a fever?

______ ______________________________

L Does the pain go down your arm?

______ ______________________________

L Is your headache pounding?

______ ____________________

L Do you have a lack of appetite?

______ ____________________

L Is the bleeding bright red?

______ ____________________

L Are you bleeding a lot?

______ ____________________

L Is the symptom worse?

______ ____________________

L Are you allergic to pollen?

______ ____________________

L Does walking make it better? Does rest make the pain worse?

______ ____________________

EXERCISE 3: REFINING COMMUNICATION SKILLS EXPLAINING MEDICAL TERMS IN LAY LANGUAGE

OBJECTIVE: To practice explaining medical terms in lay language and encourage the use of lay language in triage work.

METHOD: Translate the following medical terms to lay language as in the example below using a separate sheet of paper. Then compare your definitions with those found in a medical encyclopedia or a medical dictionary for accuracy and conciseness.

EXAMPLE:

Medical term	Lay language
Impetigo	Small yellow crusty sores with or without surrounding redness. Skin infection. Highly contagious.

EXERCISE: Lethargy
Jaundice
Dehydration
Anemia
Angina
Herpes
Ectopic pregnancy
Otitis media
Gastroenteritis
Pneumonia
Reye's syndrome
Sciatica
Projectile vomiting
Dyspnea
Anaphylaxis
Migraine
Sprain
Menopause
Pleurisy
Hemorrhoids
Lice
Tinnitus
Corneal laceration
Petechiae
Palpitations
Hives
Epistaxis
Dysmenorrhea

EXERCISE 4: MATCHING KEY CONCEPTS

OBJECTIVE: To match key concepts with examples.

METHOD: Match Column A key concepts with Column B examples. There is only one answer per item.

COLUMN A	COLUMN B
1. Open-ended question	______ Epistaxis
2. Leading question	______ "Go to the nearest emergency room."
3. Medical term	______ "What makes you think you're in labor?"
4. Lay language	______ "I'm using more than one pad per hour."
5. Pertinent negative	______ Nosebleed
6. Eliciting hidden agenda	______ Do you have any other questions or concerns?
7. Intervention	______ No shortness of breath
8. Working diagnosis	______ "From what you describe, it sounds like the flu."
9. Quantitative severity	______ "I have a splitting headache."
10. Qualitative severity	______ "Are you having crushing chest pain?"

EXERCISE 5: MATCHING INTERVIEW TECHNIQUES WITH EXAMPLES

OBJECTIVE: To link interview techniques with sample phrases.

METHOD: Match statements in Column B with objectives in Column A.

EXAMPLE: Disclaimer = Remember, I cannot diagnose by phone. If you do not feel comfortable managing this problem at home, you are welcome to come in.

COLUMN A		COLUMN B
OBJECTIVES		STATEMENTS
_____ Clarifying	A	Let me make sure I have this correct. Is that clear? Do you understand?
_____ Restating	B	Then, your plan is to . . . Let me see if I have this straight . . . Let me summarize . . . Your main concern is . . .
_____ Validating	C	Is there anything else bothering you? Do you have any questions or concerns?
_____ Exploring	D	I can see why you're anxious. You sound discouraged.
_____ Empathizing	E	Uh-huh. I hear you. I understand.
_____ Problem facilitation	F	Anytime you have further questions or if the symptoms become markedly worse or fail to improve with this treatment, please call. Call me back in one hour.
_____ Eliciting hidden agendas	G	Have you considered . . . ? What have you tried in the past? What are your options? What do you mean by that?
_____ Contracting	H	Repeat back my instructions. What is your plan of action?
_____ Working diagnosis	I	From what you've told me, it sounds like . . . My impression is . . . Going on the assumption that this is the flu . . . My working diagnosis for this problem is . . .
_____ Follow-up instructions	J	Tell me more about . . . And . . . ? Um hmm . . . ? You gave the Tylenol and then . . . ?

ANSWER KEY

EXERCISE 1: DIFFERENTIATING BETWEEN OPEN-ENDED AND LEADING QUESTIONS

O How are you feeling?
L Is it getting worse?
L Have you ever had a bladder infection before?
O Have you ever had anything like this before?
L Did the pain begin suddenly?
O How did the pain begin?
O Where exactly is the pain located?
L Is the pain above your pubic bone, in your pubic area?
O How are you feeling in general?
L Do you feel run down, fatigued?
O Tell me about the pain.
L Is your pain sharp?
L Are you having difficulty breathing?
O How is your breathing right now?
O Do you have any other symptoms going along with this?
L Are you having shortness of breath, sweating, dizziness?
O Give me a rating on a scale of 10, if 10 is the worst pain you've ever had.
L Is this the worst pain you've ever had?
O How many stools have you had today?
L Have you had severe diarrhea?

EXERCISE 2: FORMULATING OPEN-ENDED QUESTIONS

L Is this pain in your lower abdomen?
O Where is your pain?

L Does it look like chicken pox?
O Describe the rash.

L Do you have a fever?
O What is your temperature?

L Does the pain go down your arm?
O Do you have pain anywhere else?

L Is your headache pounding?
O Describe your headache.

L Do you have a lack of appetite?
O How is your appetite?

L Is the bleeding bright red?
O Describe the bleeding.

L Are you bleeding a lot?
O How many pads have you used?

L Is the situation worse?
O Is the symptom getting better, worse or staying the same?

L Are you allergic to pollen?
O Do you have any allergies?

L Does walking make it better? Does rest make the pain worse?
O What makes it better? What makes it worse?

EXERCISE 3: REFINING COMMUNICATION SKILLS

Compare definitions with a medical dictionary or encyclopedia for lay persons for accuracy and conciseness.

EXERCISE 4: MATCHING KEY CONCEPTS

3 Epistaxis
7 "Go to the nearest emergency room"
1 "What makes you think you're in labor?"
9 "I'm using more than one pad per hour."
4 Nosebleed
6 Do you have any other questions or concerns?
5 No shortness of breath
8 "From what you describe, it sounds like the flu."
10 "I have a splitting headache."
2 "Are you having crushing chest pain?"

EXERCISE 5: MATCHING INTERVIEW TECHNIQUES WITH EXAMPLES

OBJECTIVE	STATEMENT
1 Clarifying	A
2 Restating	B
3 Validating	E
4 Exploring	J
5 Empathizing	D

6	Problem facilitation	G
7	Eliciting hidden agendas	C
8	Contracting	H
9	Working diagnosis	I
10	Follow-up instructions	F

SECTION 2

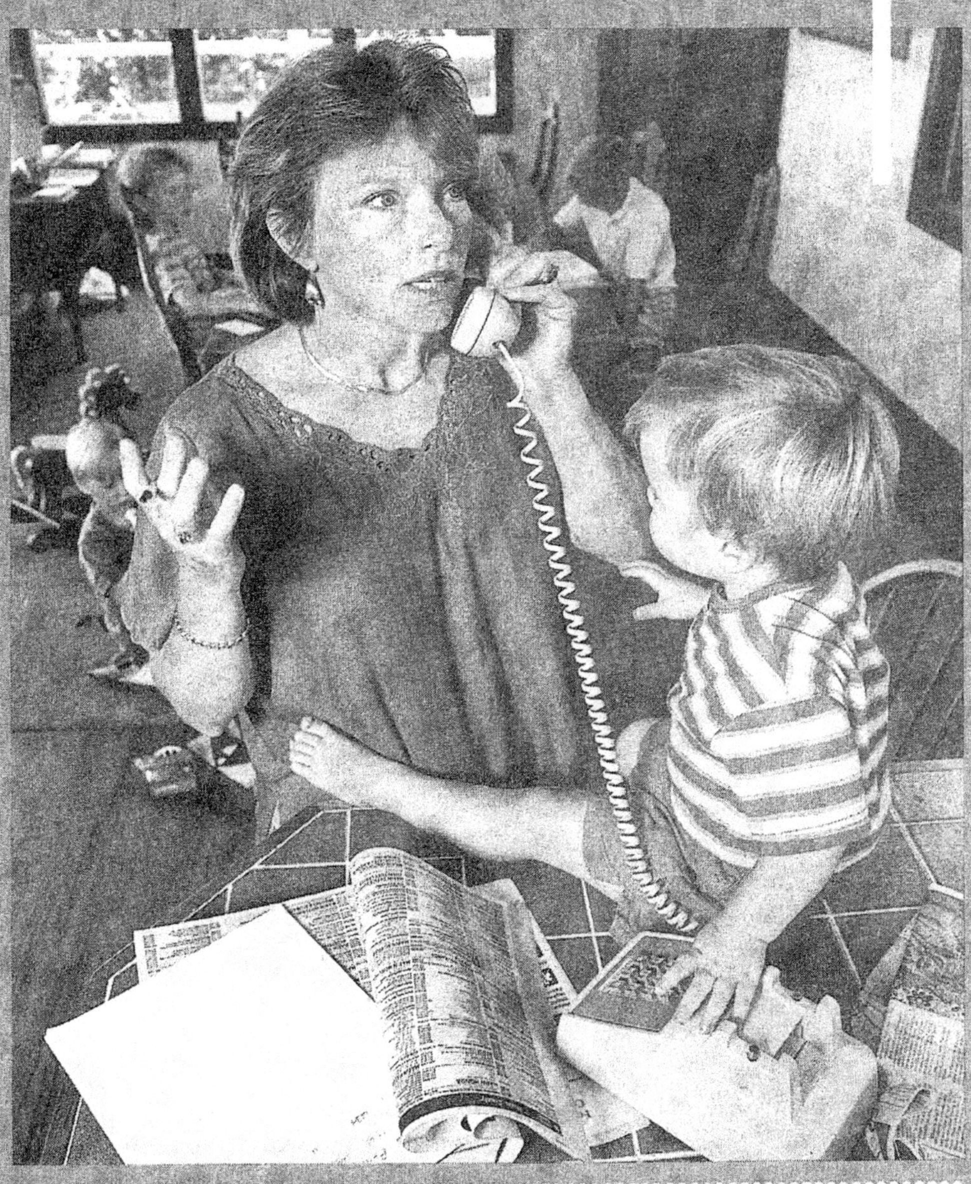

(Photo on previous page) *Parents of young children call frequently for telephone advice. (Richard Wheeler, Photographer)*

CHAPTER 4

Telephone Triage and the Nursing Process

"Nurses can function according to defined purposeful expectations or by intuition. A nursing system can operate in a designated manner or haphazardly. Patient care can be delivered by design or by impulse and habit. Standards either exist or they do not. If they exist, they must be detailed, consistent and comprehensive or they will be shallow, irrelevant and worthless." (Marker, 1988)

THE GOAL OF TELEPHONE TRIAGE

The scope of telephone triage practice is wide and the spectrum of presenting problems can be complex. Calls may involve information dispensing, referral, education or counseling. Individual callers and specific problems require a variety of intellectual, verbal, and emotional skills. The seasonal and daily ebb and flow of callers and symptoms constantly challenges the vigilance and standards of nurses, who must be alert to hidden agendas, misdiagnosis, and ill-timed calls.

As with all nursing care, the goal of telephone triage is to ensure *safe, effective, appropriate* care (Smith-Marker, 1988). One approach to problem solving is the nursing process: assessment, diagnosis, planning, implementation and evaluation. The nursing process is a standardized, yet flexible approach to problem management, on the phone or at the bedside. There are differences, however. For example, at the bedside, assessment is facilitated by verbal, visual, tactile and auditory cues; on the phone, assessment is limited to auditory, verbal and emotional cues. At the bedside, nurses formulate a nursing diagnosis, while on the phone, diagnoses are limited to impressions or working diagnoses. Instead of taking place over a period of hours or days, the telephone triage process is accomplished within an average of 5 to 8 minutes. Instead of formulating a plan, the nurse utilizes protocols and adapts them to the specific client. Finally, in telephone triage, the last two steps of the nursing process—intervention and evaluation—are carried out by the client rather than the nurse. The telephone triage nurse instructs callers to treat, monitor and self-evaluate symptoms.

The nursing process is an "organized, systematic and deliberate" (Yura & Walsh, 1978 p. 1) approach to the practice of nursing. Its purpose is to guide nursing care as well as provide for continuity of care. Among other goals, Christensen & Kenney (1990) state that the nursing process is "dynamic" and "adaptable to any practice setting or specialization" and that the "components may be used sequentially or concurrently" (p. 10). Thus, many telephone triage experts have adapted the practice of telephone triage to the nursing process (McGear & Simms 1988; Matherly & Hodges, 1990; Scott & Packard, 1990). This approach makes sense—the nursing process is familiar to nurses and provides a structure which promotes logical problem solving. Telephone triage practice is fraught with difficulty and common errors abound, partly due to its collaborative nature. The arbitrary and variable quality of the workload makes the nursing process important. This chapter examines common errors and suggests a problem solving approach based on the nursing process.

Common Practice Errors

As evidenced by studies over the last 20 years, telephone triage practice has been traditionally intuitive and informal. Without accountability or standards many false assumptions and practice errors have arisen. As noted at the opening of the chapter, nursing practice (which includes telephone triage) must not be erratic or impulsive. Until recently, most telephone triage nurses learned by trial and error. This section illustrates common practice errors, hopefully preventing novice practitioners from repeating the mistakes of their predecessors.

Using Leading Questions. The most common practice error is probably that of using leading questions. Leading questions contain the answer and require a simple yes or no response. Soliciting responses rather than eliciting information fosters an authoritarian attitude and discourages collaboration. Leading questions are everything but descriptive: 1. they cut down on the amount and variety of information and yield minimal new information; 2. they foster client passivity by encouraging the client to follow the nurse's lead in data gathering; and, 3. they can lead to stereotyping or mistriage of problems.

Successful communications depend as much on receiving and maximizing information received as sending it. Bates (1991) recommends that questions "proceed from the general to the specific" (p. 17). Start with general questions or directives such as "Can you describe your pain? Tell me about the rash" and proceed to more specific questions such as "When did it start? Where is it located? What happened before it started?" Bates also recommends asking questions which "require a graded response" (p. 18). Graded responses include questions like "How many wet diapers? How many stools? How much pain on a scale of 1–10?" As mentioned in chapter 2, some clients are poor historians. Rather than using leading questions, offer the client multiple-choice answers like "Is the pain better, worse, or the same as two days ago?" Finally, in order to avoid confusion, ask one question at a time.

Using Medical Jargon. Successful communications require the exchange of information between two people using the same medium—the same language. However, to the client, medical terminology is another language. Thus, for maximum information exchange, all communications (including written protocols and verbal utterances) must be in lay language and aimed at a 5th to 12th grade reading level.

Inadequate Data Collection. The most common cause of faulty triage is inadequate data collection. Seemingly inconsequential calls require unswerving patience. Vague symptoms such as abdominal pain require careful and time-consuming assessment.

> *A mother called regarding her 5-year-old daughter's bee sting. The nurse asked if there were any signs of allergic reaction, and the mother's response was negative. The nurse advised applying ice and meat tenderizer. Two days later the child was brought to the emergency department with symptoms of acute chemical conjunctivitis and possible blindness. The nurse had failed to determine the location of the bee sting, which turned out to be near the eye (Wheeler, 1989).*

Many illnesses are hidden below the surface. Clients may not be educated observers. Their method of reporting may be scattered, rambling, and vague. Confused elderly persons may be especially poor historians. Some callers underestimate the significance of chronic illness when discussing current problems. Thorough data collection is a basic prerequisite and lays the groundwork for appropriate disposition.

Inadequate "Talk Time." The least studied but most easily remedied deficiency is that of inadequate "talk time," the time spent processing the call. Most institutions either have no standards for talk time, while others are unrealistically brief. In fact, some gatekeeper systems require that nurses process 20 calls per hour (3 minutes per call). When it comes to telephone triage, *proficiency and efficiency are not synonymous.* If *efficiency* is defined as the speed with which an act is performed, *proficiency* should be defined as the effectiveness and expertise with which the act is performed. A study of medical students' telephone triage skills revealed an inverse relationship between efficiency and proficiency—as efficiency increased, proficiency decreased (Smith & Fischer, 1980). The authors suggest the training programs stress proficiency first and efficiency later, after a high level of proficiency is attained.

It is common for physicians to interrupt without hearing the client out (Curtis & Evans, 1983; Sloane, et al, 1985). This may be the result of training, work setting, and a predisposition to make quick decisions. However, failure to listen and elicit information can lead to inappropriate dispositions. Furthermore, a brusque manner may alienate clients and result in noncompliance.

A key study (Perrin & Goodman, 1978) compared nurse practitioners with pediatricians. Among other findings, researchers found that physicians averaged 3 to 5 minutes while nurses spent 5 to 7 minutes per call. Nurses were found to be equally or more proficient than physicians in call management. Researchers felt that the extra time spent in each call was an *indicator of quality and effectiveness* rather than a result of inefficiency. The Group Health Cooperative of Puget Sound, a leading HMO, adheres to a standard talk time of 5 to 7 minutes per call. Although no studies exist to validate the optimum call length, most have found that an *average* of 6 minutes per call is sufficient for safe, effective, and appropriate dispositions.

Stereotyping Clients or Problems. Inadequate talk time, as well as failure to remain open to new or discrepant information, can lead to stereotyping of symptoms or clients. Surprisingly, this is a common pitfall of *experienced* nurses, who often jump to conclusions. Often, critical pieces of data are revealed at the end of the call, necessitating a new working diagnosis and management plan. Emphasizing thorough data collection rather than split-second decision making would avoid this pitfall. Two case histories illustrate this point:

> *A client called and asked "Will gas kill you?" The nurse quickly responded that the caller could take Maalox and see a physician if there was no improvement. Several minutes later, the nurse realized that the client intended to use gas for a suicide attempt.*

In this case, a few extra minutes spent probing for additional information could have produced a different outcome.

> *A 65-year-old woman called complaining of "burning on urination and possible vaginitis." She asked repeatedly about whether the condition was "contagious." (Curtis, 1983)*

The physician ignored the repeated concerns about contagion, jumping to the conclusion that the symptoms were related to a urinary tract infection. However, the hidden agenda was an underlying fear of sexually transmitted disease, a valid fear in view of the fact that many elderly clients have active sex lives. In this case, the physician stereotyped the symptoms *and* client, assuming that elderly clients are not at risk for sexually transmitted diseases.

Failure to Talk Directly with Client. Telephone triage nurses are sensorily deprived—unable to observe body language or directly verify signs or symptoms. Talking directly with the client helps to minimize confusion, cuts down on potential errors, facilitates data collection, and expedites the process. Sometimes a direct conversation is impossible, with children or aphasic clients, for example. In general, however, children over the age of eight give accurate information. Therefore, with children eight and above, talk with both child and caregiver. Be aware that if clients cannot or will not come to the phone, this behavior may indicate high acuity.

Client Self-Diagnosis and Second-Guessing. Beware of placing too much or too little faith in the client's history. Sometimes clients form erroneous self-diagnoses. They, too, may stereotype symptoms, deciding beforehand that "it's the flu" or "the same old back problem." Resist the impulse to accept self-diagnoses. Always form an independent assessment based on newly collected data.

> *A mother called regarding her 5-month-old infant, stating that the infant was acting fretful. She felt the irritability was due to hunger and asked the nurse if she could begin to add solids to the diet. The nurse failed to explore the problem further, concurred with the mother's assessment, and recommended starting solids. Several days later, the mother brought the infant to the hospital and a diagnosis of meningitis was made.*

On the other hand, placing too little faith in the caller could produce tragic results, especially in an emergency. "If a caller says it's an emergency, the burden of proof is not his" (Turner, 1981). This example illustrates:

> *A mother called regarding her 25-year-old daughter who was complaining of severe chest pain. When the nurse advised the mother to come to the emergency department immediately, the mother stated she needed an ambulance. The nurse called the paramedics, even though she "knew" it was not a life threatening cardiac problem. The diagnosis was myocardial infarct. (Wheeler, 1989)*

Second-guessing the client is a dangerous practice. This power struggle could be described as the "you're not sick until I say you are" syndrome. This nurse heeded the client's distress, even though her instincts told her the symptoms could not possibly be life threatening. Be aware of impulses to blindly trust the client's self diagnosis and to second-guess callers—two dangerous pitfalls.

Don't Devaluate Reassurance Calls. A major motive for calls is reassurance. Such calls play a large role in compliance and public relations. Clients seeking "hand-holding" usually call to test the system, for emotional support, or for information gathering or elaboration. For example, new parents may call to "test" the system as well as to obtain reassurance and information. They want assurance that someone is readily accessible. New parents are often are so emotionally overloaded at the hospital or office that they fail to hear instructions, or they have new questions. In many cases, the number and length of these calls is probably inversely proportional to the amount and effectiveness of patient education.

Expect calls anytime there is a major change in the client's condition, treatment, or lifestyle such as a new baby, a new illness, a new medication, or a change in the client's health status. The number of reassurance calls may also be increased by seasonal illness such as flu or chickenpox. Finally, media coverage of epidemics such as Legionnaires' disease or meningitis can increase the call volume.

Learn to distinguish between the need for hand-holding and the need for an appointment. Increasingly frequent calls or calls which do not diminish within a few weeks or months may signal the need for an appointment. Some feel that any caller requiring 10 minutes or more of reassurance should have an appointment. Hand-holding calls serve an important public relations function and may mean the difference between compliance and noncompliance, between client satisfaction and seeking another provider.

Hidden agendas are ulterior motives or emotions driving callers to seek advice. When the symptoms seem minimal or the history is cloudy, look for hidden agendas. For example, if parents call regarding their child's illness sounding desperate and mention that they've been up for five nights with the child's coughing, the hidden agenda may be the parent's sleep deprivation and desperation rather than the child's illness. These calls alleviate parental stress caused by the child's illness and should not be underrated.

Other hidden agendas or motives for calls include fears (rational or irrational), resolving arguments, sharing responsibility, or reluctance to make a decision. Some parents are very sophisticated but simply need to assure themselves that they have covered every base so they can settle down for the night. Most callers need reassurance at some point. This is an appropriate use of telephone triage and enhances the management of illnesses at home. When it eliminates the need for *unnecessary* appointments, it saves time and money for both parties, leading to a more cost-effective system.

Overreacting, Underreacting, and Fatigue. Telephone triage work is ambiguous at best, and limited sensory input makes decision making difficult. Overreacting, underreacting, and fatigue are human foibles. Some nurses may have overactive imaginations and a tendency to panic, while others have blunted perceptions and a tendency toward denial. Individual mind-sets color perceptions, leading to denial or alarmist reactions.

Denial is a strong psychological defense in coping with any illness or crisis. One way to avoid this pitfall is to confer with colleagues or physicians to raise suspicions or quiet fears appropriately. Expert nurses can be resources for novices and can lessen isolation through a team approach. Ideally, telephone triage services should be located in the emergency department, affording face-to-face consultation with colleagues 24 hours a day.

Nurses working 8 hour shifts in high-volume systems find the last few hours mentally exhausting and tedious. Frequent breaks help to cut down on tedium. Peak periods (morning and late afternoon) or seasonal peaks (flu season) should be anticipated and staffed accordingly. For example, one HMO increases staffing when the call volume reaches more than seven calls per nurse per hour. Finally, shorter shifts (2, 4 and 6 hours) act as a quality assurance measure by helping to alleviate fatigue caused by long shifts and high call volume.

STEP ONE: ASSESSMENT AND DATA COLLECTION

This section focuses on the the process of telephone triage—comparing and contrasting it to the nursing process. The assessment phase is the most difficult and time consuming part of the triage process. Diagnosis, treatment and disposition rest upon the comprehensiveness of this phase. The nurse must listen actively, intently, and for a sufficient length of time. In contrast to face-to-face assessments, the first step and overall objective of the telephone triage process is *to describe rather than to diagnose.* Reminding clients of this potential pitfall lessens their chances of forming erroneous self-diagnoses.

Interviewing and history-taking activities rely on intuitive and systematic approaches (protocols) as well as clients' charts (if available). The data collected should be "comprehensive, multifocal, recorded and communicated properly" (Christensen and Kenney, 1990, p. 55). Ideally, this stage of the process comprises about 40–50 percent of the "talk time." Assessment entails ongoing data collection. Yura and Walsh (1978) state: "The nurse sorts, organizes, groups categorizes, compares, analyzes and synthesizes the data about the client obtained up to this point." They add: "The nurse decides what to ask, when to ask it and how to ask it. She decides when to listen, how to listen and how long to listen" (p. 111). During the data collection process, every attempt must be made to altar the data as little as possible.

There may be times when protocols are either unavailable or inadequate. In such cases, rely on the steps of the telephone triage process and use the generic protocol as a guide with special attention to the assessment phase.

Interviewing by phone is difficult because clients are rarely trained observers and may inadvertently convey inaccurate impressions about themselves or their symptoms. Perceptual distortions abound. Clients may "sound 45" and yet actually be 25 or vice versa. Flat affect or hysteria make accurate assessment difficult. In addition, high call volume can lead to overload and slipshod interview techniques. It is imperative that nurses use a systematic approach. Skillful interviewers ask questions in a manner which is logical, systematic, and personable. Effective interview skills will produce sufficient diagnostic information to formulate a working diagnosis. Assessment objectives include:

1. To elicit data in sufficient quantity, quality, and detail.
2. To establish a sequence of events relating to the presenting symptom(s).

Research suggests that a major telephone triage pitfall is failure to collect enough data (Verdile et al, 1989; Levy et al, 1980; Perrin & Goodman, 1978). Obviously, every call does not require in-depth assessment. Clients presenting with clear-cut, nonurgent problems such as symptoms of earache or strep throat require little additional data collection and in many cases can be given an appointment after determining that an urgent situation does not exist. Scheduling an appointment eliminates the need for further data collection, but a record of the call should still be kept. Calls which require crisis intervention also short circuit the assessment process.

Elicit and Document Significant Data. Face-to-face assessment differs from telephone assessment in both purpose and scope. For example, the purpose of a history and physical may be either comprehensive, problem specific, or follow-up. On the phone, assessment is restricted to problem specific and/or follow-up. In person, the scope of data collection is broad and may include a history of the present illness (HPI) as well as supportive data—the patient medical history (PMH), a review of systems (ROS), family history (FH), and psychosocial history (PSH). On the other hand, telephone assessments are problem specific and the scope of data collection is narrow. For example, it would be impractical and unfeasible to perform a review of systems by phone; however, inasmuch as it is problem specific, telephone triage *assesses the presenting symptom in detail and in the light of relevant supportive data* (specific data about patient, family, and psychosocial history). Thus, telephone triage data collection focuses on the history of the present illness (HPI) and specific elements of supportive data which serve as determinants in client disposition (pregnancy, allergies, medications, previous medical problems, emotional status).

In telephone triage, assessment means data collection by proxy. The area of data collection is still controversial. What must be documented? Nurses often ask what constitutes sufficient and significant data; the answer varies with each call. In some cases it might be to collect enough data to determine if an urgent or emergent situation exists, at which point a disposition is formulated. For more routine problems, address each item of data in some way, either by documenting the client's response or noting pertinent negatives. Thus, for example, to formulate a disposition for chest pain in a 45-year-old man requires collecting a minimum of three pieces of data; a disposition for vague abdominal pain may require 16–20 pieces of data.

Data are limited to callers' observations of symptoms. Nurses synthesize significant data to form a working diagnosis, using *symptom-based* protocols. Protocols are general guidelines used to evaluate, classify, advise, educate, and dispose of client health problems. They have two major functions: assessment (evaluation and classification) and disposition (advice, education, and treatment). Protocols determine the significance and scope of data collection. Data collection questions provide a systematic method to extract and organize data. A data collection method which is used consistently provides QA by standardizing the interview and documentation process. No method, however, is without limitations, and conscientious and judicious data collection will prevent a mechanistic approach.

In telephone triage work, the data collection system must be comprehensive and yet concise, and key information must be collected efficiently. Whatever the approach, it should not be too time consuming. The acronyms SAVED, SCHOLAR, PAMPER, and ADL, explained below, are both comprehensive and concise. They may be used separately or together to gather data effectively and efficiently.

Global Assessment

Factors such as **S**everity of symptoms, **A**ge, **V**eracity, **E**motional state and **D**ebilitation and **D**istance (SAVED) may singly or collectively trigger the decision for an appointment (see Figure 4.1). This global assessment approach has several advantages. It serves as an early warning system, alerting the nurse to clients who are at high risk. It expedites data collection and decision making and quickly establishes acuity. However, be aware that relying too heavily on the global approach may lead to stereotyping or jumping to conclusions. In general, clients with several risk factors must be treated more conservatively (i.e., by appointment rather than advice).

If a client presents with several risk factors, the question becomes not *whether* but *how soon* they will be seen. For example, a frail elderly 65-year-old with hourly diarrhea and vomiting for 12 hours and a history of heart problems requires an automatic appointment, provided the symptoms are not emergent. Emergent-level calls necessitate immediate transport to an office or emergency department.

Severity. A major difficulty lies in defining what constitutes "severe." Two ways are to quantify or qualify symptoms. For example, pain described as an 8, 9 or

FIGURE 4.1 "SAVED"—Global Data

SEVERITY
- Quantitative or qualitative severity of symptoms
- Compound symptoms or a complex of symptoms which represent a classic picture.

AGE
- Below the age of 6 months
- Above the age of 55
- Female between the ages of 12 and 55
- Males over 35

VERACITY
- Second- or third-party caller
- Speaks no English
- Aphasic or confused elderly
- Drugged or confused state

EMOTIONAL STATE
- Anxiety or denial
- Previous psychiatric history
- Severe reaction to current illness

DEBILITATION/DISTANCE
- Clients with chronic disease
- Clients living at great distance or traveling at peak traffic time

10 on a scale of 1–10 (10 being the worst pain ever experienced), is quantitatively severe. Admittedly, this scale is imperfect. Children and individuals from some cultures have difficulty quantifying pain. However, this method works in most cases. Other examples of quantitative severity are:

> Vaginal bleeding of more than 1 pad per hour
> Urine output less than one scantily wet diaper per 8 hours
> More than 6–8 large watery stools in 8 hours

Qualitative severity refers to descriptive terms or characteristics. A headache described as splitting, throbbing, or blinding is considered qualitatively severe. Other examples are:

> Crushing chest pain
> Barking "seal like" cough
> Sudden, localized, sharp abdominal pain

Age. *The most important piece of data collected is the client's age.* This is true for several reasons:

1. Some diseases are age related. For example, women of reproductive age have a higher incidence of ectopic pregnancy, birth control side effects, and sexually transmitted diseases.
2. Extremes of age increase vulnerability to "routine" illnesses. All infants under six months (especially newborns and premature infants) as well as "frail elderly" over 55 years of age are more vulnerable to communicable disease and common infections. Document the age of infants and newborns in days, weeks, or months.
3. Some middle-aged people sound very young; some young people sound old. Eliciting the age at the beginning of the call expedites the process, preventing embarrassment and confusion, as shown by this example:

> *A mother called to make an appointment for her son, who complained of symptoms of a possible sprained ankle. The nurse scheduled an appointment in pediatrics. It was later revealed that the son was 40 years old.*

Veracity. Some callers are unable to state the facts accurately. In the case of severe language barriers or aphasia, the ability to receive or give accurate information is impaired. In such cases, ascertain if any emergency exists, if possible. If none exists, give an appointment and document that the caller has a "severe language barrier." It is more expeditious and legally less risky to give appointments than to attempt to evaluate symptoms by phone.

Information relayed through **second** or **third parties** is almost always distorted in some way. This risk is often associated with calls about children. Third-party calls occur when the working parent receives a report of the child's condition from the caretaker, a situation often requiring an appointment.

Emotional Status. Emotional status is a major factor in assessing acuity. One study of calls to medical dispatchers showed two factors to be related to actual cardiac arrests. In 96% of the cases regarding cardiac arrest, *callers were highly emotionally distraught and victims were 50 years of age or older* (Eisenberg, 1986).

Assess carefully the *immediate* emotional state. If possible, determine if emotions (signs of hysteria, panic, confusion, unusually flat affect, or denial) are a temporary reaction to the current illness or chronic, long-standing emotional patterns. Like acute illness, extreme emotional reactions upgrade the call acuity. For example, if a caller known to be normally calm, exhibits extreme panic, it indicates high acuity. On the other hand, panic in a caller known to be an alarmist may be a "normal" reaction. However, all callers exhibiting extremes of emotion must also be handled with care. Overanxious parents, drug abusers, chronic callers, and psychiatric patients may confound the most conscientious of interviewers. Having heard the client's story once too often, nurses resist what seems to be merely attention-getting behavior. Yet an urgent situation may exist. Severe anxiety is a red flag signaling the the need for an appointment. Signs of severe anxiety can include multiple phone calls within a short period of time, client statements, tone of voice, rapid speech, and extremes of affect.

Always document client hostility, legal threats, system abuse, inappropriate affect, confusion, multiple phone calls, extremes of affect, and client statements of emotional state to assure that calls are placed within the proper context and not disregarded.

Debilitation. Chronic disease and debilitation upgrade acuity. For example, "flu symptoms" might prove life threatening in clients with AIDS, cancer, hemophilia, congenital defects, alcoholism, drug abuse, or multiple surgeries.

Distance. Distance is a risk factor that applies mainly to rural areas but may also apply to urban settings where rush hour gridlock may impede paramedic transport. Time and distance to medical aid always upgrades acuity in borderline cases.

> *A 75-year-old male was discharged following coronary artery bypass surgery. Following a 2-hour drive home, he experienced shortness of breath and fatigue. He lived 2 hours from the nearest hospital.*

Thus, using the global approach, an example of a high risk client might be a male over 35 with chest pain, whose wife is calling for him. Without even consulting a protocol, it is clear that he qualifies in three out of five categories: severe symptoms (chest pain), age and sex (35 year old male), and veracity (second party call). On this basis alone, such a client requires immediate transport to the nearest emergency department.

The Generic Protocol

Protocols are general guidelines (questions and advice) for the evaluation, classification, advice, education, and disposition of problems. For purposes of this discussion, protocols are divided into generic and specific. The generic protocol as described here, consists *only* of questions which elicit the history and details and *common* aspects of the present illness (HPI) as well as relevant supportive data about the client's medical history (PMH), family history (FH), and psychosocial history (PSH). Specific protocols, on the other hand, contain *both* questions and advice *specific* to the present illness (see Appendices P, Q, R).

Primary Questions. The second level of data collection is comprised of primary questions that explore the chief complaint and provide a brief history of the presenting problem. Most chief complaints are characterized by pain, abnormal function, change from a normal state, or observations by the client. The SCHOLAR list of questions asks what, how much, when, where, and how often. (See Figure 4.2.)

FIGURE 4.2 "SCHOLAR"— Primary Data

SYMPTOMS AND ASSOCIATED SYMPTOMS
Pulse, temperature, recent blood pressure

CHARACTERISTICS
Qualitative and quantitative descriptors of severity

COURSE
Are the symptoms better, worse, or same? Effect on daily routine?

HISTORY OF SYMPTOM(S) IN PAST
What was done? By whom? When? Results?

ONSET
When did it start? How long has it existed? (Try to get in time frames of 8, 16 or 24 hour periods) Gradual or sudden? (Sudden onset tends to be more serious)

LOCATION
Strive for precise location. Radiation? Localized vs. diffuse? (Localized tends to be more serious)

AGGRAVATING FACTORS
What (food, medications, activities, positions) makes it worse?

RELIEVING FACTORS
What (food, medications, activities, positions) makes it better? What has the client done thus far to relieve symptoms and was it successful?

Secondary Questions. The third level of data collection is comprised of secondary questions which *briefly* explore certain elements of the client's previous medical history (PMH), relevant family history (FH), and psychosocial history (PSH). This supportive data provides additional information about the client that may expedite the decisionmaking process. The acronym for this is PAMPER. If global or primary data is sufficient in quantity and quality, form a working diagnosis and choose a specific protocol. Always collect secondary data if primary data is insufficient, if the chart is unavailable, or if the client is unknown to the nurse. (See Figure 4.3)

FIGURE 4.3 "PAMPER"—Secondary Data

PREGNANCY STATUS/BREAST FEEDING?

All sexually active women between ages 12 and 50. Ask: "Are you sexually active? What method of birth control do you use and have you used it consistently?"

ALLERGIES

Food, chemicals, drugs, and pollen?

MEDICATIONS

Current over-the-counter, birth control pills, recreational drugs, alcohol, vitamins (e.g., megadoses of B vitamins have been known to cause alarming side effects)

PREVIOUS HEALTH

Chronic illness, surgery? Family history of disease? Eating disorders?

EMOTIONAL STATUS (relates to previous emotional state rather than immediate emotional state)

Recent (job, family, relationship) emotional stress? Psychiatric history?

RECENT INJURY, INFECTION, ILLNESS OR INGESTION

Recent communicable illness or exposure? Injury or ingestion? (Ask for time frames)

Use SCHOLAR and PAMPER before referring to specific protocols. This has certain advantages:

1. It is a quick way to establish urgency.
2. It pinpoints the correct specific protocol when clients present with multiple or conflicting symptoms.
3. It incorporates many of the same questions as specific protocols, ultimately saving time.
4. It serves as a generic protocol when no specific protocol exists.

Synthesizing intuitive and standardized approaches combines the best features of both. This cumulative approach starts with intuitive questions and follows up with standardized ones. Generally, it is best to start with SCHOLAR and PAMPER, followed by more detailed, specialized questions from specific protocols. In the case of multiple symptoms, focus on the most acute symptom or one which is most likely to lead to an appointment (Schmitt, 1980, p.3). For example, a frail elderly caller with a history of multiple abdominal surgeries presents symptoms of sore throat and dizziness. Dizziness is the most acute symptom in view of client age, history, and symptom severity. Thus, this protocol is the best choice.

Medication-Related Calls. Not surprisingly, a large percentage of advice calls are about medications (refills, possible side effects, and interactions) and many of these callers are elderly women (Curtis & Talbot, 1980). Overmedication, drug interactions, or side effects are common underlying causes for presenting symptoms in the elderly.

> *A middle-aged woman called. She was concerned about a possible interaction between her antidepressant and an over-the-counter decongestant. The directions on the box of decongestant warned against combining it with MAO inhibitor antidepressants. The nurse checked and discovered that the decongestant was contraindicated and could have caused a serious reaction.*

Before advising any medication, prescription or over-the-counter, *always* check breastfeeding and pregnancy status, allergies, and current medications. To avoid confusion when refilling medications, have clients spell out the name while reading directly from the label.

The FDA is moving quickly to approve many prescription drugs for over-the-counter (OTC) status. One expert, Fred Weissman, Pharm.D., J.D., compares it to "putting a film on video when theater sales dry up" (Gray, 1991 p. 1). Although it seems progressive, this new policy has significant implications for telephone triage nurses, raising new questions about nursing autonomy and the limits of practice. It will have serious repercussions if standards are not formulated concurrently. Some warn that OTC access can lead to delayed diagnosis, flawed triage, and possible complications. Experts recommend the following guidelines:

1. Determine if the client is taking any OTC medication.
2. Educate clients about when symptoms require an appointment.
3. Instruct clients to follow up if symptoms fail to improve on medication.
4. Instruct newly pregnant women about the potential danger of OTC medications, (Gray, 1991).

Always explore and document current medications, including birth control pills and OTC medicines. Ask all women of reproductive age: "Is there any possibility that you might be pregnant? What is your method of birth control? Have you used it consistently?" Determine the breastfeeding status as appropriate.

Pharmacists are invaluable but underutilized sources of information. Because medication questions are a large portion of calls, responding directly may take up valuable time. Some nurses refer these callers to a pharmacist. Answering medication questions directly requires access to current drug references written in lay language. Finally, educate clients about the role of the pharmacist, and instruct them to establish a relationship with a pharmacist for future medication questions.

Recent Illness, Infection, Injury, or Ingestion. Concurrent illness, injury, or possible ingestions cloud the picture and increase acuity. The following example illustrates how a recent head injury superimposed upon routine symptoms of an upper respiratory infection and drowsiness complicated the diagnostic picture:

> *A mother called regarding her child, who had hit his head and seemed cranky and drowsy. He had also been on a decongestant for a recent upper respiratory infection. The mother wanted to know if the drowsiness was due to the medication or the fall.*

The nurse advised the parent to observe the child over the next few hours after giving head injury instructions. The caller was also instructed to call back if there was any marked change in condition or failure to progress.

Activities of Daily Living (ADL)

With children and frail elderly, SCHOLAR and PAMPER may be ineffective. Clients may be poor historians, confused, or preverbal. In these cases, the best barometer of health is activities of daily living (ADL): how the client is eating, drinking, sleeping, playing, working, and eliminating (urine output and bowel movements) general appearance and demeanor. Activities of daily living provide a surprisingly concrete picture of the client when other data are sketchy.

Activities of daily living focus on certain "vegetative functions"—general mood and normal routine patterns. This assessment is compared with the client's normal baseline state. This baseline state can also be evaluated by a second party. Ask these specific questions:

1. How much and what food has the person eaten? (Intake)
2. How much in clear fluids (not milk)? (Intake)
3. What is the quantity and quality of bowel movements? (Output)
4. What is the quantity and quality of urine output? (Output)
5. What is the client's current activity level? Did the person stay home from work or school? Are they following their usual routine? (Activity)
6. How well and how long did the person sleep? More than usual or less than usual? (Sleep)
7. What is the person's general appearance—color and mood, compared to their usual temperament? How sick do they seem? (Appearance/Mood)

Ideally, data should be collected about two sources—the client and the symptom (see Figure 4.4). The data collection methods (SAVED, SCHOLAR, PAMPER, and ADL) elicit a range of information from global (or generic) to specific. They should precede specific protocols which elicit specific information about the client or the symptom. For example, SAVED asks generic questions. With the exception of Severity (which pertains to the symptom), the remaining questions pertain to the client (Age, Veracity, Emotional Status, and Debilitation or Distance). The generic protocols are data collection tools which elicit primary and secondary information. SCHOLAR (primary) elicits specific information about the symptom(s), while PAMPER (secondary) collects specific data about the client. Finally, ADL is a data collection tool which, in the absence of a specific symptom, focuses on the client condition.

FIGURE 4.4 Data Collection Methods

SYMPTOM DATA		
S(AVED)	SCHOLAR	SPECIFIC PROTOCOLS
Global Data	Primary Data	Specific Data
CLIENT DATA		
(S)AVED	PAMPER	ADL
Global Data	Secondary Data	Specific Data

Facilitate Client Self-Assessment

In telephone triage, the nurse must enlist the aid of the client who performs self-assessment and self-evaluation. In fact, some studies suggest developing better methods to get clients to describe their symptoms accurately (Levy et al, 1980). In telephone triage, the nurse uses the methods of auscultation, inspection, palpation, and the sense of smell to assess symptoms. The nurse can perform some auscultation by phone (gross respirations, emotional tenor, speech patterns, background sounds). However, the client must serve as eyes, nose, and hands to the nurse who then elicits data about what the client sees, smells, and feels.

Assessment by proxy includes visual, auditory, tactile, and olfactory data. For example, a visual assessment of a possible fracture includes comparison of extremities (fingers, hands, feet, ankles) for swelling, discoloration, or deformity (How do the wrists compare?), as well as tactile information (Is there point tenderness?). In the case of a possible chemical ingestion, elicit olfactory data (What does the child's breath smell like?). To determine whether pitting edema is present, ask the client to press on the ankle for 5 to 10 seconds and then note whether there is a deep indentation which fails to disappear quickly (visual and tactile data).

Pain is a common presenting symptom and may be sudden or gradual, severe or mild, diffuse or localized. If the client can point with one finger to the location, it may indicate localized pain, whereas if they cannot, it may indicate diffuse pain. Landmarks help to identify the location of pain or other symptoms. The elbows, knees, nipples, sternum, umbilicus, and pelvic bones can serve as landmarks to aid clients in self assessment. Use a clock analogy to determine location of a foreign body in the eye or a lump in the breast. (See Appendix J for additional examples).

It may be helpful to formally acknowledge to the client the collaborative nature of the telephone encounter. With certain exceptions, clients are subject to many of the same errors as the nurse—stereotyping, inadequate data collection, erroneous self-diagnosis, overreacting, underreacting, and fatigue. Making clients aware of these pitfalls can facilitate the process.

Use Time Frames

Time frames are another self-assessment tool. They aid in clarifying symptom duration as well as home treatment and disposition instructions. Use them at the following points:

1. When eliciting symptoms ("How many wet diapers in the last 24 hours?")
2. When stating disposition and advice ("You must be seen within 2 hours. Can you be in the emergency department within 2 hours?")
3. When giving advice ("This flu usually lasts for 24 hours. If there is no improvement within 36–48 hours, please call back for an appointment.")

Asking clients to place symptoms within time frames of 8, 16, 24, or 48 hours helps establish acuity. Obviously, a 24-hour episode of hourly vomiting and diarrhea is more serious than a 4-hour episode. Time frames help establish the seriousness of symptoms. Finally, follow-up instructions eliminate confusion, including when to expect improvement or when to report failure to progress. In all of the above cases, time frames help achieve client compliance by clarifying symptoms, treatment, and when to call back.

STEP TWO: THE WORKING DIAGNOSIS

In telephone triage, as well as the nursing process, diagnosis requires analysis and synthesis of data. The nurse categorizes data, filling in gaps and "identifying incongruencies" (Christensen and Kenney, 1990, p. 133), using the protocols, medical expertise, and, often, intuition. In telephone triage, diagnosis is highly collaborative and the nurse is more dependent upon the caller's assessment than in a face-to-face encounter. As with all assessments, it helps to ask the client what they think their symptom means. The nurse formulates a working diagnosis rather than a nursing diagnosis. This working diagnosis is more descriptive than diagnostic—measuring seriousness rather than determining causes. Thus, nurse *and* client must always remain open to new information and be alert to the need to upgrade the diagnosis as the illness develops.

Yura and Walsh (1978) divide nursing judgments into 10 categories. Six of these apply to telephone triage. Thus, the telephone triage nurse must determine:

1. whether a problem exists;
2. whether a potential problem exists;
3. whether the client is handling it well or needs help;
4. whether the problem needs to be studied further;
5. whether the problem sounds serious; and
6. whether the problem is urgent or emergent.

These categories form the basis for triage decisions. Answering these questions is what telephone triage is all about.

Medical, Nursing, and Working Diagnoses

The issue of nursing diagnosis is fraught with controversy, and making assessments over the telephone is even more controversial. Although most nurses and physicians agree that diagnosis by phone is a dangerous practice, most argue that they are not diagnosing. However, they may fail to transmit this information to callers, who may believe that they are being diagnosed. If clients are to give informed consent, it is critical that they be made aware of the presumptive nature of the diagnosis. Thus, formally point out to the caller, at the beginning or end of the call, that this is a working diagnosis—a "rough estimate" of the problem.

It is important to distinguish among medical diagnosis, nursing diagnosis, and working diagnosis. Webster's New Collegiate Dictionary (1975) defines *diagnosis* as the "art or act of identifying a disease from its signs and symptoms, a statement or conclusion concerning the nature or cause of some phenomenon" (p. 313). Only physicians can make medical diagnoses. Likewise, only nurses can make nursing diagnoses. Nursing diagnosis is defined as a "concise phrase or term summarizing a cluster of empirical indicators . . . ." (Roy, 1982, p. 4). Both medical diagnoses and nursing diagnoses are *empirical,* which Webster's defines as, "capable of being verified or disproved by observation or experiment" (Webster, 1975, p. 373). Empirical assessment is impossible to perform by phone.

Thus, empirical diagnosis is possible when the client is physically present and tests are performed, but telephone triage diagnoses are restricted to a presumptive or working status. Webster, (1975, p. 1351) defines *working* as "adequate to permit work to be done; assumed or adopted to permit or facilitate further work or activity." Thus, the working diagnosis is not "written in stone." Rather, it is fluid, a "work in progress." This approach can be facilitated by formulating a new list of approved terminology which is different from both previous medical and nursing diagnostic terminology and approved by the institution in which it is used.

To formulate a working diagnosis, several components must be present: a symptom-based, generic protocol title (abdominal pain, nose bleed) and/or optional classifiers (severe, moderate) as well as presumptive terminology (possible, apparent). Thus, terminology also must be symptom-based, generic, classified, and presumptive. These terms create the basis for a list of approved working diagnostic terms for telephone triage use (see Appendix L). When no protocol exists, as is often the case, this terminology can help nurses to formulate a working diagnosis.

Nursing Diagnostic Terms

Unfortunately, most nursing diagnostic terms are unusable, because they are empirically based and too unwieldy for telephone triage practice. However, terms such as knowledge deficit, pain, communication deficit, noncompliance, spiritual distress, self-care deficit, and emotional distress can be used. Finally, risk factors (SAVED) are part of the working diagnosis. They not only aid in determining the disposition but also help to defend dispositions for appointments which may later be disputed.

Classifiers. Classifying terminology may include nursing diagnostic terms such as ineffective, potential for, altered, and impaired. In addition, terms such as severe, moderate, acute, nonacute, new, and chronic are useful.

Presumptive Terms. Old standbys such as etiology unknown, possible, and apparent are medically based and establish that the diagnosis is presumptive. Thus, a bare bones diagnosis might read *"nosebleed,"* the generic symptom-based title. The nursing diagnostic terms "emotional distress, communications deficit," further delineate the acuity of the symptoms. The classifier "severe" and the presumptive term "etiology unknown" complete the working diagnosis. Thus the final working diagnosis becomes *"Severe nosebleed, etiology unknown. Emotional distress/communication deficit"* describes a high acuity client.

Nurses must determine whether the symptoms are serious, if so, how serious; and if not, how to best manage them using protocol advice and their own best judgment. Any caller with serious-sounding symptoms must be seen within a safe time. Severity of symptoms has many facets. Some symptoms, although solitary, are usually considered severe, such as chest pain. Other examples of severity include multiple, conflicting, or confusing groups of symptoms (dizziness, nosebleed, possible pregnancy, recent back injury). An example of a symptom complex or classic picture might be chest pain associated with shortness of breath and diaphoresis. Another example of severity is sudden onset of mild chest pain in a 45-year-old man, a high-risk client. The cause of the chest pain—angina, myocardial infarct, pericarditis, pulmonary distress, or esophagitis—is less important than insuring safe, expeditious transport to the emergency department. Because chest pain is always considered serious, as are severe headache, abdominal pain, dizziness, and loss of consciousness, and there is no differential home treatment for different diagnoses, then the most important issue becomes the disposition—when and where the client will be seen.

Mild symptoms can be treated on a presumptive basis, provided the need for an appointment has not been clearly demonstrated, the nurse and client feel comfortable monitoring and treating at home, and the caller agrees to call back if treatment fails to work or symptoms persist. Most treatments are based on the premise that simple first aid measures or home remedies are relatively harmless but provide comfort or relieve symptoms (first-aid, food and fluids, OTC medications, rest, fever control, baths). Then even if the working diagnosis proves erroneous, little or no harm can come to the client, from the home treatment itself. However, harm can come from both the nurse and client underestimating the problem.

STEP THREE: INTERVENTION

According to Yura and Walsh (1978), "the planning phase begins with the nursing diagnosis" (p. 115) and "once the plan has been developed, the implementation phase begins" (p. 129). In telephone triage, planning and implementation are melded into intervention. The working diagnosis precedes the protocol advice or treatment plan. Rather than implement the treatment, the nurse educates and instructs the client how (or where) the symptom is to be treated. The nurse contracts with the client to carry out the treatment, which usually takes place after the call is over. In certain cases, the nurse may remain on the line and coach the client while he or she carries out and evaluates the treatment.

Disposition

At the bedside, intervention refers to treatments and medications administered by the nurse. In telephone triage, intervention becomes disposition: advice for treatment and medication (*what* and *how*) and directives about *where* and *when* treatment should take place. For example, clients may be treated at an emergency department, clinic, or at home within minutes, days, or weeks. Advice may include home treatment, referral (hot line numbers, self-help groups, community resources), reassurance, and counseling.

Contracting

An important aspect of the disposition is a verbal contract between client and nurse. Although they are not legally binding, contracts foster client ownership of problem and solution, enhance collaboration, and promote mutual understanding and compliance. It may not be realistic to have clients document instructions; however, most can repeat back the plan to assure understanding. For example, if Ms. Byrnes, an elderly client, calls complaining of severe vomiting, diarrhea, and dizziness, the nurse might reply: "Remember that I cannot diagnose by phone. Your problem could cause dehydration. At your age, dehydration can be very serious. My advice is that you come to the Emergency Department within one hour. What do you plan to do?" Ms. Byrnes agrees and the nurse writes: "Client states 'husband will drive her to ED in one hour.' " In this case, the time frame makes the disposition more concrete, decreasing possible denial and avoiding confusion.

STEP FOUR: EVALUATION

According to Christensen and Kenney (1990), "evaluation is a planned, systematic comparison of the client health status with the desired expected outcomes" (p. 220). In telephone triage, the client rather than the nurse, becomes the "agent of evaluation" (Yura & Walsh, 1978, p. 141). The nurse instructs the caller how to evaluate the effectiveness of the treatment or the progress of the illness. Thus, the final step is to educate the caller how to self-evaluate their symptoms. In most cases, the client then hangs up, performs the treatment, and evaluates the results. The client may then place a follow-up call to the nurse as needed.

Yura and Walsh (1978) postulate four possible evaluation outcomes. Three of these apply to telephone triage: improvement as expected, failure to progress, and evidence of complications or new problems. Information about desired outcomes must be passed on to the client in order for them to adequately evaluate progress at home.

Client Education and Self-Evaluation

Most clients want to "do the right thing" and call to find out what that is. It is the task of the nurse to facilitate this process. Unfortunately, many nurses and physicians fail to provide adequate instruction about how to treat the problem, including a full explanation of symptoms, how to treat them, and what to expect as a normal course of illness. One study showed that both nurses and physicians fail to ensure that clients understand their assessments, advice, and the impact of possible complications (Perrin & Goodman, 1978). To ensure the safe practice of telephone triage, clients must be taught how to monitor their progress effectively and to call back if the symptoms fail to improve. Although no pertinent studies exist, it seems self-evident that thorough and explicit instructions will decrease repeat phone calls, enhance system efficiency and patient compliance, and reduce client anxiety. Thus, at the bedside, all evaluation is carried out by the nurse; on the phone, nurses *instruct* clients to perform self-evaluation.

To treat illness at home safely the client must be reliable. One way to test reliability is to ask the client what they have tried thus far. Some clients will have tried common home remedies prior to calling, thus demonstrating a level of sophistication. Another way to assess reliability is to have clients repeat back the instructions. If they seem confused or lack confidence, schedule an appointment.

Follow-Up Instructions

Self-evaluation includes a follow-up plan composed of instruction the three areas:

1. What to expect as a normal course of events in the next few hours or days
2. Possible complications
3. A time frame within which to call back if there is failure to improve.

Always instruct clients to call back if further questions arise, symptoms worsen, or home treatment fails to work.

Closure

The final step in the telephone triage process is closure: addressing hidden agendas and making disclaimers. Some callers are embarrassed at their "irrational fears" or "stupid questions"—often the underlying motive for calls.

Exploring hidden agendas is a good way to wrap up a call. Such questions as "Is there anything else you wanted to ask me?" or "Is anything else bothering you?" can elicit the caller's true motive.

Many clients have misconceptions about the function and purpose of telephone advice. They misconstrue the role of the nurse, often thinking that they can be diagnosed by phone. Some callers are unaware that decision making is their responsibility. Informed consent requires that clients be apprised of the limitations inherent in telephone triage by the nurse.

Disclaimers serve two purposes: they disavow legal responsibility for the outcome and they bolster informed consent to clients. Disclaimers are vital in any gatekeeper system and all *routine* calls should include them. Always document any refusal to follow advice. Crisis-level calls, psychological or medical, are exceptions to the disclaimer requirement. In crises, disclaimers are inappropriate and even dangerous. Callers in a crisis are highly emotional, have impaired judgment, and may be incapable of making decisions. Disclaimer statements might be interpreted as abandonment. Clawson advises emergency medical dispatchers that "the caller in crisis becomes our responsibility" ("60 Minutes," December 25, 1989). This seems a reasonable and prudent practice for telephone triage nurses as well.

DOCUMENTATION TECHNIQUES

A governing principle of all nursing practice is, "If it wasn't documented, it wasn't done." In telephone triage, documentation is vital. However, serious deficiencies still exist. Documentation serves as a vehicle for communication between caregivers as well as a record of advice and treatment. All medical records are considered legal evidence of the care given and the quality of that care.

As with all other aspects of telephone triage, documentation standards are underdeveloped and controversial. Some feel generic forms are sufficient and less likely to lead to problems of liability (D. J. Tennenhouse, personal communication, March 26, 1992), while the author favors a more structured, specific documentation form. Both approaches have advantages and disadvantages. However, because the field is relatively untested regarding the ideal form for documentation it remains highly speculative at this point.

Even though documentation is performed in a short time, standards can be set forth and maintained. Charting must be concise and concrete. Notes should be written in appropriate and approved phraseology and terminology using standard abbreviations. To that end, each program must develop approved terms and abbreviations. (See Appendices K and L) The following illustrates examples of effective and ineffective charting.

EFFECTIVE: c/o abd pain x 3 days. Denies N, V, D.
INEFFECTIVE: Patient states she has had severe abdominal pain for 3 days. She denies any nausea, vomiting or diarrhea.

The second example is long-winded. Streamline charting by using explicit, concrete terms. Avoid ambiguity, remembering that what you write may be used against you in a court of law. Detailed, concrete data demonstrate the nurse's efforts:

EFFECTIVE: 8 loose watery green stools × 16 hours.
INEFFECTIVE: Diarrhea.

Elicit Pertinent Negatives

Pertinent negatives are documentation which help establish acuity. In general, all documentation must include complete, accurate, timely observations including *normal as well as abnormal findings*. Findings which are normal and significant are called "pertinent negatives." For example, when the presenting symptom is abdominal pain, the notation of "no black or bloody stools" demonstrates that the nurse asked the question and the client responded negatively.

EFFECTIVE: Cheesy, white vag. discharge, itching, sl. odor. Denies abd. pain, fever, malodorous discharge.
INEFFECTIVE: Yeast symptoms.

Be Concise

Thorough documentation supports the nurse's advice and dispositions. The more concrete the better. Use measurable terms such as pads per hour, diapers per hour, numbers of diarrhea or vomiting episodes. Also, use time frames. One possible guideline for triaging minor, uncomplicated symptoms is to allow sufficient time to pass for symptoms to reveal themselves, as appropriate. Clients often do this, "watching and waiting" to see if the symptom will go away. Thus a symptom placed within the context of 8, 24, or 48 hours affords a more comprehensive baseline picture of the client than those which have arisen in the last hour or two.

EFFECTIVE: 2 lg., watery stools/24 hrs.
INEFFECTIVE: Diarrhea × 24 hours.

Clients on antibiotics should always be instructed to evaluate themselves within 24 or 48 hours to measure drug effectiveness. They must be instructed to call back if symptoms persist after 24 to 48 hours.

EFFECTIVE:	On PCN 500 mg. QID × 48 hours.
INEFFECTIVE:	Taking antibiotics.

Use specific adjectives (qualitative) to describe symptoms. Although generic descriptions may seem more concise, they are generally too vague and are to be avoided.

EFFECTIVE:	"Worst headache I've ever had, splitting, throbbing."
INEFFECTIVE:	Severe headache.

Quote the client as appropriate:

EFFECTIVE:	Screaming, "I want to die!"
INEFFECTIVE:	Hysterical.

Define the emotional tone concretely:

EFFECTIVE:	Voice is breathless, high pitched, speech rapid. Called 3 × in 2 hours.
INEFFECTIVE:	Seems anxious.

Some data are best written out; other information is better suited to a checkbox approach. Thus, documentation forms may incorporate blank spaces as well as checkboxes. If allowed to do so, clients will freely describe the presenting symptom and its history. Most nurses start out by writing a description of symptoms, then review to see if any data are missing by using SCHOLAR as a checklist. PAMPER works better as a series of checkboxes or blank spaces adjacent to "trigger words" to facilitate the collection of secondary data (see Figure 5.15). Most nurses prefer to document in this way, incorporating both blank line and checkbox formats.

Another approach to documenting calls is audiotaping. This approach works best in the dispatch setting. However, taping has certain advantages if time is of the essence and calls are of high acuity. In addition, wording and intonation can be reproduced precisely. Nonetheless, audiotaping has several drawbacks. Tapes are not always admissible as evidence in a court of law. Nurses are required to inform all callers that they are being recorded. For caller and nurse alike, taping may inhibit self-disclosure, preventing intimacy and trust. Unlike written records, tapes are not readily accessible for relaying information to other providers and insuring continuity of care.

Always document the client's age, the emotional state, any threats of litigation, the presence of a language barrier, and any extenuating circumstances (recent death in the family, loss of job, recent car accident, possible child or elder abuse, etc.). Like a chart, telephone triage records may include a "mini-history," working diagnosis, self-care plan, client self-evaluation (if appropriate), and follow-up progress note.

The telephone triage process is much like the nursing process with some modifications (see Figure 4.5). It involves precise, conscientious and thorough data collection and formulating a working rather than a nursing diagnosis. The nurse can neither directly implement nor evaluate the plan, but must educate the caller to follow through on the treatment plan and evaluation steps. Finally, informed consent requires that the caller be notified of the presumptive status of the diagnosis, and accept final responsibility for the disposition. The work of telephone triage—history taking, documentation, and advice—is facilitated by the tools of the trade: protocols, forms, and standards.

ADDITIONAL GUIDELINES

Telephone triage is "client driven" meaning that clients call at times and for reasons of their own choosing. For example, a client may delay calling about a new symptom, hoping that it will improve. Later, their anxiety prompts a late evening call to the doctor. Some clients may wait even longer if the symptom is a familiar one, again, hoping it will go away. This is not an entirely unreasonable approach considering that the client may be trying to save money or may be reluctant to "bother" the doctor or nurse.

Understanding the client's perspective promotes a proactive rather than a reactive stance and reduces irritation and frustration. Thus, anticipating clients' needs can reduce repeat phone calls, improve client satisfaction and enhance overall practice. The following examples illustrate common scenarios and possible solutions.

After-Hours Calls

Telephone management involves monitoring routine illnesses (fever, upper respiratory illness, gastrointestinal upset) for brief periods of time, during which the client implements the advice and evaluates progress or improvement to determine if an appointment is needed. Telephone management is a common practice in gatekeeper systems, particularly after normal business hours 5 P.M. to 8 A.M.) The goal of after-hours telephone management is to spare clients and

FIGURE 4.5 Procedural Analysis of Telephone Triage

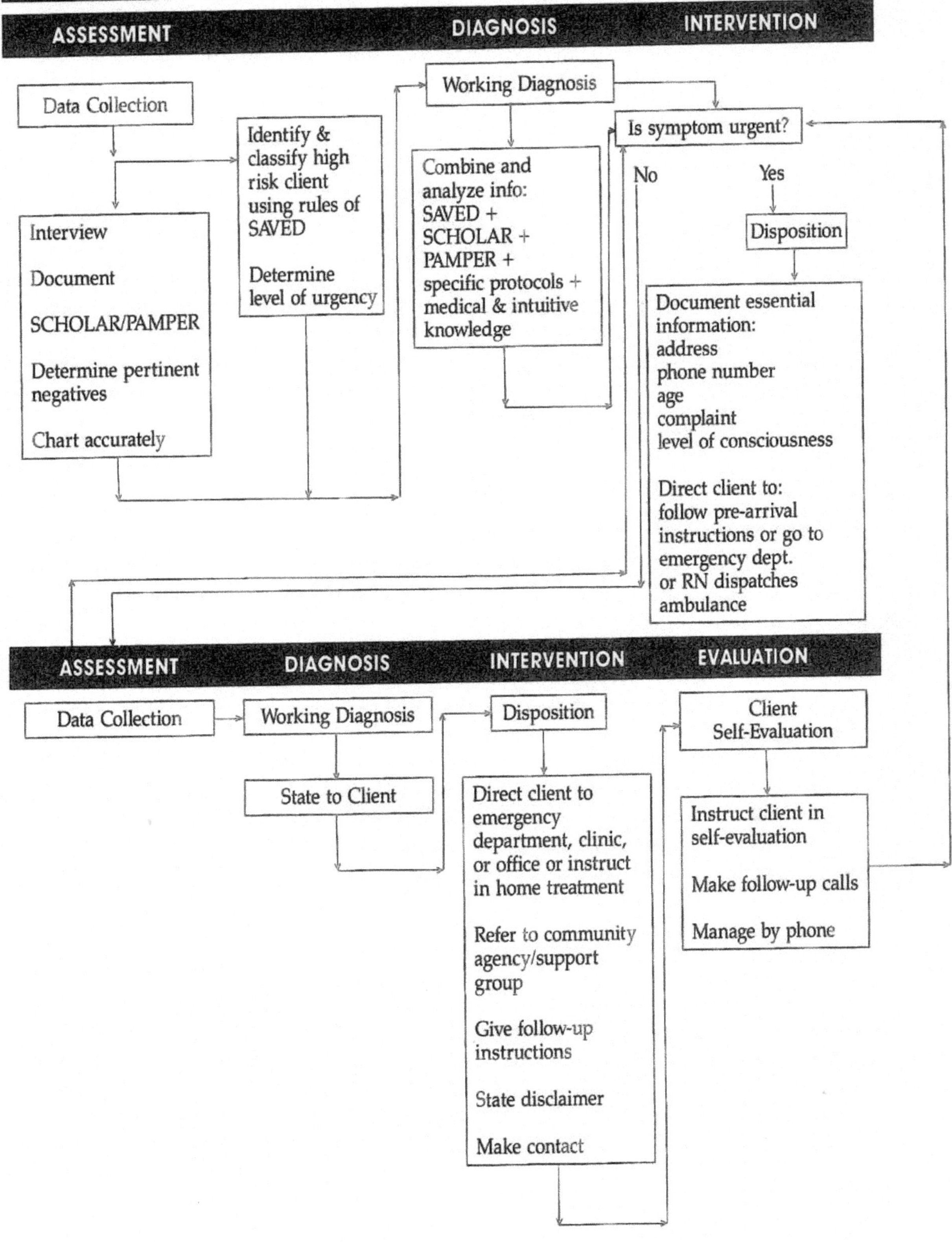

staff unnecessary night visits. Frequent consultations between nurse and client insure that problems are still safely managed at home. Again, self-evaluation instructions must be concrete, placed within time frames, and easily understood. Client reliability must be weighed against the inconvenience of an office visit.

Two types of compliance problems arise with after hours calls: people who want to come in but don't need to, and those who won't come in but should. In the first case, because nurses cannot refuse appointments, document the client's intention to come in. In the second case, take the call to the next highest authority.

Follow-Up Calls

Follow-up calls have two functions: public relations and case management. Currently, welcome-mat (marketing) systems include these calls as a routine part of the interaction, and they are considered the ultimate public relations gesture. Not surprisingly, managers have found that such calls demonstrate concern and create a lasting, favorable impression on callers.

One study showed that follow-up calls increased patient satisfaction and compliance following emergency department visits (Jones, Clark, Bradford, & Dougherty, 1987). A surprising finding was that these calls only took an average of 70 seconds to complete. Researchers also discovered that 42% of the clients required further clarification of their discharge instructions. A majority of the calls resulted in direct medical intervention because the client's condition had worsened. The authors concluded that follow-up calls reinforce instructions, demonstrate concern, provide feedback, and enhance risk management and quality assurance. Based on their findings, follow-up became a permanent part of their ED quality assurance program. The cost-benefit ratio includes unidentified savings through risk management, marketing, and effective public relations. Although the above study was performed in the ED setting, telephone triage programs in any area can benefit by routinely making follow-up calls.

Beware of Early and Late Calls

Indecisiveness afflicts callers as well as professionals. It is not unusual for clients to wait until 5 P.M. to call after hoping the symptom will improve. Likewise, transition times—early morning and late afternoon—are periods when emergencies often occur. As 5 P.M. approaches, nurses are anxious to shut down lines or turn them over to the next shift. The case study below illustrates how calls get lost during the transition time—change of shift.

A mother called, extremely irate, 90 minutes after originally contacting an HMO emergency department. She had called regarding her 8-year-old daughter who had fallen from a tree and was complaining of severe lower back pain and could not move her legs. The child had now become cold and clammy. The call had been "lost in the shuffle" between the ED nurse and physician during the change of shift.

Bureaucratic Snags

The solution to the unfortunate situation described below shows what can happen when guidelines for home deaths (covering body removal, autopsy, and pronouncing policies) are ignored by family members.

A hospice nurse received a call from the family of a client who had recently died. Although prior arrangements had been made for the client to die at home, the family had notified the police department. The police regulations did not permit the deceased to be removed from the home without approval from a physician. As a result, the body had to remain in the home for 24 hours.

Prescription Refill Tapes

Nonnursing, clerical tasks can be avoided by installing a voice-activated telephone answering machine for refill requests. Answering machines enable callers to make refill requests 24 hours a day. Specific information is collected on the tape, transcribed by a secretary, and then, with the chart, reviewed and approved by the physician. Specific questions might include pregnancy and breastfeeding status, allergies, medications, and previous medical history.

Telephone Abuse

Over a period of several years, a group of emergency departments received several anonymous calls from a man requesting castration. It was later discovered that these calls coincided with rape cases.

Although not directed at the nurse personally, many calls are bizarre and frightening—rape, bomb threats, homicidal and suicidal threats, and child abuse. Novice practitioners may find these calls especially disturbing if they have not been adequately prepared. Debriefing sessions help to alleviate the staff's anxiety.

An occupational hazard of telephone triage nurses is telephone abuse. Emergency department nurses relate that they occasionally receive hostile and obscene calls. At some institutions, staff work under assumed names to protect themselves against the intrusiveness of obscene or harassing calls. With experience, nurses can become familiar with obscene callers and recognize voice and speech patterns early in the conversation. One may confront the caller or disconnect with or without warning. Confrontation requires time and emotional energy. It is acceptable practice to disconnect and go on to the next call. Finally, chronic callers can also be problematic. A "problem caller file" on the client's background (drug abuse, alcoholism, psychiatric problems, or obscene or abusive calls) may prove helpful.

Animal First Aid

A man called, insisting on talking to the physician. He wanted him to diagnose whether or not his dog had kennel cough. To facilitate the process, he had the dog bark over the phone.

A young woman called, frightened and crying, because her cat had run into the coffee table and "popped its eye out."

A woman called asking for CPR instructions for a cat that had drowned.

A farmer called about his "sick chickens."

Surprisingly, many emergency nurses relate that people often call seeking first aid advice for pets. The nurse's first priority is to the community. Attempting to field these calls is not recommended; however, it is not difficult to prepare a list of local veterinarians who can manage these problems.

Humorous Calls

"My boyfriend wanted to play Santa Claus and used superglue to glue on his eyebrows. How do I remove them?"

"Is the electricity running the heart AC or DC?"

"My bedroom is full of bees. What do I do now?"

Newlyweds called for instructions on how to cook their first Thanksgiving turkey.

Not all nuisance calls are malicious or upsetting. Humorous calls provide nurses with a good laugh and a way to gain perspective.

INFORMATION AND REFERRAL BROKERING

Because of its role as gatekeeper, telephone triage has given new meaning to access—a key issue for the 1990's. Broadly defined, access includes both the ability of the client to obtain an appointment as well as the ability to obtain needed information, referral, or resources. Access to resources (information, support groups, classes, or counseling) that promote health or prevent disease can decrease the need for access to appointments, crisis intervention, or emergency care. Nurses and physicians have largely ignored their role as educators, information brokers, enablers, and consumer advocates. Informational skills flesh out and enhance the service, making it sophisticated and comprehensive.

Self-Care and Self-Help

In America, self-care is an old and revered concept. Self-care is the concept that health consumers can and should assume responsibility for their own health. Common examples of self-care programs are smoking cessation and weight loss programs, diabetic education, and parenting and birthing classes. Closely aligned to the self-care concept is that of information brokering. The "information age" is here, and telephone triage nurses have a key role in this revolution (Curtis & Talbot, 1981). To remain credible, nurses must respond in increasingly diverse, complex, and sophisticated ways to challenges posed by populations that are also diverse, complex, and sophisticated. Attempts to bluff a sophisticated AIDS client, for example, may damage an institution's credibility and foster mistrust. Therefore, telephone triage nurses must either know the answers or know where to find them quickly. Current, accurate lists of contact persons for self-care and self-help groups are among the important resources that should be readily available.

Self-help or support groups are a natural offshoot of the self-care concept. Self help groups are small, voluntary groups of people with a common problem. They meet regularly for mutual support in bringing about personal change. Self-help is built upon the concept that those who help are helped the most. They focus on diverse problems such as adjustment to chronic disease, single parenting, cocaine addiction and surviving a child's death. Since the early 1970s, self-help and support groups have proliferated and grown to 500 thousand in number. (Leerhsen et al, 1990).

Self-help groups have several common characteristics. They are peer-run and members both give and receive support from other members. They emphasize day-to-day victories—another day without a drink, without bingeing, without giving in to depression. In most groups, family involvement is encouraged. Peers act as role models and identify with each other. Groups are nonprofessional, encourage responsibility and self-knowledge, and rely on preventive medicine.

For some clients, self-help groups are an ideal option because they are *free, accessible, and designed to address chronic problems,* in contrast to a health care system which is expensive, less accessible, and designed for acute problems. Self-help groups are highly accessible, affordable and some offer telephone support 24 hours a day, in contrast to expensive weekly psychiatrist or counselor visits.

Marion K. Jacobs, adjunct professor of psychology at U.C.L.A. and Codirector of the California Self-Help Center, states "there is still a huge amount of resistance in medicine to incorporating self-help as part of health care" (Leerhsen et al, 1990). Self-help is a form of preventive medicine, providing social support and strengthening coping skills through shared experience and solutions. Members are self-selected and can come and go as they please. For some, self-help can be a substitute for traditional therapy; for others, it can be an adjunct to it.

Assessing Support Groups. Not all self-help groups are successful. Some fail because of the problems inherent in any group process—lack of effective leaders, inability to involve members in a meaningful way, and attrition. Assess groups before including them on the referral list. For example, Alcoholics Anonymous (AA) is one of the oldest and most successful support groups addressing one of civilization's oldest problems—drug and alcohol abuse. Because of its scope, longevity, and reputation, AA has become the standard by which to measure similar groups.

Information and Referral Systems

Information brokering and referral are a large part of the work of telephone triage. Increasing numbers of hospitals are setting up information and referral "mini-systems" for the sole purpose of public relations and to increase revenue. Even small services can be surprisingly complicated and time-consuming to implement. For this reason, the aid of an expert resource person—the medical librarian—is invaluable.

High-quality information is concrete, complete, and current. Dispensing faulty information undermines client trust and weakens program credibility. For example, outdated hot line phone numbers are useless. For the system to be effective, each element of the informational product, from books to hot line numbers to resource persons, must be of the highest quality.

Developing Referral Services. Medical librarians are experts in data bases and search techniques, skills that take years to develop. Cultivate a collaborative relationship with the local medical librarian—usually found in a hospital setting. Collaboration saves time, effort and money. Develop a range of resources—books and magazines, advocacy groups, experts, and audio and video tapes. Remedying knowledge deficits is a large part of telephone triage work. Keep a tally of question topics. Add categories as needed. Every three to six months, update your "informational protocols," including problem definition, common causes, signs and symptoms, duration and acuity, and support groups or hot lines. See Appendices E, F, G, and H for lists of informational protocols, support groups, resources, and file card sample.

THE PHYSICAL SETTING

Nowhere is the primitive status of telephone triage more clearly reflected than in the work space in which most nurses practice. Many nurses state that they work in "airless closets," noisy hallways, or dark, windowless rooms with fluorescent lighting. There is often little regard for comfort, safety, or privacy, adding stress and creating less effective systems. Workstations should be comfortable, spacious, airy, and aesthetically pleasing, with desks large enough to accommodate a computer screen and yet provide ample writing space. A small file cabinet and reference library should be within easy reach. Chairs should be ergonomic and headsets lightweight and comfortable with clear sound reception and transmission. Soundproof partitions or carrels cut down on noise and distraction. Openable windows looking onto relaxing views can cut down on sensory deprivation. Plants can soften and beautify the environment.

Mirrors can make the cubical appear more spacious. They also allow nurses visual feedback on their emotional state, helping staff to regain composure after stressful calls. Muted pastels are restful, rejuvenating colors. Ambient noise level can be reduced by wall coverings, drapes, carpet, and plants as well as low-level, classical or easy-listening music to buffer extraneous sounds. Items such as framed photographs of significant others, a religious icon, or a small object from nature (stone, shell, or flower) can act as triggers for relaxation. These items can be removed at day's end and placed in a drawer, leaving the work space clear for the next nurse to personalize.

Workstations will rely increasingly on computer, telemetry, and telephone technology. In the future, "video windows" may comprise one entire wall, allowing nurses to see callers. Telemetry equipment will be routinely used to monitor high-risk mothers, cardiac patients, and the elderly. Computers will be the workhorses of the system, eliminating the drudgery of working with cumbersome protocol books and documentation by hand. Information and referral systems will be incorporated into the computer memory, producing powerful information banks offering instantaneous recall of support groups or definitions of medical terms in layman's language.

A new technological twist is the use of both electronic "beepers" and call forwarding by telephone triage nurses, who are then able to take call, much like physicians currently do. The advantage is obvious—flexible staffing. The disadvantage is the possible loss of quality through distractions, failure to use protocols, and reduced privacy for callers who find the background noise an intrusion. These situations can be remedied through use of a private home office, and mandatory use of protocols at all times.

STRESS REDUCTION

There are five major sources of stress for telephone triage nurses—poor self-image, high call volume, lack of feedback, physiological tension and abusive calls—all of which lessen a sense of control. Because telephone triage is still gaining acceptance as a subspecialty, telephone triage nurses report that they feel like stepchildren in the nursing field. Lack of standards and inadequate training increase anxiety and denial.

One way of improving morale is to upgrade training and standards through certification. Certification is common practice and demonstrates institutional commitment to standards while validating and rewarding staff efforts. Another stressor is lack of feedback. In the clinical setting it is possible to observe firsthand the client's progress or deterioration. In telephone triage, nurses operate in a vacuum. One solution is to follow up on questionable calls, but this is not always feasible. Another solution is to eliminate 8-hour shifts by staggering shifts and cross-training staff. Thus, 8-hour shifts are split into 4 hours in the clinical setting and 4 hours on the phone. This affords three benefits:

1. Increased clinical skills and constantly updated knowledge
2. Feedback from clients when they arrive
3. Reduction of the intensity and monotony of telephone work

In other settings, the work load is intense or monotonous or the acuity is high. In some high-volume systems, practitioners are required to answer 160 calls per shift, about one call every 3 minutes. This mentality reduces nurses to clerical workers. It downgrades nursing expertise and judgment, reducing the work to menial, repetitious appointment giving. It also can result in making the system less cost effective, because nurses will be forced to triage less stringently. In order to err on the side of caution they will be forced to give out higher numbers of appointments.

It is stressful to listen attentively and analyze for 8 hours. Paradoxically, the work itself creates a sort of mental and auditory overload combined with visual and tactile sensory deprivation. Video display terminals (VDT) create eye strain and increase x-ray exposure, leading to "technostress"—physical ailments such as headaches, neck, back and shoulder pain, and carpal tunnel syndrome related to long hours of work at a VDT. The solutions to many of these problems are shorter shifts and better staffing. Setting lower expectations for call volume (6 minutes per call or 80 calls per shift) requires additional staff but may enhance public relations as well as raise productivity, system effectiveness, and morale.

CHAPTER 4

EXERCISE 1: SETTING PRIORITIES

OBJECTIVE: To identify risk factor using a global approach (SAVED).

METHOD: Assuming that all other things are equal, choose the client who is *least* at risk.

A. Mild chest pain in:

______ non-English-speaking elderly woman

______ AIDS patient

______ healthy 5-year-old

______ 55-year-old male (second-party call)

B. Sudden onset of abdominal pain in:

______ 11-year-old

______ sexually active female teenager

______ 65-year-old woman

______ 25-year-old male

C. Headache in:

______ 25-year-old woman with history of migraines

______ 45-year-old woman with history of hypertension

______ child with recent head injury

______ in elderly man who feels it is due to eyestrain

D. Confusion in:

______ 19-year-old college student, calling from party

______ 65-year-old, daughter calling from convalescent home

______ 5-year-old, hysterical mother calling

______ AIDS client, friend calling from home

E. Dehydration symptoms, fever 102 degrees in:

______ healthy 25-year-old male

______ 6-week-old infant

______ 2-year-old toddler

______ 65-year-old frail male

EXERCISE 2: DOCUMENTATION: AVOIDING VAGUE TERMINOLOGY

OBJECTIVE: To practice making precise descriptions of symptoms.

METHOD: Rephrase the following list of generic descriptions in more precise quantitative or qualitative terms. Any answer in the severe range will be correct.

VAGUE DESCRIPTION	PRECISE DESCRIPTION
EXAMPLE: Severe headache	10 + , splitting unable to get out of bed
1. Severe vaginal bleeding	______________________ ______________________
2. Severe diarrhea	______________________ ______________________
3. Severe nausea and vomiting	______________________ ______________________
4. Severely dehydrated infant	______________________ ______________________
5. Severe fever (1-year-old child)	______________________ ______________________
6. Severe shortness of breath	______________________ ______________________
7. Severe fever (adult)	______________________ ______________________
8. Severe abdominal pain, woman of child-bearing age	______________________ ______________________
9. Severely infected wound	______________________ ______________________

EXERCISE 3: DATA COLLECTION

OBJECTIVE: To practice identifying and classifying categories of data.

METHOD: Identify and classify data using SAVED, SCHOLAR, PAMPER, and ADL. Place number of each piece of information from each case next to the correct category or categories of the classification lists.

EXAMPLE:

SAMPLE CASE

1. 30-year-old
2. Woman
3. 2 weeks postpartum
4. UTI symptoms × 1 day
5. Hematuria
6. Breastfeeding
7. Denies pregnancy
8. History of recent UTI's

List according to numbers:

High risk factors

SAVED

- S
- A—1, 2
- V
- E
- D

ADL

- Pertinent Negatives—7

SCHOLAR

- S—4, 5
- C
- H—8
- O—4
- L
- A
- R

PAMPER

- P—7, 6
- A
- M
- P—3
- E
- R—8

CASE 1

1. 28-year-old
2. Woman
3. 38 weeks pregnant
4. c/o low back pain
5. Noted swelling in arms, legs, face × 3 days
6. Abdominal tightening
7. Denies headache, visual problems
8. Feels sluggish
9. Uncomfortable
10. Felt faint yesterday
11. Contractions q 15 minutes × 3 hours yesterday
12. Drinking a lot
13. Anorexia
14. Unable to wear shoes or rings
15. Increased water discharge × 1 day
16. Bedrest × 1 month

List according to numbers:

High risk factors

SAVED

S

A

V

E

D

ADL

Pertinent Negatives

SCHOLAR

S

C

H

O

L

A

R

PAMPER

P

A

M

P

E

R

CASE 2

1. 15-month-old boy
2. Acting tired, unusually sleepy, whiny
3. Mom wants to go to the ED
4. Temp 101 degrees (scan)
5. Large watery stools 4 × day × 3 days

List according to numbers:

High risk factors

SAVED

S
A
V
E
D

ADL

Pertinent Negatives

SCHOLAR

S
C
H
O
L
A
R

PAMPER

P
A
M
P
E
R

CASE 3

1. 2-month-old boy
2. URI symptoms
3. Wakeful nights × 3
4. "Crackly cough" × 3 weeks
5. Vaporizer, syringe have not helped
6. Nursing well
7. Alert
8. "Rosy cheeks"
9. History of ventricular septal defect (VSD)
10. Has appt with cardiologist tomorrow

List according to numbers:

High risk factors

SAVED

S

A

V

E

D

ADL

Pertinent Negatives

SCHOLAR

S

C

H

O

L

A

R

PAMPER

P

A

M

P

E

R

CASE 4

1. 26-year-old woman
2. 38 weeks pregnant
3. Many contractions last night, now 4 to 5 per hour, 30 to 60 secs long
4. Last fetal movement at 10 P.M. last night
5. Drank ice water to stimulate baby without results

List according to numbers:

High risk factors

SAVED

S

A

V

E

D

ADL

Pertinent Negatives

SCHOLAR

S

C

H

O

L

A

R

PAMPER

P

A

M

P

E

R

ANSWER KEY

EXERCISE 1: SETTING PRIORITIES

A. Mild chest pain in healthy five year old
B. Sudden onset of abdominal pain in 25-year-old male
C. Headache in 25-year-old woman with migraine history
D. Confusion in AIDS client
E. Dehydration, fever in healthy 25-year-old male

EXERCISE 2: DOCUMENTATION: AVOIDING VAGUE TERMINOLOGY

The answers provided here are only examples of possible symptoms.

VAGUE DESCRIPTIONS	PRECISE DESCRIPTIONS
1. Severe vaginal bleeding	Vag. bleeding > 1 pad/hr.
2. Severe diarrhea	8+ loose, watery stools/8 hrs
3. Severe nausea, vomiting	Vomiting hourly × 12 hours, unable to retain fluids
4. Severely dehydrated infant	1 scantily wet diaper/8 hr, sunken fontanelle, no tears
5. Severe fever (1-year-old child)	T 105.6 rectal
6. Severe shortness of breath	Audible wheeze, unable to complete full sentence without catching breath
7. Severe fever (adult)	T 103.5 po
8. Severe abdominal pain, woman of child-bearing age	Sudden onset, sharp pain, LLQ, 9+
9. Severely infected wound	Wound is hot, red, painful to touch, foul smelling discharge

EXERCISE 4: DATA COLLECTION

CASE 1

SAVED
S—4
A—1,2

ADL—16
Pertinent negatives—7
SCHOLAR
S—4, 5, 6, 8, 9, 10, 11, 12, 13, 14, 15
O—5, 11, 15
L—4, 5
PAMPER
P—3
R—16

CASE 2

SAVED
S—4
A—1
V—1
E—3, 2
ADL—2, 5
SCHOLAR
S—2, 4, 5
O—5

CASE 3

SAVED
A—1
V—1
D—9
ADL—3, 6, 7, 8
SCHOLAR
S—2, 4, 8
O—3, 4
R—5
PAMPER
P—9, 10
OUTCOME: Congestive heart failure (for reader's information)

CASE 4

SAVED
S—3, 4, 5
A—1, 2
SCHOLAR
S—4, 5
C—3, 4, 5
O—3, 4, 5
A—6
PAMPER
P—2

CHAPTER 5

Protocol and Form Design and Development

"Quality happens when everyone everyday does the best they can to do their job." (Skillicorn, 1980)

Protocols, whether computerized or in book form, are at the heart of telephone triage practice. Without protocols, practice remains undefined and unprofessional. Protocols guide the nurse in making decisions and giving advice. They are usually composed of questions and advice for a range of symptoms.

The field of telephone triage is still developing standards and quality assurance measures. Thus, standards for this new field must be extrapolated from those developed for the clinical setting. Guidelines developed by the California Board of Registered Nurses (1989) state that "protocols are rules and/or procedures to be followed in performing a clinical function or service authorized by the policy." Another major function of protocols is to define dependent, independent, or interdependent roles.

The primary goal of telephone triage protocols is the safe, effective, and appropriate disposition of client health problems. Protocols are a sorting or prioritizing tool designed to eliminate common practice errors. For example, in one study of system utilization in a pediatric setting (Ott, 1974), physicians tended to "over-triage" (gave too few appointments) while pediatric health aides (equivalent of nurse's aides) tended to give more "unnecessary" appointments. Researchers concluded that the imbalance occurred because physicians are able to recommend treatments and prescribe medications more liberally than health aides. The study concluded that protocol use would result in more appropriate triage decisions.

In telephone triage, most difficulties arise because of the lack of firsthand information. For this reason, protocols must be written to err on the side of caution. In reality, "welcome mat" or marketing systems tend to be conservative (liberally offer office visits). On the other hand, HMOs or "gatekeeper" systems are less conservative and offer fewer visits. In all settings, even with protocols, nurses must remain autonomous (free of undue institutional pressures) and maintain a conservative stance when in doubt.

Telephone triage is both art and science, a synthesis of human intuition and artificial intelligence. Artificial intelligence (AI) parallels the thought processes, logical steps, rules, and intuition used in problem solving. The same process is used in "computer diagnostics" to help physicians think through diagnostic and treatment decisions (Kalikowski, 1985; Korcok, 1983). Like artificial intelligence systems, protocols help to analyze and classify symptoms. Like AI, they have several functions:

1. *Problem solving:* Protocols are *expert systems* on paper or computer that guide nurses through the processes of interview, assessment, and decision making, comparable to having an expert nurse at one's side.
2. *Structure:* Protocols organize vast amounts of information for consideration by the decision maker. They determine what constitutes *significant* information.
3. *Risk Management Safeguard:* Protocols show the interrelationship of various data, forcing consideration of *all* possible decision choices and safeguarding against stereotyping.
4. *Reconstructive:* In some institutions, especially gatekeeper systems, nurses must defend their dispositions. Protocols can help to reconstruct the decision-making process.

PROTOCOL STANDARDS

Protocols must be well designed, comprehensive, standardized, and actively used by staff—very few sets achieve this standard. Thus, high-quality, comprehensive sets of protocols are in great demand. Protocols are designed to:

1. Promote the client's physical and psychological comfort
2. Prevent possible complications
3. Promote rehabilitation as appropriate
4. Facilitate self-care activities (Marker, 1988)

These goals provide a basis for protocol design and development. Standards must be built into the protocol structure. The following key components are common to all protocol design:

1. *Quality assurance mechanisms:* Problem disposition must be effective and appropriate.

2. *Risk management mechanisms:* Dispositions must be safe, based on community standards, and delineate dependent, independent, and interdependent roles.
3. *Self-care mechanisms:* Instructions must be designed to bolster client self-reliance while acknowledging the limited resources of low-income populations.

Protocols should also be:

- **Comprehensive**—most current systems cover 50 to 150 problems or symptoms
- **Current**—based on information collected within the last five years
- **Authoritative**—written by nurses, and approved by physicians, nurses and administration
- **User-friendly**—concrete, concise information in lay language, well formatted
- **Symptom-based**—working diagnosis in lay language
- **Effective**—act as a working tool to classify common symptoms, provide high-quality information, and appropriate referrals.

CONSIDERATIONS IN PROTOCOL DEVELOPMENT

Many factors influence telephone triage protocol content: community standards, advances in medical technology, practice setting, changing philosophy of client care, and the increasing knowledge base of nurses (Thompson, Jones, Cox, & Levy, 1983). For example, health care rationing, unthinkable 20 years ago, is now a dominant force in the health care industry, and approaches to the prevention, diagnosis and treatment of AIDS have been redefined many times over the last ten years.

Although several books of protocols have been written, protocol writing is still a new field and until now, no text existed which described how to develop and design telephone triage protocols. According to some experts (Scott & Packard, 1990), protocols are extremely labor intensive to develop—100 protocols require approximately 800 to 1000 hours of work or 8 to 10 hours per protocol. As a result, many institutions have found it preferable to adapt existing books of protocols rather than reinventing the wheel. (See Appendix V)

Protocols must be easy to use or they may not be used consistently. The best set is worthless if it sits idle while staff field calls. Many protocols contain design flaws that make them difficult to use and impede data collection.

One common mistake is developing protocols with little or no input by the nurses who must use them. Nurses' and physicians' perspectives are different.

On the other hand, it is not adviseable for a single nurse, lacking the necessary expertise, to develop an entire set. Protocols are best developed as a collaborative process using a task force of at least six expert level nurses, then reviewed by a task force of physicians. Final approval must come from administration, physicians and nurses. To enhance risk management, the task force must clearly define independent and interdependent roles on such issues as advising prescription and nonprescription drugs or ordering and reporting of lab test results.

The way in which protocols are designed and developed is influenced by the creator's view of the client, problem, and the practitioner. Protocols are modeled upon typical or classic symptoms and tend to be generic rather than specific. They cannot be relied upon to account for individual and situation variability. Thus, they must always be used judiciously. Finally, in instances where no protocol seems to fit the presenting symptom(s), the nurse must rely on the generic protocol (SCHOLAR, PAMPER) and the nursing process.

Some, however, have tried to create *"nurseproof"* protocols designed to be reliable even when used by untrained, underqualified, inexperienced nurses. Simplistic protocols using leading questions and yes/no checkboxes create confusion and lead to flawed data collection.

Protocols are a tool. In the hands of poorly qualified nurses, however, they could become lethal weapons. Thus, performance standards and qualifications must be rigorous and staff must be articulate, professional, and reliable. Finally, staff must be able to function with autonomy, knowing when to override protocols. Experience, training, and common sense are prerequisites. Protocols must never be used in a mechanical or mindless way and should *never* be designed for unqualified or untrained users.

Practitioners' intuitive and cognitive skills complement the mechanistic approach of the protocol. Protocols prompt or trigger standardized questions and advice for an array of symptoms. Nurses discriminate, synthesize, analyze, modify, and sometimes override protocols—a more difficult and complex task of human intellect and intuition than a mindless, mechanical approach.

Some predict that in the future, nurses will be replaced by computers. This scenario is highly unlikely. Artificial intelligence can never completely replace the subtleties of human intellect and nuances of human emotion. The human voice, like the human touch, will never be replaced by audiotapes, however sophisticated. Humans in distress seek out human comfort. Machines can never replace the emotional support of the receptive, understanding, compassionate human heart.

Preparation

After choosing a task force, decide the scope, that is, the range of symptom titles for the collection. For example, many collections start with about 10 titles and build to a maximum of 150 protocols. (See Appendices C, D, E) Most protocols use a vertical layout and are listed in alphabetical order in lay terms.

Next, gather raw materials and resources, including recent research, existing protocols, specialty reference books, periodicals, diagnostic references, community resource lists, and in-house program lists. One of the first major tasks is to create lists for approved abbreviations, support groups, over-the-counter and prescription drugs, and lab tests that can be ordered independently. (See Appendices K, L, M, N.) Protocols must contain current information (less than 5 years old) and be authoritative (based on reliable, reputable sources). State of the art information ensures that protocols will have a long shelf life, an important quality in any reference.

After gathering the raw materials and determining the scope, establish ground rules for the creative process. Protocol development is labor-intensive, controversial, and intellectually challenging. A playful, spontaneous, open, and nonjudgmental atmosphere fosters creativity. Activities such as thinking out loud and brainstorming are common problem-solving techniques which make expertise conscious and accessible to the group (Corcoran, Narayan, & Moreland 1988).

Where appropriate, incorporate rules of thumb and "tricks of the trade." Examples of rules of thumb are the following:

- Give automatic appointments to clients who call more than twice in 2 to 3 hours.
- Females of childbearing age are pregnant until proven otherwise.
- Chest pain is cardiac until proven otherwise.

Tricks of the trade are based on home remedies and first aid measures. For example:

- For a cut lip, use a Popsicle™ to soothe the child as well as cut down on bleeding and swelling.
- Use the BRAT diet for diarrhea: bananas, rice, applesauce, and white toast. (See Appendix I for additional examples.)

The protocol design is made up of two parts: format and content. Format means the graphic presentation, the way things are laid out on the page or screen (when protocols are computerized). The words of advice and assessment questions make up the content. For the protocol to work, both format and content must be well designed.

Before content can be developed, a sort of skeletal framework or format must be designed for the questions and advice for each protocol. The format is generic, standardized, and less variable, while the content is specific and variable. Format determines the form (presentation on the page or screen) and breadth for the prototype (first protocol). The prototype becomes the standard upon which all subsequent protocols are modeled. For example, if the task force decides that the standard number of dispositions for a prototype will be four, then all subsequent protocols will have four dispositions. But generally speaking, it would be confusing to vary the number of dispositions from protocol to protocol although nurses are free to individualize dispositions as appropriate within each time frame.

DEVELOPING A PROTOTYPE

Most nurses have a general sense of the community in which they serve. However, this knowledge may be superficial. Thus, in-depth knowledge of the community may require an epidemiological assessment. Mortality, morbidity, and disability statistics are indicators that provide evidence of disease trends, while interviews of representative clients (i.e. women, elderly, students) provide a more personal view of the concerns and health problems of the client population. Statistics on mortality, morbidity, and disability are available from the National Center for Health Statistics, Centers for Disease Control, and local and state health departments. Texts such as *Health Promotion and Planning* (Green and Kreuter, 1991) provide guidelines for priority setting and problem identification. Current editions of *Health: United States 1991* (U.S. Department of Health and Human Services) contain epidemiological information and trends. Measure consumer awareness by surveying knowledge about patients rights, informed consent, alternative therapies, and second opinions.

Collectively speaking, clients' strengths and weaknesses play a part in the content, format, literacy level, and selection of protocols. For example, clients of an HMO are of a more "ideal" population. They are probably currently employed, high school educated, and by virtue of having passed an employee physical, relatively healthy. On the other hand, as a group, low-income families present more of a challenge for a community clinic. They may be unemployed, read at a 5th grade level and have many health problems. Due to poverty and lack of resources, there *may* be more risk factors, drug abuse, and little consumer awareness.

Protocol content and selection varies with the client population. A clinic exclusively serving women or children will probably not need as wide an array of protocols as that of an ED setting or an HMO. Clients in a hospice setting will need informational, consumer-oriented protocols while clients from a university setting (student health center) will need comprehensive STD, AIDS, and drug abuse protocols aimed at a more sophisticated audience.

Step One: Community Assessment

In telephone triage, the community is the client (Higgs & Gustafson, 1985). Thus, the first step in protocol design is to assess the surrounding community (Figure 5.1). Such factors as age, educational level, alcohol and drug abuse,

FIGURE 5.1 Community Assessment Checklist

1. Type of Community
   - ☐ Suburb
   - ☐ Inner City
   - ☐ Rural
   - ☐ Small Town
   - ☐ Other
2. Age Groups
   - ☐ Elderly
   - ☐ Young Families
   - ☐ Young Adults (college population)
   - ☐ Other
3. Socioeconomic Resources
   - ☐ Lower Class
   - ☐ Middle Class
   - ☐ Upper Class
4. Educational Attainment
   - ☐ 4th grade or less
   - ☐ 8th grade or less
   - ☐ 12th grade
   - ☐ College level
   - ☐ Graduate
5. Drug Use
   - ☐ Alcohol abuse
   - ☐ Crack
   - ☐ Tranquilizers
   - ☐ Other
6. Endemic Diseases/Risk Factors
   - ☐ High-risk mothers/babies
   - ☐ Sickle cell disease
   - ☐ AIDS
   - ☐ Other
7. Cultural and Religious Factors and Resources
   - ☐ Religious practices (diet, attitudes)
   - ☐ Religious prohibitions
   - ☐ Sexual practices
   - ☐ Other
8. Consumer awareness (patient rights, health options, informed consent, second opinion, etc.)
   - ☐ Low
   - ☐ Medium
   - ☐ High
9. Language Barriers
   - ☐ Non-English speaking
   - ☐ Bilingual community
   - ☐ Other
10. Community Resources
    - ☐ Poison control
    - ☐ Suicide prevention
    - ☐ Rape hot line
    - ☐ Child abuse hot line
    - ☐ Drug abuse hot line
    - ☐ *Trained* medical dispatchers
11. Environmental Dangers
    - ☐ Toxic waste dumps
    - ☐ Nuclear waste/accidents
    - ☐ Coal mining
    - ☐ High crime rate
    - ☐ Other

and language barriers may determine protocol design and content. Synthesizing demographics, resources, and needs with common symptoms and health problems produces protocols which are user-friendly and reality based.

Step Two: Select Common Symptoms

Developing protocols may seem overwhelming at times. Break the task into manageable segments. For instance, to determine the scope of the collection, keep a 3-month log of the volume and acuity of problems. Remember to factor in seasonal volume increases (flu, recurrent summer or winter problems, volume flurries related to media reports, etc.)

Remember, "when you hear hoof beats, don't think of zebras." The object is not to diagnose exotic diseases but to describe and sort out serious sounding symptoms. So think of common presenting symptoms (GI upset, URI, and abdominal pain) and emergencies (CPR, Heimlich, childbirth). Select the most common 10 to 20 problems to develop first. This bare bones or starter set serves to bring the task force up to speed while addressing the most urgently needed protocols first. The ultimate goal is to create a comprehensive set of 50 to 150 protocols.

Design Flaw—Overly Specific Cross-Reference Section

Attempting to get too specific is a common design flaw. It forces nurses to spend enormous time and effort to cross-check each subheading. Limit all symptoms, and especially major symptoms like abdominal pain, chest pain, headache, dizziness, and shortness of breath, to five or six subtitles each. This eliminates the flaw of overly specific protocols and the possibility of straying into medical diagnosis.

For example, in a protocol for abdominal pain, the cross-reference section might look like this: *Appendicitis symptoms, ectopic pregnancy symptoms, hemorrhage symptoms, peritonitis symptoms, pelvic inflammatory disease symptoms, abdominal trauma.*

Consider how time consuming it would be to check more than six cross-references. Keep it simple; think generic, not specific. Collections of more than 200 protocols are too specific and not user-friendly. The cross indexing becomes unwieldy. Thus, the flow of data collection proceeds from generic protocols (SCHOLAR, PAMPER, ADL) to a specific protocol (abdominal pain) and if needed, to a cross-referenced protocol—abdominal trauma.

Design Flaw—Use of Medical Terminology

Major protocol titles and protocol content are more accessible when written in lay language, although of necessity, some subtitles may be in medical terms.

(See Effective list, Figure 5.2) Mixing medical and lay terminology (see Figure 5.2) is confusing and leaves nurses open to charges of making medical diagnoses. Instead, compile a *symptom-based* list using lay terms such as "eye problem," "headache," and "vaginal discharge."

Some nurses object to this approach. They feel that developing protocols with the client rather than the nurse as end user eliminates expertise and makes telephone triage seem very elementary. However, protocols aimed at nurses and written in highly technical language may resemble nursing texts. Such protocols

FIGURE 5.2 Design Flaw: Use of Medical Terminology

EFFECTIVE	INEFFECTIVE
EAR, NOSE, AND THROAT PROTOCOLS	OTOLARYNGOLOGY PROTOCOLS
1. Dizziness	1. Bell's Palsy
2. Ear problems A. Trauma, foreign body, hearing loss, B. Pain, discharge, ringing, ear lobe problems, auricle	2. Can I fly? 3. Earache 4. Ear congestion/Hearing Loss 5. Ear Lobe, Auricle 6. Epiglottitis
3. Facial paralysis	7. Foreign Body in Nose 8. Foreign Body in Throat
4. Nose problems A. Trauma, foreign body, bleeding B. Discharge, congestion, sinus problem	9. Hearing Aid Problems 10. Hoarseness 11. Lump in Throat 12. Nasal Pain, Infection
5. Throat problems Trauma, foreign body, difficult breathing, epiglottitis symptoms, difficult swallowing, hoarseness, cough, soreness	13. Nasal Fracture 14. Post Tonsillectomy 15. Sinus Complaint 16. Sore Throat 17. Stuffed up Nose 18. Tinnitus 19. Vertigo
PATIENT INSTRUCTION 6. Tonsillectomy 7. Flying 8. Hearing aid problems	

require nurses to translate to make the information usable to the caller, a skill which varies from nurse to nurse.

In fact, the best protocols are dual purpose tools for expert-level analysis and classification, while simultaneously providing information in lay language for teaching, coaching, and advising. This approach synthesizes the best aspects of both types of protocols.

Step Three: Select Data Collection Method

All protocols have two main sections—data collection and advice. However, some protocols have data collection sections which are haphazard and arbitrary, varying from one protocol to the next. The lack of a systematic approach leads nurses to combine intuition and a shotgun approach to collect data—highly informal, erratic, and subject to human error. Formal data collection methods range from the generic to specific, and many in current use are not suitable to telephone triage practice. For example, the SOAP method (subjective, objective, assessment, and plan) assumes that clients always present objective data. Also, this approach is too generic, providing too few triggers to help gather significant information. The PQRST approach is limited to the parameters of pain (pain, quality, region, severity, timing). However, pain is often only one of several presenting symptoms, making this approach too narrow. The physiological systems approach is based on the physical exam model (GU, GI, dermatology, neurology, CV, resp, ENT). This method is too wide-ranging, time-consuming, and cumbersome. Focusing on the *presenting symptom(s) and history* makes more sense than attempting to assess every system. Data collection should be based on symptoms, not systems.

Clearly, these data collection methods fail to gather enough of the right information. Furthermore, they often overlook supportive data which might clarify symptom acuity such as previous medical history, accidents, communicable disease, emotional status, and activities of daily living. In *The Common Symptom Guide* (Wasson, Walsh, Tompkins, Sox, & Pantell 1984) the authors suggest collecting the following symptom data: age, onset, coincidental events, past episodes, manner of onset, duration, location, character, radiation, precipitating or aggravating factors, relieving factors, past treatment or evaluation, course, and effect of activities on daily living.

The generic SCHOLAR/PAMPER protocol detailed in Chapter 4 synthesizes the above approaches, defines 15 to 19 generic parameters of symptoms, and serves as a QA tool. It is generic enough to be efficient yet specific enough to be proficient. This component can be incorporated into documentation forms and the body of the protocol. In documentation forms it acts as a list of open-ended trigger questions. In the body of the protocol it becomes a list of leading questions, designed to explore a specific symptom.

Step Four: Select a Format

Generally speaking, protocol formats have varied little over the years. Most are based on an algorithm or decision tree concept. An algorithm is a step-by-step procedure for solving a problem or accomplishing some end. In general, strict algorithmic approaches are too simplistic and rigid. The algorithm shown in Figure 5.3 is an excellent example of a protocol designed for the layperson. However, for the professional, the narrowly defined set of questions in this decision-tree format is too specific and oversimplified.

Strict algorithmic formats are more appropriate for crash cards (adult and child CPR, Heimlich, and childbirth coaching) where the user is limited to a few decision choices (Figure 5.4). To manage callers in crises effectively, when establishing instant human contact and trust is vital, crash cards must be very regimented. They are coaching aids to be read verbatim to callers. The type of call (high acuity and highly specific), the caller (emotionally distraught) and the user (medical dispatchers) make this format ideal. For routine calls, however, the algorithm concept must be more generic. Narrow decision-tree branches must be converted into decision boxes. Instead of each question leading to a separate disposition, each box contains several questions about emergent, semi-urgent and routine symptoms, and leads to one of three or four possible dispositions. (see Figure 5.8)

The decision box may be placed on the page either vertically or horizontally, whichever works best (see Figure 5.7 for an example of vertical placement and Figure 5.18 for horizontal placement). In order to be graphically pleasing, information must be neither too plentiful nor too sparse. Divide lengthy protocols into several protocols. Place the major heading first and follow it with the subheading, e.g. Abdominal Pain: Ectopic Pregnancy Symptoms; Abdominal Pain: Pediatric. Combine or eliminate sparse protocols.

Step Five: Formulate Dispositions Section

The guiding principle behind the algorithmic approach and all telephone triage practice is to address urgent symptoms first. This principle forms the basis for the hierarchy of acuity in Figure 5.5. This model ranks specific symptoms in order of severity and groups them into three categories: emergent, semi-urgent, and routine. Further defining these categories with a predetermined time frame helps form the basis for dispositions—a time and place where symptoms will be treated. Establishing *when* symptoms will be treated often determines *where* treatment will take place. The hierarchy of acuity prioritizes different symptoms and/or one specific symptom (fracture symptoms—simple or compound) into levels of urgency.

The pyramid shown in Figure 5.5 signifies the relative frequency and volume of each type of call. Note that emergent/urgent symptoms are rare;

FIGURE 5.3 Algorithmic Format for Dizziness/Fainting Protocol

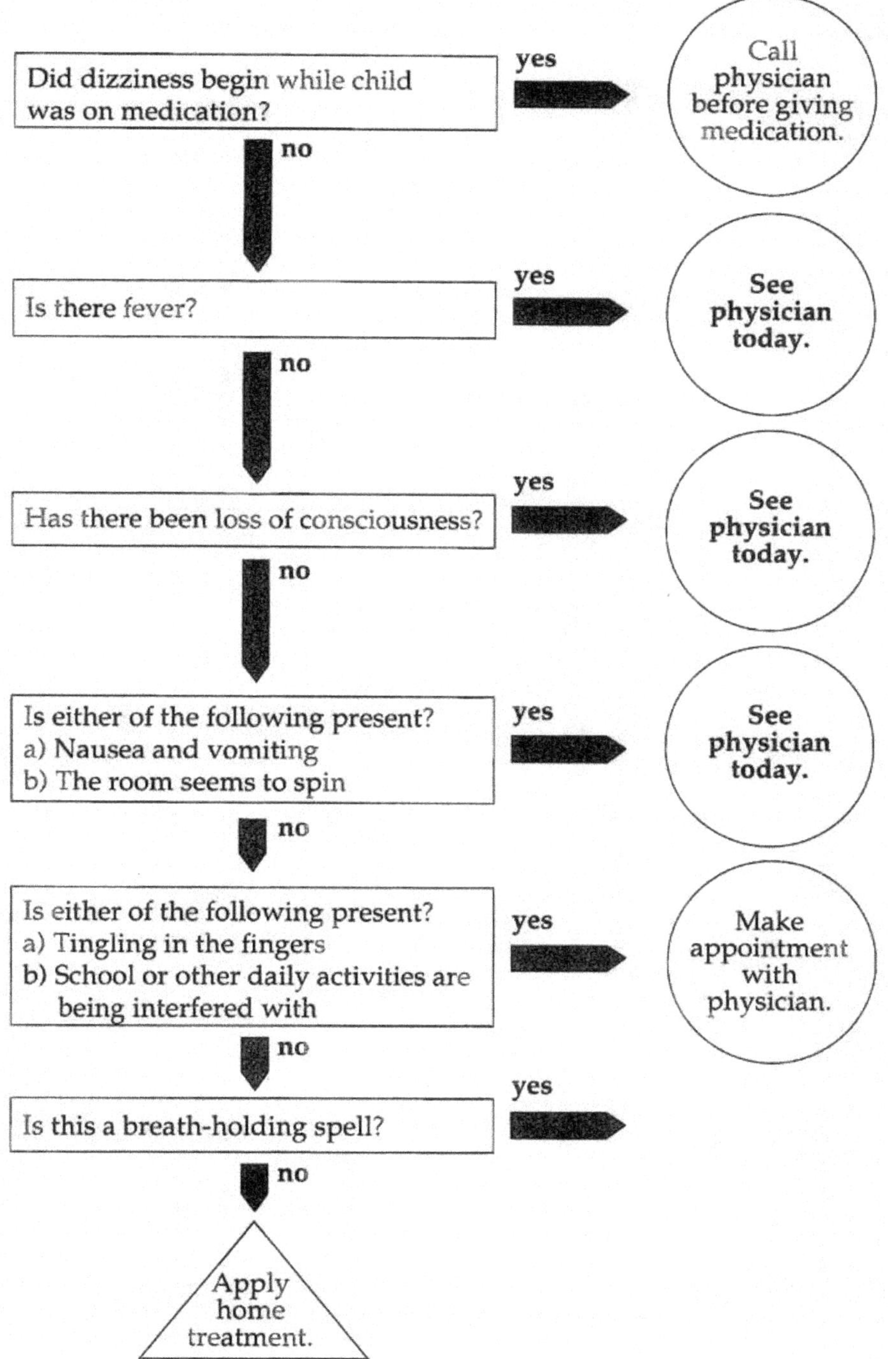

(From Pantell, Fries, Vickery, *Take Care of Your Child*, copyright 1990, by Addison-Wesley Publishing Company, Inc. Reprinted with permission of the publisher)

FIGURE 5.4 Pre-Arrival Instruction (Crash Card)

B ARREST – CHILD

For use through Exclusive License only Pat. Pend. ©8/90 Medical Priority

DISPATCH LIFE SUPPORT™

PRE-ARRIVAL INSTRUCTIONS

1 PATIENT TO PHONE

Listen carefully. I'll tell you how to help your child. **Get him/her as close to the phone as possible.** I'm going to tell you how to do CPR. **Don't hang up. Go do it now.**

WHERE is the child now?

→2

2 CHECK AIRWAY

Listen carefully. **Lay him/her flat on his/her back on the floor.** Remove any **pillows**. Now place your **hand** under the **neck** and **shoulders** and **tilt** the **head** back. Then **look** in the **mouth**. **Go do it now** and come right back to the phone.

Is there VOMIT in the mouth?

NO→3 YES→13

3 CHECK BREATHING

I want you to see if s/he is **breathing**. Put your **ear** next to his/her **mouth**. See if you can **feel** or **hear** any breathing, or if you can **see** the **chest rise**. **Go do it now** and come right back to the phone.
(If I'm not here, stay on the line.)

Can you FEEL or HEAR any breathing?

NO/UNCRTN→4 YES→16

4 START M-TO-M

I'm going to tell you how to give Mouth-to-Mouth. Place your **hand** under the **neck** and **shoulders** and **tilt** the **head** back. **Pinch** the **nose** closed. Completely **cover** his/her **mouth** with your **mouth**.

→5

5 GIVE BREATHS

Blow **2 soft breaths** of air into the lungs just like you are blowing up a balloon. **Watch** for the **chest** to **rise** with each breath. When you have done this come right back to the phone. **Don't hang up. Go do it now.** ***(If I'm not here, stay on the line.)***

Can you FEEL the air going in?
Did you SEE the chest rising?

NO→14 YES→6

6 CHECK PULSE

I want you to **check** his/her **pulse**. **Place** your index and middle **fingers** over his/her left nipple. **Feel carefully for a pulse.** Don't press too hard. Feel for **5 seconds**. **Go do it now** and come right back to the phone. ***(If I'm not here, stay on the line.)***

Can you FEEL a PULSE?

NO→7 YES→17

7 RECHECK PULSE

I want you to **check** for a **pulse** again on his/her upper arm. Use your index and middle **fingers** to feel on the **inside** of his/her **upper arm** for a pulse. Feel carefully for **5 seconds**. **Go do it now** and come right back to the phone.

Do you FEEL a PULSE now?

NO→8 YES→17

8 CPR LANDMARKS

Listen carefully. I'll tell you what to do next. Put the **heel** of **one hand** on the **breast-bone** in the **center** of his/her **chest**, right between the **nipples**.

→9

9 COMPRESSIONS

Push down with your hand **1½ inches** with only the **heel** of one hand touching the chest. Do it **5 times**, just like you are **"pumping"** his/her chest **twice** a second. When you have done this come right back to the phone. **Don't hang up. Go do it now.**

→10

(Reprinted with permission of Jeff Clawson, M.D.)

routine symptoms comprise the majority of calls. One expert states that of all pediatric calls "3% are emergencies, 47% need appointments (urgent) and 50% are helped by telephone advice" (Schmitt, 1980). Experts in emergency medical dispatch estimate that only about 10% of 911 calls are true emergencies (B. MacMurray, personal communication, 1992). Thus, the bulk of calls either require an appointment or advice. Dispositions for routine problems can range from reassurance, information, teaching, and referral to counseling and advocacy.

Placing routine symptoms first or erratically is a common design flaw which leads to faulty assessment and prioritizing techniques. When setting up the format, address the most acute symptoms first so they can be quickly identified and disposed of. Placing acute symptoms last creates an inverted hierarchy of acuity (Figure 5.6).

FIGURE 5.5 Hierarchy of Acuity

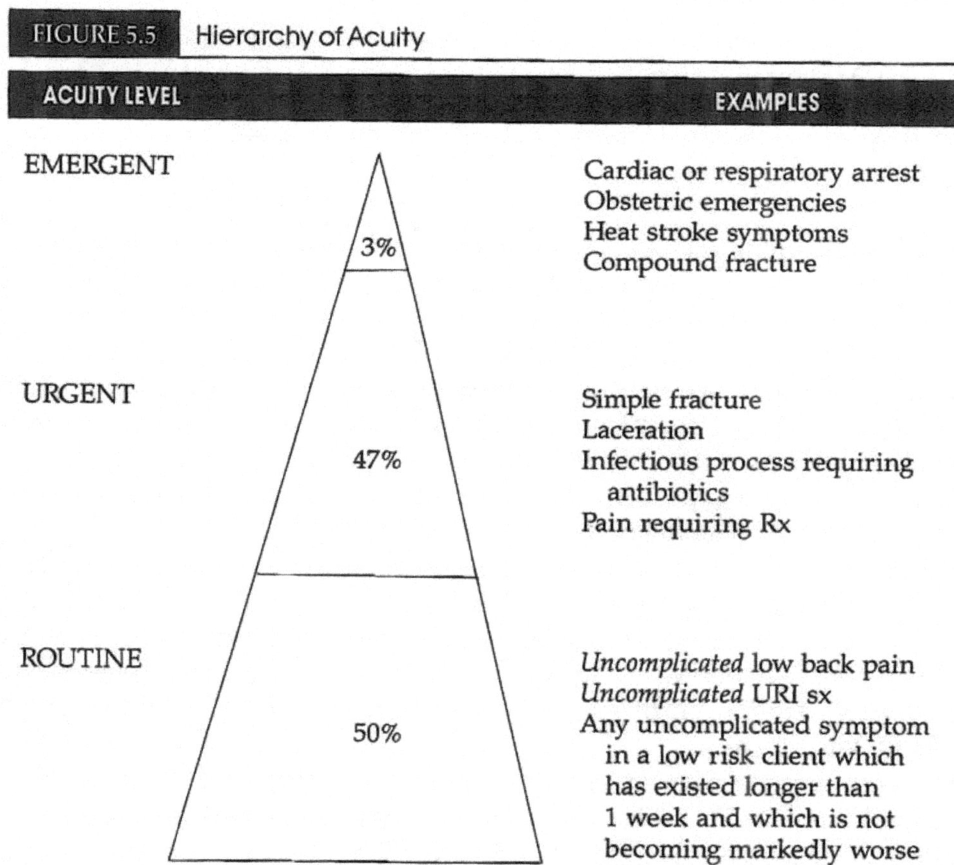

FIGURE 5.6 Inverted Hierarchy of Acuity for Chest Pain Protocol

1. Symptoms/Criteria
   - ☐ Assoc. URI symptoms
   - ☐ Pain worsened by cough, deep breath, twisting, touch
   - ☐ 30 years or under

   } Office visit

2. Symptoms/criteria
   - ☐ Assoc. SOB
   - ☐ ED request
   - ☐ History of Pneumothorax

   } ED visit

3. Patient wants to speak with MD re: chest pain
   - ☐ MD available → Message to MD
   - ☐ MD unavailable
   - ☐ Panic calls

   } Transfer to ED

Some symptoms may be further subdivided into different time frames. For example, symptoms of simple and compound fractures have different dispositions. Failure to designate dispositions in a consistent and concrete way is a common design flaw (Perrin & Goodman, 1977; Brown, 1980; Greitzer et al, 1976, Ott et al, 1974). Evidence for the need to establish time frames comes from the "golden hour" concept used to determine optimum time elapsed for successful treatment. Existence of this time frame lends credence to the concept of establishing other time frames. Even though it may be difficult to determine, general categories should be established in which to sort symptoms.

It may be difficult to form a consensus about what constitutes safe, appropriate and effective dispositions (times and places) for specific symptoms, because it means creating categories which may not always hold true. Admittedly, it is difficult to determine dispositions with great precision over the phone. Many protocols are flawed by dispositions which are vague, overly restrictive, or which leave large gaps.

Protocol formats should contain dispositions that include time as well as place. The format in Figure 5.7 separates symptoms into three levels of acuity. The place of treatment is clearly defined. Time frames overlap, eliminating gaps.

Once the disposition has been chosen, the master format is ready to be fleshed out (see example, Figure 5.7). The master format provides the skeletal structure for the prototype with sections for advice, teaching, referral, and cross-reference.

FIGURE 5.7 Master Format (Courtesy of Wheeler and Associates)

SPECIFIC DATA	DISPOSITION/ADVICE
EMERGENT/URGENT SYMPTOMS	**ED/MD IN 0–2 HOURS**
SEMI-URGENT SYMPTOMS	**MD/APPT IN 2–24 HOURS**
• "SAVED"? • *Any infectious process requiring antibiotics?* • *Painful conditions requiring prescription drugs?* • *Failure to improve after 48 hours on antibiotic?*	
ROUTINE SYMPTOMS	**MD/APPT IN 24 HOURS–2 WEEK**
• *Self-limiting symptoms existing over 1 week but not becoming markedly worse?*	• *Remain at home and begin treatment* • *Call back if symptoms become markedly worse or fail to improve with treatment within 48 hours*
CROSS-REFERENCE	**BASIC TEACHING**

FIGURE 5.8 Prototype: Burns (Thermal—First, Second, Third Degree) (Courtesy of Wheeler and Associates)

SPECIFIC QUESTIONS	DISPOSITION/ADVICE
EMERGENT/URGENT SYMPTOMS	**ED/MD IN 0–2 HOURS**
THIRD DEGREE • Absence of pain, loss of skin? • Third degree in excess of 10% body surface? • Third degree in excess of 3% body surface–child? • Third degree of face, hands, feet, or groin? • SECOND DEGREE in excess of 20%–child, 30%–adult? • White, dark, charred appearances? • *Degree, Percentage, Location, Complications, Age?*	• **Immed. cool (not ice) water × 10 min** • Wrap in clean wet sheet or saran wrap • Transport to ED
SEMI-URGENT SYMPTOMS	**MD/APPT IN 2–24 HOURS**
SECOND DEGREE • Red, mottled color, blisters, extreme pain? • Facial, neck, genitals, hands, feet? • Deep sunburn? • Uncomplicated second degree of 10-20%–child? • "Moderate Burn" + High Risk Factor (SAVED)? • AGE - 0-5 yrs, 60+ yrs. = Thin skin, low immunity? FIRST DEGREE (Poss. fatal if 2/3 surface involved)? • *Degree, Percentage, Location, Complications, Age?* • *Infectious process requiring antibiotics?* • *Painful conditions requiring prescription drugs?* • *Failure to improve after 48 hours on Antibiotic?*	• **Immed. cool (not ice) water × 10 min** • Wrap in clean wet sheet or saran wrap
ROUTINE SYMPTOMS	**MD/APPT IN 24 HOURS - 2 WEEK**
FIRST DEGREE: • Red, mild swelling, moderate pain, no blisters? • Sunburn?	• **Immed. cool (not ice) water × 10 min** • *Remain at home and begin treatment* • *Call back if symptoms become markedly worse or fail to improve with treatment within 48 hours*
CROSS REFERENCE	**BASIC TEACHING**
INHALATION BURNS ELECTRICAL BURNS	RULE OF NINES–ADULT–Head/Neck–9, Post. Trunk–1 Ant. Trunk–18, Arm–9, Perineum–1, Legs–18 CHILD–Head–18, Post. Trunk 18, Ant. Trunk 18, Arm–9, Leg–14 • COMPLICATIONS: Airway problems, pain/anxiety or fluid loss leading to shock, swelling, infection • SA TECH: Measure using hand = 1%

Step Six: Develop Protocol Content

Prototype development can challenge task force members who are learning new skills as well as learning to work together as a group. It is helpful if a secretary and computer expert are available in the initial stages to produce rough drafts.

Choose a specific protocol to develop. Some protocols, like abdominal or head pain, are too wide-ranging to use as prototypes. Rather, start with one which is simple and specific, like nosebleed. The task of protocol writing is more manageable when broken into major segments such as questions, advice, referral, teaching, title, and reference. Farm out these sections to be developed by two or three team members. Titles and subtitles should be generic and symptom-based. Dispositions and general guidelines are standing policies and often routinely included as part of the master format (see Figure 5.7). Data collection questions should be specific, leading questions which relate directly to the presenting symptom. Referral sections should include specific names, agencies, hot line numbers, support groups, book titles. (See Appendices F, G, H)

Make the best use of protocol space by combining symptoms. For example, it is not necessary to create three separate protocols for first, second, and third degree burns. Rather, create one protocol called "Burns, Thermal" with sections for first, second, and third degree (see Figure 5.8).

Design Flaw: Medical Terminology and Lay Language

Key components are instruction and teaching sections. Avoid undisciplined, unedited, and long-winded instruction in medical jargon—a common design flaw. Writing succinct, readable instructions which are both efficient and proficient requires discipline and skill. Microteaching sections of protocols should be conversational, directive, lucid instructions written in "cookbook" style. Home treatment instructions, definitions of medical terms, and self-assessment instructions should be written in this way. For example, instructions for a fever in a child might include:

- Give Tylenol®
- Give tepid bath/shower
- Wet head while in the tub/shower (to speed up cooling process)
- Give clear fluids
- Recheck temperature 1 1/2 hours after Tylenol®

The following examples contrast the use of lay language versus medical terminology in describing side effects to the same medication.

> *Example A: Side Effects: Redness, blistering, peeling or loosening of skin; unusual bleeding or bruising; unusual tiredness or weakness; aching of joints and muscles (U.S.P. Dispensing Information, 1985)*
>
> *Example B: Adverse Reactions: epidermal necrolysis, purpura, serum sickness, anaphylactoid reactions, urticaria (Huff, 1988)*

Example A is more readable, concrete, and conversational and could be easily adapted into a teaching section. Teaching sections contain advice and definitions of common terms. For example, a chest pain protocol might include a definition of angina.

Medical jargon alienates callers and reinforces authoritarian attitudes, whereas lay language builds a communication bridge and breaks down role stereotypes. Well-written, well-designed teaching sections demonstrate the institution's efforts to make the service more usable and accessible.

> *Example A - Vertigo: The room seems to spin around, caused by a disturbance of balance in the inner ear. (Vickery & Fries, 1978)*
>
> *Example B - Vertigo: Sensation of dizziness, caused by cerebral anemia or congestion; reflex irritation, as in gastric disturbances, eyestrain, uterine disease, constipation. (Taber, 1962).*

Advice for home treatment of yeast infection can be concrete and useful (Example A) or technical and verbose. (Example B):

> *Example A - To relieve itching: A compress of cool damp washcloth or baking soda. (Baking Soda Bath- Place 1/2 cup baking soda in tub of warmwater.) (Vickery & Fries, 1978)*
>
> *Example B - To alleviate the pruritis: Application of cold compresses to the vaginal area or use oatmeal baths. In the case of normal bowel flora compromise, recurrences are expected. Further advise the client to consume active culture yogurt to assist in reestablishing a more normal condition.*

Final Touches

Perform "dry runs" by role-playing with the protocols before implementing them. Obtain physician, nursing, and management approval. Initially, new protocols should be reviewed and updated every 12 months. To be current and reliable, HIV protocols and medication advice sections must be updated at least every 6 months. As a final step, perform a patient satisfaction survey to determine if protocols reflect client needs. Include questions about call length, disposition appropriateness, nurses' interpersonal skills, information usefulness, education, and follow-up calls. The protocol checklist is a QA tool to evaluate each completed protocol (see Figure 5.9).

FIGURE 5.9 Protocol Checklist

The following checklists are standards for evaluating protocols both individually and as a collection. Use them to refine existing protocols or to assess newly created protocols.

PROTOCOL TITLE ________________

1. FORMAT	YES	NO
Effective, consistent hierarchy of acuity?	________	________
Overlapping time frames?	________	________

Comments____

____

____

Person responsible for revision:____

2. DATA COLLECTION METHOD	YES	NO
Comprehensive?	________	________
Consistent?	________	________

Comments____

____

____

Person responsible for revision:____

3. TEACHING/ADVICE SECTIONS	YES	NO
Advocacy/consumer information?	________	________
Self-help and support groups?	________	________
Informationally sound?	________	________
Follow-up advice?	________	________
Includes time frames for self-evaluation	________	________

Comments____

____

____

Person responsible for revision:____

4. USER FRIENDLY?	YES	NO
Lay language?	________	________
Cookbook approach?	________	________
Lay language/symptom based titles?	________	________
Well presented graphically?	________	________
Easily accessed?	________	________
Quick cross-reference system?	________	________

Comments______________________________

Person responsible for revision:____________________

5. ENHANCEMENTS

	YES	NO
Reference section?	______	______
Follow-up mechanism?	______	______
Computer adaptable?	______	______

Comments______________________________

Person responsible for revision:____________________

6. CONSUMER FEEDBACK

	YES	NO
Contact made?	______	______
Numbers of contacts?	______	______
Consumer satisfaction?	______	______

Suggestions______________________________

Person responsible for revision:____________________

THE COLLECTION

1. CREDIBILITY/AUTHORITATIVE

	YES	NO
Collaborative effort (task force of six expert nurses)?	______	______
Approved by MDs/Administration?	______	______

Comments______________________________

Person responsible for revision:____________________

2. PROTOCOL COLLECTION	YES	NO
Current?	________	________
Comprehensive? (50–150)?	________	________
Pediatrics section?	________	________
"Crash cards" (optional)?	________	________
Informational protocols (optional)?	________	________

Comments____

____

____

Person responsible for revision:________________________________

3. QUALITY ASSURANCE FEATURES	YES	NO
Used 95% of the time?	________	________
Time tested?	________	________
How old is the collection?	________	________
Annual review and revision?	________	________
8- to 10-hour development time?	________	________
Formal training program?	________	________
Telephone triage certification?	________	________
Standards to describe correct use?	________	________

Comments____

____

____

Person responsible for revision:________________________________

Although it seems unimportant, graphic presentation is an important factor in making the set user-friendly. Copy which is poorly laid out and print which is difficult to read will make telephone work difficult. Is the product easy to use? For example, a Kardex™ or Rolodex™ is easier to use than a book or binder, which are cumbersome and bulky. A Rolodex™ leaves the nurses' hands free for writing, typing, or skimming other references. If the set is to be computerized, protocol content will be limited to a certain number of words per screen.

CRASH CARDS

Crash cards or pre-arrival instructions as they are called by emergency medical dispatchers (Clawson, 1988), are special instructions for rare but predictable life-threatening symptoms. They are analogous to the crash cart, now standard equipment on every floor of a hospital. A basic set of crash cards includes adult and child CPR and Heimlich maneuver instructions as well as childbirth coaching. Crash cards are less diagnostic and more mechanistic than protocols. They are algorithmic, action oriented, geared to split-second decision making and first aid implementation. They contain more leading questions and specific actions to prevent further injury or death.

All crash cards contain specific instructions that are usually read verbatim. Although this technique may seem elementary at first glance, a recent study (Eisenberg, 1986) shows that standardized instructions read verbatim produce better outcomes than coaching from memory. Medical dispatchers who have used them find standardized instructions bolster confidence. The best examples of pre-arrival instructions for medical dispatchers are those created by Clawson (1988). Nurses may use them in their existing form or may use them as a basis for creating their own crash cards.

FORM DESIGN

No system or protocol collection is complete without a complementary documentation form. After training, standards, and protocols, forms are the last line of defense in telephone triage practice. Use of protocols without documentation of calls is risky and most systems document calls as a minimal standard of practice (see Figure 5.10). In telephone triage, documentation serves as legal proof of assessment and advice and should be kept in the client's permanent record. Documentation forms have three major benefits:

1. They provide QA by standardizing data collection.
2. They complement protocols by facilitating and expediting data collection, helping to validate protocol use or filling in gaps.
3. They can be used to provide statistics on call volume, acuity, peak hours and peak days, and are especially helpful in validating staffing needs, or in training program development.

FIGURE 5.10 Charting Standards

1. Chart information in chronological order
2. Keep entries brief and concise
3. Use approved abbreviations only
4. Include pertinent negatives
5. Avoid vague expressions (quantify where possible)
6. Include date, time, first initial, last name, and title
7. Use quotes when possible

(Adapted from *Nurses' Legal Handbook*, Springhouse, 1985)

The best forms are simple, complete, and efficient. The best designs facilitate data collection, insure data comprehensiveness, and minimize error (Rowland, 1987). Telephone Triage forms in current use range from blank sheets of paper to forms that combine protocol and data collection sections. The best forms are easy to use and complement the protocol set. Include information and demographic data such as age, address, and phone number. For some data collection, checkboxes may be sufficient to assure documentation. In other cases, information must be written out. For emergency departments where charts are rarely available, the log format is most effective.

As with protocols, many current documentation forms have design flaws or are poorly conceived, making them confusing to use. One common design flaw is creating forms which are too abbreviated or generic. For example, a form used in a pediatric clinic contains the following information: date, time, patient name, age, phone number, a few lines for the problem and eight possible disposition check boxes (ED, advice, ambulance called, etc). It is $8\frac{1}{2} \times 4$ inches in size. The size is inadequate to allow sufficient writing space, and the data collection approach is too generic. It contains no space to write the advice given, protocol used, or working diagnosis. The quantity and generic quality of data required decrease the form's usefulness. This form could be improved through larger size and more specific data collection. Other common design flaws include forms which are too generic or specific, too short or long. The guidelines in Figure 5.11 can help to avoid these common design flaws.

Final Touches

All forms require a form description (Figure 5.12 and Figure 5.13) and standards for use (Figure 5.14). Use the form checklist (Figure 5.15) for QA. See Figures 5.16 and 5.17 for examples of different forms. Please note that the actual size of Figure 5.17 would be 11 × 17 inches.

The final step is to create a rough draft of the form. Use a small number of photocopied forms until the final version is refined and ready to print. Obtain final approval from the task force and administration. Finally, produce the new form and *destroy all old forms.*

FIGURE 5.11 Design Guidelines for Forms

1. INTEGRATE: Design forms, logs, or stamps which complement and integrate well with existing protocols and documentation systems.
2. CONSOLIDATE: Generic forms or logs are most effective for several reasons. All forms are expensive to produce. Generic forms cut costs by eliminating the need for several forms. A good general rule is to consolidate forms wherever possible. It is impractical and expensive to create different forms for each group of patients.

If *feasible*, rubber stamps can be used on existing forms rather than creating a new form (i.e., one generic form with stamps for Ob/Gyn, pediatrics, and emergency department calls). However, remember that rubber stamps eliminate the possibility of using duplicates or triplicates.

3. SIZE: The best size for forms is 5 by $8\frac{1}{2}$ inches. The size provides ample documentation space and yet does not create voluminous charts.

4. COPIES: Triplicate forms aid QA review, job performance evaluation, and client follow-up.

5. HEADING: Choose a simple, descriptive title and use bold type for headings.

6. ABBREVIATE: Develop a list of approved abbreviations specific to telephone triage and include in standards manual (see Appendix K).

7. LOGICAL SEQUENCE: Use a logical sequence for task performance and data collection. The conventional flow for data collection is top to bottom and left to right. Group similar types of data on the form or log. Divide the form into six sections:
   a. Demographic information
   b. Data collection
   c. Working diagnosis/impression
   d. Advice/disposition (treatment, teaching, appointment)
   e. Verbal contract/disclaimer
   f. Follow-up

8. CHECKBOXES/SLOTS: Where possible, use boxes to expedite and facilitate data collection:
   - CHECKBOXES
     - Disclaimer—Yes/No
     - Protocol deviations—Yes/No
     - Pregnancy status—Yes/No
   - SLOTS
     - Age
     - Plan of action
     - Protocol number or name
     - Consultations and initials of colleague/MD
     - Phone numbers (home/work)
     - Working diagnosis/impression
     - Follow-up call
     - Medications

9. DATE OF LAST REVISION: Always include date of the most recent revision and approval

FIGURE 5.12 Basic Documentation Form (Courtesy of Wheeler and Associates)

SOON/WK

TO 1 | FROM 2 | DATE 3 | TIME 4 | CHECKED BY 5 MD

NAME 6 | AGE 7 | WT 8 | CALLER 9 | PHONE HOME 10 | WORK 11

SX. CHAR/COURSE/HX/ONSET/LOC/AG.FX/REL.FX

12

TEMP 13 O R AX

ADL 14

PREG/BRSTFDG 15 ☐ Y 16 ☐ N LNMP 17

ALLERGIES 18

MEDS 19

PREVIOUS CHRONIC ILLNESS 20

EMOTIONAL STATUS 21

RECENT INJURY, ILLNESS OR INGESTION 22

Telephone Triage Data Form

WORKING DIAGNOSIS 23

ADVICE/PROTOCOL 24

DEVIATIONS 25 ☐ 26 VERBAL CONTRACT

☐ 27 DISCLAIMER

DISPOSITION 28 ☐ ED ☐ UCC ☐ ADVICE ONLY ☐ APPT.

FOLLOW-UP CALL 29 TIME 30

Rx 31

PHARMACY 32

OUTCOME: 34 | PHONE 33

SIG 35

FIGURE 5.13 Telephone Triage Form Description

Numbers refer to those in the Generic Form in Figure 5.12:

1. Physician to whom the message is addressed
2. Party writing the message
3. Today's date
4. Time of call
5. Physician reviewing message or consulting on call
6. Name of client or victim
7. Age of client
8. Weight of client (as appropriate)
9. Name/relationship of caller, if different from patient (i.e., friend, neighbor, daughter)
10. Home phone number (reachable time)
11. Work phone number (reachable time)
12. Data collected by SCHOLAR
13. Temperature. Circle route—axillary, oral, rectal
14. Activities of Daily Living
15. Pregnancy/breastfeeding status
16. Circle yes or no and draw line to related item in #15
17. Last normal menstrual period
18. Allergies
19. Medications—over-the-counter, vitamins, birth control pills, prescriptions, recreational
20. Previous chronic disease. Pediatrics—recurrent illnesses, multiple surgeries
21. Emotional status of child, caregiver, or client
22. Recent exposure to communicable illness, possible injury or ingestion
23. Working diagnosis
24. Protocol title or number (e.g., advised per protocol for chest pain)
25. Deviations from standard protocol advice
26. Check off if verbal contract obtained
27. Check off if disclaimer stated
28. Check one disposition (ED—emergency department; UCC—urgent care clinic; appt—appointment)
29. Follow-up calls (telephone management of routine illness—patient tries treatment and reports back or is called by nurse for progress report)
30. Time of follow-up call(s)
31. Prescription instructions (any prescription medications recommended by physician or advised per protocol)
32. Pharmacy name
33. Pharmacy phone number
34. Outcome information
35. Signature and title of nurse

FIGURE 5.14 Standards for Documentation Form Use

When using the documentation form, please remember that leaving spaces blank on this form or using abbreviations other than approved abbreviations may be interpreted as failure to collect adequate data or a faulty assessment. Please observe the following guidelines:

1. The telephone triage form is designed to provide documentation of all calls and advice, referrals, and information dispensed. Collect data in any order which seems appropriate to elicit key information quickly.
2. When clients present with multiple symptoms, rely on the symptom which has the best chance of leading to an appointment. If this is not workable, ask the client which symptom is most bothersome and rely on that protocol.
3. State the working diagnosis in client's own words and use approved classifying terms to clarify it.
4. Further clarify the disposition by adding method of transport and expected time of arrival or appointment.
5. Disclaimers should include the following information:
   a. That this is a "working diagnosis" or "impression"
   b. That treatment is based on that "working diagnosis"
   c. That the final disposition to use home treatment rests with the client. If clients disagree with the working diagnosis, then they are to be given an appointment.
   d. That if symptoms become markedly worse or fail to respond to the home treatment, they will call back within a specific period of time.
6. Client Plan of Action—Elicit and document what the client plans to do following the conversation.
7. All calls must be documented.
8. Use only approved terminology and abbreviations.
9. All charting is to be performed at the time of the call and must include the client's age, phone number, date, time and signature, as well as appropriate demographic information.
10. Standard pertinent negatives must be charted (allergies, pregnancy status, medications).
11. All forms must be checked by MD prior to posting in chart. For triplicate forms, the white copy is sent to MD prior to posting; yellow copy is for pharmacy; and all pink copies are saved for stats and peer review purposes.

12. Leave no blank spaces (i.e., if the client states they have no allergies, write "none known").
13. If clients answer negatively to items 18, 19, 20, 21, 22, write "denies" or "none" or a "zero" with a slash above it to fulfill the pertinent negative charting requirement.
14. Always collect data on items 7, 10, and 11.
15. Always collect items 15, 16, 17, 18, 19 when advising any OTC medication.

FIGURE 5.15 Documentation Form Checklist

	YES	NO
1. INTEGRATED WITH PROTOCOL	______	______
2. GENERIC	______	______
3. ADEQUATE SIZE	______	______
4. DUPLICATE/TRIPLICATE	______	______
5. HEADING	______	______
6. ABBREVIATIONS	______	______
7. LOGICAL SEQUENCE	______	______
a. Client demographic information	______	______
b. Data collection	______	______
c. Working diagnosis/impression	______	______
d. Advice/disposition (treat, teach, appt)	______	______
e. Verbal Contract/Disclaimer	______	______
f. Follow-up	______	______
8. CHECKBOXES/SLOTS		
Age	______	______
Pregnancy status	______	______
Medication	______	______
Allergies	______	______
Risk management safeguards:		
Protocol number or name	______	______
Disclaimer	______	______
Contracts	______	______
Protocol override/deviations	______	______
Pertinent negatives	______	______
Working diagnosis/impression	______	______
9. SUFFICIENT SPACE	______	______
10. DATE OF LAST REVISION	______	______

FIGURE 5.16 Maternal/Child Form (Courtesy of Wheeler and Associates)

NAME:
CALLER
DATE PHONE
TIME: AM PM WORK

MATERNAL	AGE:
SYMPTOMS	
	TEMP
CHARACTERISTICS	
COURSE	
HX (PAST)	
ONSET	
LOCATION	
AGGRAVATING FX	
RELIEVING FX	
PREG.STATUS	
ALLERGIES (FOODS, MEDS)	
PREVIOUS ILLNESS	
EMOTIONAL STATUS	
RECENT INJ/ILLNESS/INGESTION	

BREASTFEEDING ONLY	POSSIBLE LABOR
REST	CONTRAC: FREQ/LENGTH
WORK	ONSET
FLUIDS	SHOW
	FETAL ACTIVITY
DIET	
	MEMBRANES
FMO	

ASSESSMENT
ADVICE
DISPOSITION
RX
PHARMACY
PHONE

CHILD	
AGE	PREMATURE
WEIGHT	
BIRTH: DISCHARGE:	CURRENT:

SX	TEMP/ROUTE
CHARACTERISTICS	
COURSE	
HX (PAST)	
ONSET	
LOCATION	
AG/REL FX	
PREV. CHRONIC ILLNESS	
ALLERGIES (FOODS, MEDS.)	
MEDS	
EMOTIONAL STATUS	
RECENT INJ/ILLNESS/INGESTION	
SLEEP	
PLAYING	
COLOR	
FOOD/FLUID INTAKE X 24 HRS.	
VOMITUS/URINE/STOOLS X 24 HRS.	

BREASTFEEDING ONLY	
#FDG/24 HRS.	#MINUTES/FDG
FDG TERM BY: MOM BABY	
#WET DIAPERS & CHAR./8-24 HRS.	
#STOOLS & CHAR. X 24 HRS.	
#EMESIS & CHAR. X 24 HRS.	

FOLLOW UP TIME:

SIG.

FIGURE 5.17 Emergency Department Log (Courtesy of Wheeler and Associates)

					"Red Flags"					Primary Data							Secondary Data				Plan				Eval.	
Date	Time	Ca/Cl Name/ Address	Phone Home & Work	Age	Sev	Age	Ver.	Emo	Deb	Sx/Assoc Sx/Char/Hx	B/W/S Course	# Hrs S/G Onset	Loc	Aq. Fx.	Rel. Fx.	Temp.	Preg. Yes/No LMP	Allergies	Meds	Rec. Inj./Ill./Inf.	Protocol #/Advice	Disp.	Plan	Disc.	F.U. Eval.	MD/RN Init.

CHAPTER 5

EXERCISE 1: PROTOCOL DESIGN AND DEVELOPMENT

OBJECTIVE: To understand principles of protocol design and development.

METHOD: Choose the answer or answers which are most correct.

_____ 1. The most comprehensive data collection tool is:
   a. the acronyms SCHOLAR and PAMPER
   b. the acronym SOAP
   c. the acronym PQRST

_____ 2. SCHOLAR is used to collect:
   a. primary data relating to the presenting symptoms
   b. secondary data relating to the client and his or her medical history
   c. the parameters and characteristics of pain

_____ 3. Protocols should be used:
   a. instead of common sense
   b. instead of intuition
   c. judiciously

_____ 4. The ideal protocol:
   a. reflects population's characteristics plus common problems
   b. is sophisticated, holistic, and accurately reflects community needs
   c. forces consideration of several common decision choices

_____ 5. Protocols are most useful for:
   a. standardization of documentation
   b. provision of standard advice and questions for a range of problems
   c. decision making

_____ 6. The nurse is best at:
   a. remembering advice for 150 different problems
   b. emotional support
   c. synthesizing, analyzing, making fine discriminations, and decision making

_____ 7. The hierarchy of acuity
   a. states that many injuries lie below the surface
   b. acts as a "rough sort" for symptoms
   c. separates symptoms into time frames

_____ 8. Documentation procedural safeguards include:
  a. a form which includes checkboxes for disclaimer, contracts, and protocol deviations
  b. holistic elements—support groups and referral agencies
  c. pertinent negative checkbox

_____ 9. Protocols should:
  a. be time-tested, user-friendly, and use lay language
  b. use medical terms when possible, contain 300–400 symptoms and contain "crash cards"
  c. include comprehensive referral components and follow-up mechanism when possible

_____ 10. Protocols and documentation forms are:
  a. not a valuable product in today's telephone triage marketplace
  b. are admissible in a court of law
  c. a waste of time and effort because they are rarely used

EXERCISE 2: PROTOCOL AND FORM COMPONENT ANALYSIS

Assessment, diagnosis, treatment/advice, and referral are the major aspects of telephone triage interview and documentation. They are also major components of the protocol and documentation forms. All protocols and forms should include four sections: 1. assessment/data collection, 2. working diagnosis, 3. plan/disposition (treatment/advice, teaching), and 4. demographic information. Forms which lack space for a working diagnosis are seriously flawed.

OBJECTIVE: To identify and analyze protocol and form components.

METHOD: Using colored marking pens or hatchmarks to match key, circle each section of the following protocols (Figures 5.19–5.25) and forms, as appropriate. After identifying and delineating the components of each of these protocols and forms, use the Protocol and Form checklists (Figures 5.26 and 5.27) to evaluate Figure 5.18, fever in children, and Figure 5.19, the Basic Documentation Form. For additional practice, duplicate these checklists and evaluate your own or other protocols and forms included here.

COLORS	HATCHMARKS	
Red	▧	Assessment (data collection)
Yellow	▨	Working diagnosis
Green		Plan/disposition/treatment/advice/teaching
Purple		Demographics (name, address, time, etc.)
Pink	▤	Client self-evaluation (per follow-up call)
Blue	▥	Referral (MD, NP, self-help, hot line, book)

EXAMPLE:

FIGURE 5.18 Fever in Children (Newborn–16 years) (Courtesy of Wheeler and Associates)

SYMPTOMS/HISTORY			BASIC TEACHING
EMERGENT-URGENT	SEMI-URGENT	ROUTINE	
1. Accompanied by: seizure; difficult breathing; high-pitched or continual cry; stiff neck; sunken Fontanelle; Floppy Infant; purple spots; confusion; difficult to arouse, Dysuria; dry lips & tongue and/or sunken eyes; frequent nausea and/or vomiting; marked behavior change? 2. Any infant less than 6 months with fever over 100°F? 3. Any infant/child over 6 mo. with fever over 104°F? Medical History: • History of immunocompromising disease (e.g. leukemia, sickle cell disease, etc.) • a history of splenectomy • utilization of immuno-suppressive drugs (e.g. prednisone)?	1. Recent exposure to communicable disease associated with serious complications (e.g. meningitis)? (see 1) 2. Are parents extremely anxious: transients or homeless; or unable to contact medical help by phone if the infant/child's condition worsens? (see 2) 3. Persistent high fever x 24 hours? Unresponsive to treatment? 4. Failure to improve during the past 48 hours, or the parents think the infant/child looks ill? (see 3)	Any self-limiting symptom which is not becoming markedly worse. Recurrent fever after afebrile x 24 hours. Fever x 72 hours - Fever without evidence infection x 24 hours "Worried Parent"	FEVER in Infant - 6 mo. ________F ________C in child ________F ________C in Adult ________F ________C DEHYDRATION: Dry lips & tongue and/or sunken eyes; extreme sleepiness or inability to awaken, vomiting more than __ times in 4 hours. Unwilling to take any fluids for more than 4 hours. Less than 1 scantily wet diaper in 8 hours. Lack of tears. FEBRILE SEIZURES: Causes . . .

DISPOSITION			REFERRAL:
E.D. OR M.D. WITHIN 2 MINUTES - 2 HOURS	M.D. WITHIN 2-8 HOURS	M.D. WITHIN 8-48 HOURS	
CROSS REFERENCE • Earache • Symptoms of poss. ear pain (rubbing of his/her ears) • cold symptoms • abdominal pain • skin rash • severe vomiting and/or diarrhea • urinary frequency? SEE SPECIFIC PROTOCOLS Recent immunization within the past 24-48 hours? SEE IMMUNIZATION PROTOCOLS	1. Some communicable diseases have serious complications, such as meningitis. 2. Appointment within 8 hours. 3. Further evaluation to determine underlying fever lab tests and/or therapy.	REMAIN AT HOME BEGIN TREATMENT ADVICE: 1. Instruct parents to take temperature. If anxious or unsure, review process. Advise axillary temperatures in infants especially if parents are anxious. 2. Take infant's/child's temperature, if not already done; again 11/2° after initiating home treatment (baths, etc.). 3. Fever control–*warm* bath/shower, get head wet. Acetominophen (see dosage table), fluids (breastmilk, formula, juices, popsicles, water, Jello, ice chips, 7-Up). 4. Call back anytime infant's/child's condition worsens or he/she does not respond to home treatment. Signs of worsening condition: SEE DEHYDRATION & FEBRILE SEIZURES & #1 under EMERGENT/URGENT	1. PHYSICAL REFERRAL: Referral to ________ as appropriate for clients not being currently followed by M.D. 2. HOSPITAL REFERRAL-CLASSES/GROUPS/PROGRAMS ________ Refer to in-house as appropriate. 3. COMMUNITY-RESOURCE REFERRAL (Low income or anyone interested) Refer to free classes available through ________ (see Info Referral Section) Refer to free support group ________ 4. HOTLINES: Refer to Hotline: ________ for support group info.

FIGURE 5.18 Fever in Children (Newborn–16 years) (Courtesy of Wheeler and Associates)

SYMPTOMS/HISTORY			BASIC TEACHING
EMERGENT-URGENT	SEMI-URGENT	ROUTINE	
1. Accompanied by: seizure; difficult breathing; high-pitched or continual cry; stiff neck; sunken Fontanelle; Floppy Infant; purple spots; confusion; difficult to arouse, Dysuria; dry lips & tongue and/or sunken eyes; frequent nausea and/or vomiting; marked behavior change? 2. Any infant less than 6 months with fever over 100°F? 3. Any infant/child over 6 mo. with fever over 104°F? Medical History: • History of immunocompromising disease (e.g. leukemia, sickle cell disease, etc.) • a history of splenectomy • utilization of immuno-suppressive drugs (e.g. prednisone)?	1. Recent exposure to communicable disease associated with serious complications (e.g. meningitis)? (see 1) 2. Are parents extremely anxious: transients or homeless; or unable to contact medical help by phone if the infant/child's condition worsens? (see 2) 3. Persistent high fever x 24 hours? Unresponsive to treatment? 4. Failure to improve during the past 48 hours, or the parents think the infant/child looks ill? (see 3)	Any self-limiting symptom which is not becoming markedly worse. Recurrent fever after afebrile x 24 hours. Fever x 72 hours - Fever without evidence infection x 24 hours "Worried Parent"	FEVER in Infant - 6 mo. ________F ________C in child ________F ________C in Adult ________F ________C DEHYDRATION: Dry lips & tongue and/or sunken eyes; extreme sleepiness or inability to awaken, vomiting more than __ times in 4 hours. Unwilling to take any fluids for more than 4 hours. Less than 1 scantily wet diaper in 8 hours. Lack of tears. FEBRILE SEIZURES: Causes . . .

DISPOSITION			REFERRAL:
E.D. OR M.D. WITHIN 2 MINUTES - 2 HOURS	M.D. WITHIN 2-8 HOURS	M.D. WITHIN 8-48 HOURS	
CROSS REFERENCE • Earache • Symptoms of poss. ear pain (rubbing of his/her ears) • cold symptoms • abdominal pain • skin rash • severe vomiting and/or diarrhea • urinary frequency? SEE SPECIFIC PROTOCOLS Recent immunization within the past 24-48 hours? SEE IMMUNIZATION PROTOCOLS	1. Some communicable diseases have serious complications, such as meningitis. 2. Appointment within 8 hours. 3. Further evaluation to determine underlying fever lab tests and/or therapy.	REMAIN AT HOME BEGIN TREATMENT ADVICE: 1. Instruct parents to take temperature. If anxious or unsure, review process. Advise axillary temperatures in infants especially if parents are anxious. 2. Take infant's/child's temperature, if not already done; again 11/2° after initiating home treatment (baths, etc.). 3. Fever control–*warm* bath/shower, get head wet. Acetominophen (see dosage table), fluids (breastmilk, formula, juices, popsicles, water, Jello, ice chips, 7-Up). 4. Call back anytime infant's/child's condition worsens or he/she does not respond to home treatment. Signs of worsening condition: SEE DEHYDRATION & FEBRILE SEIZURES & #1 under EMERGENT/URGENT	1. PHYSICAL REFERRAL: Referral to ________ as appropriate for clients not being currently followed by M.D. 2. HOSPITAL REFERRAL-CLASSES/GROUPS/PROGRAMS Refer to in-house as appropriate. 3. COMMUNITY-RESOURCE REFERRAL (Low income or anyone interested) Refer to free classes available through ________ (see Info Referral Section) Refer to free support group 4. HOTLINES: Refer to Hotline: ________ for support group info.

FIGURE 5.19 Basic Documentation Form (Courtesy of Wheeler and Associates)

TO	FROM	DATE		TIME	CHECKED BY MD	
NAME		AGE	WT	CALLER	PHONE HOME	WORK
SX. CHAR/COURSE/HX/ONSET/LOC/AG.FX/REL.FX				WORKING DIAGNOSIS		
		TEMP O R AX				
				ADVICE/PROTOCOL		
				DEVIATIONS		☐ VERBAL CONTRACT
						☐ DISCLAIMER
ADL				DISPOSITION	☐ ED ☐ UCC ☐ ADVICE ONLY	☐ APPT.
				FOLLOW-UP CALL	TIME	
PREG/BRSTFDG	☐ Y ☐ N	LNMP				
ALLERGIES				Rx		
MEDS						
PREVIOUS CHRONIC ILLNESS						
EMOTIONAL STATUS				PHARMACY		
RECENT INJURY, ILLNESS OR INGESTION				OUTCOME	PHONE	
				SIG		
Telephone Triage Data Form						© 1990 Sheila Quilter Wheeler

FIGURE 5.20 Headache Protocol/Form (Reprinted with permission of Kaiser Permanente, San Diego, CA)

PATIENT'S NAME:________________ DOB:________ PHONE:________

M.R.# ________________ DATE:________________ TIME: ________

DR.____________ PHARMACY:____________ SPOKE WITH ____________

HEADACHE

CLINICAL ASSESSMENT | PROVIDER COMMENTS

1. Date of onset:________________
2. Duration/frequency________________
3. Location________________
4. Description________________
5. Accompanying symptoms:
   a. neck stiffness________ f. motor impairment________
   b. visual disturbances________ g. syncope________
   c. M/V________ h. lightheadedness ________
   d. aura________ i. sinus headache________
   e. fever________
6. Hx of:
   a. hypertension________ e. trauma________
   b. surgery/L.P.________ f. ↑ in normal sleep pattern________
   c. headaches________ g. recent illness________
   d. allergies________ h. ↑ stress level________
7. Current medications________________
8. Dietary habits________________
9. Date of LMP________________
10. Prescriptive lenses________ Date of last exam ________
11. Additional comments: ________________

____

SELF CARE ADVICE: SIGNATURE:________________

____ Rest in darkened room ____ OTC antipyretics as directed
____ Cold compresses to head ____ Progressive clear liq. to reg. diet
____ Warm compresses/steam vapor if known sinus headache
____ Review & instruct pt. on proper use of all medication
____ Review prescribed use of lenses
____ Food elimination if known Hx of migraine: Foods rich in Tryamine (chocolate, milk, mild products, cured pork, caffeine, MSG, alcohol)
____ Migraine - heat to neck, cool compresses to head, semi-fowlers position
____ If S/S persist or ↑ call A.M.

DISPOSITION: ○ SELF CARE ○ APPOINTMENT WITH ____________ ON ________ @________

○ OTHER ________________________________

ADVICE NURSE________________________________

FIGURE 5.21 Pediatric Advice Form (Reprinted with permission of Children's Hospital at Stanford, Palo Alto, CA)

LUCILE SALTER PACKARD
CHILDREN'S HOSPITAL AT STANFORD
725 WELCH ROAD, PALO ALTO, CA 94304

TELEPHONE ADVICE DOCUMENTATION

PATIENT NAME ______________ D.O.B. __________ M.R. # __________

DATE __________ PATIENT CALL TIME __________ CALLER __________

TELEPHONE: HOME( ) __________ WORK ( ) __________ LANGUAGE __________

PARENTAL CONCERN ______________________________

______________________________ SIGNATURE __________

ASSESSMENT: Chief complaint (Symptoms, Characteristics, Course, Onset, E.R. Follow-up request)

Historian's relationship to patient: ______________________________

CURRENT LABS:

ADVICE / FOLLOW-UP:

____

____

____

____

____

____

Standard Advice # ______________ Deviations ______________

Service / M.D. __________ Date __________ Time __________ Interpreter __________

Attempted call backs ______________ Signature ______________

MEDICAL RECORDS-WHITE • CLINIC FILE-YELLOW

8700-241(5/97)
MR8003.01.90

FIGURE 5.22 Poison Control Form (Courtesy of San Francisco Bay Area Regional Poison Control Center, San Francisco, CA)

Phone line: 800 476 8058 911 5338 3182

PCC Log Book #:
Computer Case #:

Substance 1:______ Amt 1:____ Size:____ Units:____

PCode 1: [| | | | | | |] SF Code 1: [| |]

Substance 2:______ Amt 2:____ Size:____ Units:____

PCode 2: [| | | | | | |] SF Code 2: [| |]

Units:
1 Bite 10 Swallow/Sip
2 Grains 11 Tbls
3 Grams 12 Tsp
4 lick/taste 13 Tabs/Caps
5 μgrams 14 Vial/Ampute
6 mgrams 15 Whiff
7 mliters 16 Unknown
8 Oz. 17 Other
9 Splash/Spill

Total # Subs: 1 or______

PATIENT DATA

Name:
Phone:( )
Address: ZIP:
Age:__Yr Mo UNI Unkn Infant UC2 Unkn 2-5 Y UC6 Unkn 6-12 Y UAL Unkn Adolesc UAD Unkn Adult UAG Unkn Age
Sex: M F Weight:____ Pds Kgs Unk
Route(s): _Ingestion _Ocular _Bite/Sting _Unkn _Inhal/Nasal _Dermal _Parenteral _Other____
Time since exposure: ____Min. Hr. Day or Chronic
PMHx: (mark all that apply) Pregnant?: T F Unk
_Alcoholism _Drug Abuse _Pulm-Asthma/COPD
_Allergy-Drug _Hepatic Dis. _Pulm-Other
_Allergy-Other _Medications _Renal Dis.
_Cardiac/CHF _Ment. Handicap _Seizure Dis.
_Down's Synd. _Psych./Schizoph _Other

CALLER DATA

Name:
Relation: Moth Fath Self Oth
Title: MD RN Pharm Oth
Hospital:
ZIP:____ Phone:( )
Address:
City:____ State:____
County:

Site of Caller:		Site of Exposure:
____	Residence	____
____	Workplace	____
____	Health Care Facility	____
____	School	____
____	Other	____
____	Unknown Site	____

Notes:

Call type:	Victim:	Exposure Type:
1 Exposure 3 Poison Info. 2 Drug Info. 4 Med./Other	1 Human 2 Animal	1 Acute 2 Chronic 3 Unknown

Reason for Exposure:
1 Acc Gen 5 Acc Unkn 9 Int Unkn
2 Acc Occup 6 Int Suicide 10 Adv Rxn Drug
3 Acc Environ 7 Int Misuse 11 Adv Rxn Food
4 Acc Misuse 8 Int Abuse 12 Adv Rxn Oth
13 Unk.

Initial Sx:
1 Asymptomatic
2 Symp., Related
3 Symp., Unrelated
4 Symp., Unkn if Related
5 Unkn if Symptomatic
6 Late Symptom Develop.

Symptoms:
_CNS-Coma _Gi-Minor
_CNS-Sz _Gi-Major
_CNS-Major _Met. Acid.
_CNS-Minor _Renal Fail.
_CV-Hypotens. _Rhapdo.
_CV-Hypertens. _Resp.-Major
_CV-Minor _Resp-Minor
_CV-Ser. EKG _Skin/Eye-Major
_Hyperthermia _Skin/Eye-Minor
_Other

Care Provided:
1 No therapy nec.
2 Observation only
3 Patient refused
IF THERAPY PROVIDED. LEAVE BLANK OR ENTER "0"

PCC #2? True False

Decontamination:
_Ipecac _Lavage _Fresh Air
_Act. Charcoal _Dilute _Other decon.
_Cathartic _Irrigate/Wash _Other ematic

Other Therapies:
_Acidification _Deferoxamine _NAC, IV
_Alkalinization _EDTA _NAC, PO
_Anticonvulsants _Ethanol _Naloxone
_Antihistamines _Exchg. Transf. _Oxygen
_Antivenin _Fab Fragmnts _2-Pam
_Atropine _Forced diuresis _Penicillamine
_BAL _Glucose _Perit dialys
_CPR _Hemodialysis _Physosogmine
_Char Hemoper. _Hyperbar Oxy _Pyndoxine
_Cyanide Kit _Methylene blue _Resin Hemoperf.
_Other

Patient Flow:
1 Managed on site (non HCF)
2 Patient already in/enroute to HCF
3 Treated and relased
4 Admitted for medical care
5 Admitted for psych care/eval
6 Lost to follow-up/left AMA
7 Patient was referred by PCC to HCF
8 Treated and relased
9 Admitted for medical care
10 Admitted for psych care/eval
11 Refused ref/didn't arr HCF
12 Lost to follow-up/left AMA
13 Other
14 Unknown

# of F/U:____

Outcome:
1 No effect
2 Minor effect
3 Moderate effect
4 Major effect
5 Unkn. nontoxic
6 Unkn. pot toxic
7 Unrelated effect
8 Death

Teaching Case?: (free area #1) Y N

HCF #2?______ (name)

HazMat? True False

Foreign Language? (free area #2) Y N

Signed:______ Reviewed:______

Complete?: True False

Entered in Computer:______

FIGURE 5.23 Health Access Logsheet (Courtesy of Northern Michigan Hospital, Petosky, MI)

DATE | TIME | AM PM | COOR/ RN/ TITLE

CALLER NAME | CALLER TELEPHONE | RELATIONSHIP TO PATIENT

CALLER ADDRESS | CITY | COUNTY/REGION | STATE | ZIP CODE

PATIENT'S NAME | PATIENT'S TELEPHONE | PATIENT'S AGE

PATIENT'S ADDRESS | CITY | COUNTY/REGION | STATE | ZIP CODE

HEALTHACCESS AWARENESS

REFERRALS

PERSONAL PHYSICIAN | DEMOGRAPHIC RELEASE ☐ YES ☐ NO

HEALTHACCESS CONTACT ☐ YES ☐ NO | APPOINTMENT MADE ☐ YES ☐ NO | DATE | PROVIDER NAME

NATURE OF INQUIRY/ CHIEF COMPLAINT

ASSESSMENT: SUBJ. & OBJ.

TREATMENT INSTITUTED / RESULTS

MEDICAL HISTORY (ALLERGIES, MEDICATIONS, PREGNANCY, DISEASE STATES, FAMILY HX)

NURSING DIAGNOSIS

MANAGEMENT OPTIONS ☐ EMERGENT ☐ URGENT ☐ DELAYED ☐ SELF CARE

PLAN OF ACTION

RFC PROVIDED? ☐ YES ☐ NO | CALLER REPEAT INSTRUCTIONS? ☐ YES ☐ NO | CALLER SATISFIED? ☐ YES ☐ NO

TRANSPORTATION NOTIFIED? ☐ YES ☐ NO | SERVICE USED | TIME | AM PM

EMERGENCY FAC. NOTIFIED? ☐ YES ☐ NO | CONTACT PERSON | TIME | AM PM

FOLLOW UP ☐ YES ☐ NO | ☐ HEALTHACCESS ☐ CALLER | DATE | TIME | AM PM

FOLLOW UP SUMMARY

RESOURCE MATERIALS / CONSULTANTS

TYPE OF CALL ☐ PHYSICIAN REFERRAL ☐ SERVICE REFERRAL ☐ GENERAL INFORMATION ☐ SYMPTOM - BASED

FIGURE 5.24 Head Injury Protocol
(Courtesy of Northern Michigan Hospital, Petosky, MI)

HEAD INJURY

Traumatic injury to the head resulting in a fall, high speed accident (car), great force (baseball) or possible child abuse

ASSESSMENT:

- Determine AVPU Scale: A-Alert, V-Responds to verbal stimuli, P-Responds to painful stimuli, U-unresponsive.
- Describe in detail the events of the accident:
  - time
  - area injured (laceration, bleeding, swelling, abrasions)
  - distance of fall or struck with what object
  - any loss of consciousness?
- Any of the following symptoms: headache, nausea, vomiting, blurred or double vision, unequal pupils (black circle in center of eyes), perfuse bleeding, confusion, unsteady gait, seizure activity, neck pain, difficulty moving arms or legs, swelling of head, change in speech or usual behavior, loss of appetite
- Describe skin color and temperature: pin, pale, warm, cool, clammy?
- Any drainage from the ears, mouth or nose? color? amount?
- Signs and symptoms of respiratory distress? (Shortness of breath, Cyanosis, Rapid, Labored breathing? Restlessness?)
- Any difficulty arousing from sleep?
- Prior medical history of neurological deficits, surgery, seizures?
- Present list of medications taken today.
- Treatment instituted? Effectiveness?

EMERGENT:

*IF PARALYZED, DO NOT MOVE PATIENT WITHOUT MEDICAL ASSISTANCE

- Head injury with subsequent loss of consciousness (immediate or delayed).
- Head injury with open laceration, active bleeding requiring sutures.
- Head injury associated with nausea, vomiting, and/or seizure.
- Head injury with severe neuro deficits (respiratory distress, decreased level of consciousness, change in pupils, pale skin color, change in gait, speech, affect).
- Drainage from ear, nose or mouth (not related to cold).
- Any muscle weakness, twitching, paralysis.
- Head injury with complaint of stiff-sore neck.
- Change in status, decreased level of consciousness, difficult to arouse, loss of nerve function as described above.

URGENT:

- Head trauma with:
  - minor swelling, controlled bleeding from laceration
  - headache unrelieved with home management
  - post trauma fever greater than 100 degrees

DELAYED:

Not applicable

SELF-CARE:

A head injury which causes confusion, loss of memory or a brief period of unconsciousness is called a concussion. Some person with concussions will also vomit one or more times. Children may sometimes vomit once even though they do not have a concussion. Nearly all persons with concussions will recover within one to three days. Occasionally, however, complications develop. Follow these instructions carefully and call your doctor promptly if you are concerned for any reason.

WHAT TO DO:

1. A responsible person should watch a person who has any sign of concussion carefully for signs of complications.
2. Have the person rest. He should be allowed to sleep if he wants to, but awakened every 1–2 hours for the first 24 hours to be checked. Ask person to identify familiar family members or objects.
3. Have the person drink only liquids if he is feeling nauseated.
4. Take Tylenol/Panadol, as directed by manufacturer, as needed for pain. Do not use any stronger pain medicine.

REASONS FOR CONCERN:

- Increasing sleepiness or inability to awaken
- Bleeding from ears, mouth or nose
- Close discharge from the nose (not associated with crying or a cold) or ear
- Blurred or double vision
- Garbled speech or any other difficulty that occurs in talking
- Unusual stumbling or inability to use arms or legs
- Unusual behavior, personality change or confusion, irritability, combative
- Muscle weakness in arms or legs
- Convulsions or seizures
- Unequal pupil size not present prior to injury
- Vomiting more than twice, loss of appetite
- Severe persistent or worsening headache unrelieved with home management
- Persistent fever over 100 degrees orally (101 degrees rectally)
- Any other symptoms that might seem unusual to you

NOTE: The single most important sign that a complication of head injury is developing is inability to arouse the person and get him to respond appropriately to questions or instructions.

CROSS-REFERENCE:

Balance Problems, Coma, Confusion, Convulsions, Dizziness, Headache, Nausea and Vomiting

FIGURE 5.25 Abdominal Pain Protocol (Reprinted with permission of Kaiser Permanente, South San Francisco, CA)

SUBJECT: Surgery Advice Protocols	NUMBER: 2	PAGE 1 OF
TITLE: Abdominal Pain	EFFECTIVE DATE: 10/75	
PERSONNEL APPLICABLE TO:	REVISION DATE: 8/80, 4/81, 6/90	

ABDOMINAL PAIN

1. Inquire from patient:
   a. Where is it?
   b. How long have you had it?
   c. Have you had recent surgery? If so, what and where and when?
   d. How severe is it?
   e. Have you vomited? If so, what?
   f. Do you have fever?
   g. Do you have headache or muscle aches?
   h. Do you have frequent or painful urination?
   i. Do you have diarrhea, bloody or black stools?
   j. Do you have gall stones, ulcers or chronic intestinal disease?
   k. Do you have yellow eyes or skin?
   l. For women: When was your last period? Do you have any vaginal bleeding or discharge?
2. If patient has had:
   a. Surgery recently (within one month)
   b. Is being followed for a specific problem by a surgeon, refer message to patient's surgeon, surgeon on-call, or clinic surgeon.
3. If patient complains of:
   a. Severe pain of recent onset.
   b. Vomiting of blood or coffee ground emesis.
   c. Bloody or tarry stools.
   d. High fever (over 101).
   e. Yellow eyes or skin or dark urine.
   f. Localized abdominal tenderness.
   g. Heavy vaginal bleeding.

   DIRECT PATIENT TO THE EMERGENCY DEPARTMENT.
4. If patient complains of:
   a. Pelvic pain as in menstrual cramps, abnormal bleeding (less than heavy) vaginal discharge.

   TRANSFER TO GYNECOLOGY ADVICE NURSE
5. All others transfer to Medical Advice Nurse.

FIGURE 5.26 Protocol Checklist

PROTOCOL TITLE: FEVER IN CHILDREN

	YES	NO
1. FORMAT		
Effective, consistent hierarchy of acuity?	______	______
Overlapping time frames?	______	______

Comments______

	YES	NO
2. DATA COLLECTION METHOD		
Comprehensive?	______	______
Consistent?	______	______

Comments______

	YES	NO
3. TEACHING/ADVICE SECTIONS		
Advocacy/consumer information?	______	______
Self-help and support groups?	______	______
Informationally sound?	______	______
Follow-up advice?	______	______
Includes time frames for self-evaluation	______	______

Comments______

	YES	NO
4. USER FRIENDLY		
Lay language?	______	______
Cookbook approach?	______	______
Lay language/symptom based titles?	______	______
Well presented graphically?	______	______
Easily accessed?	______	______
Quick cross-reference system?	______	______

Comments______

	YES	NO
5. ENHANCEMENTS		
Reference section?	______	______
Follow-up mechanism?	______	______
Computer adaptable?	______	______

Comments______

FIGURE 5.27 Documentation Form Checklist

	YES	NO
1. INTEGRATED WITH PROTOCOL	______	______
2. GENERIC	______	______
3. ADEQUATE SIZE	______	______
4. DUPLICATE/TRIPLICATE	______	______
5. HEADING	______	______
6. ABBREVIATIONS	______	______
7. LOGICAL SEQUENCE	______	______
a. Client demographic information	______	______
b. Data collection	______	______
c. Working diagnosis/impression	______	______
d. Advice/disposition (treat, teach, appt)	______	______
e. Verbal contract/disclaimer	______	______
f. Follow-up	______	______
8. CHECKBOXES/SLOTS	______	______
Age	______	______
Pregnancy status	______	______
Medication	______	______
Allergies	______	______
Risk management safeguards:		
Protocol number or name	______	______
Disclaimer	______	______
Contracts	______	______
Protocol override/deviations	______	______
Pertinent negatives?	______	______
Working diagnosis/impression	______	______
9. SUFFICIENT SPACE	______	______
10. DATE OF LAST REVISION	______	______

EXERCISE 3: PROTOCOL AND FORM DESIGN

OBJECTIVE: To design a protocol prototype and form.

METHOD: Use the following guidelines to aid you in the protocol and form design process.

FIGURE 5.27 Documentation Form Checklist

	YES	NO
1. INTEGRATED WITH PROTOCOL	______	______
2. GENERIC	______	______
3. ADEQUATE SIZE	______	______
4. DUPLICATE/TRIPLICATE	______	______
5. HEADING	______	______
6. ABBREVIATIONS	______	______
7. LOGICAL SEQUENCE	______	______
a. Client demographic information	______	______
b. Data collection	______	______
c. Working diagnosis/impression	______	______
d. Advice/disposition (treat, teach, appt)	______	______
e. Verbal contract/disclaimer	______	______
f. Follow-up	______	______
8. CHECKBOXES/SLOTS	______	______
Age	______	______
Pregnancy status	______	______
Medication	______	______
Allergies	______	______
Risk management safeguards:		
Protocol number or name	______	______
Disclaimer	______	______
Contracts	______	______
Protocol override/deviations	______	______
Pertinent negatives?	______	______
Working diagnosis/impression	______	______
9. SUFFICIENT SPACE	______	______
10. DATE OF LAST REVISION	______	______

EXERCISE 3: PROTOCOL AND FORM DESIGN

OBJECTIVE: To design a protocol prototype and form.

METHOD: Use the following guidelines to aid you in the protocol and form design process.

Add specific data collection and leading questions which relate directly to the presenting symptom.
Incorporate referral sections with specific names, agencies, hot line numbers, support groups, and book titles.
Add instruction and teaching sections.

Final Touches

Evaluate the protocol, using protocol checklist (Figure 5.9).
Perform "dry runs" by role-playing, using the protocol.

EXERCISE 4: FORM DESIGN

OBJECTIVE: To develop correct and useful forms.

METHOD: Use the following steps to develop a form.

1. Choose a simple, descriptive title and use bold type for headings.
2. Use a logical sequence for task performance and data collection (top to bottom and left to right).
3. Group similar types of data on the form or log.
4. Divide the form into six sections:
   a. Client demographic information
   b. Data collection
   c. Working diagnosis and impression
   d. Advice and disposition (treatment, teaching, appointment)
   e. Verbal contract/disclaimer
   f. Follow-up
5. Add Checkboxes/Slots:
   Disclaimer: Yes/No
   Protocol deviations: Yes/No
   Pregnancy status: Yes/No
   Age
   Plan of action
   Protocol number or name
   Consultations and initials of colleague or MD
   Phone numbers (home and work)
   Working diagnosis and impression
   Follow-up call
   Medication
6. Include date of the most recent revision and approval.
7. Develop directions for form use, including a form description, purpose, and standards for use.
8. Create a rough draft of the form.

ANSWER KEY

EXERCISE 1: PROTOCOL DESIGN AND DEVELOPMENT

1. a
2. a
3. c
4. a, b, c
5. b
6. b, c
7. b, c
8. a, b, c
9. a, c
10. b

EXERCISE 2: PROTOCOL AND FORM COMPONENT ANALYSIS

Refer to Figures 5.19A through 5.27A for answers.

FIGURE 5.19A Basic Documentation Form KEY

TO | FROM | DATE | TIME | CHECKED BY | MD
NAME | AGE | WT | CALLER | PHONE HOME | WORK
SX. CHAR/COURSE/HX/ONSET/LOS/AG.FX/REL.FX
TEMP O R AX
WORKING DIAGNOSIS
ADVICE/PROTOCOL
DEVIATIONS ☐ VERBAL CONTRACT ☐ DISCLAIMER
DISPOSITION ☐ ER ☐ USC ☐ ADVICE ONLY ☐ APPT.
ADL
FOLLOW-UP CALL TIME
PREG/BRST FDG ☐ Y ☐ N LNMP
ALLERGIES
MEDS
Rx
PREVIOUS CHRONIC ILLNESS
EMOTIONAL STATUS
PHARMACY
RECENT INJURY, ILLNESS OR INGESTION
OUTCOME | PHONE
SIG
Telephone Triage Data Form
© 1990 Sheila Quilter Wheeler

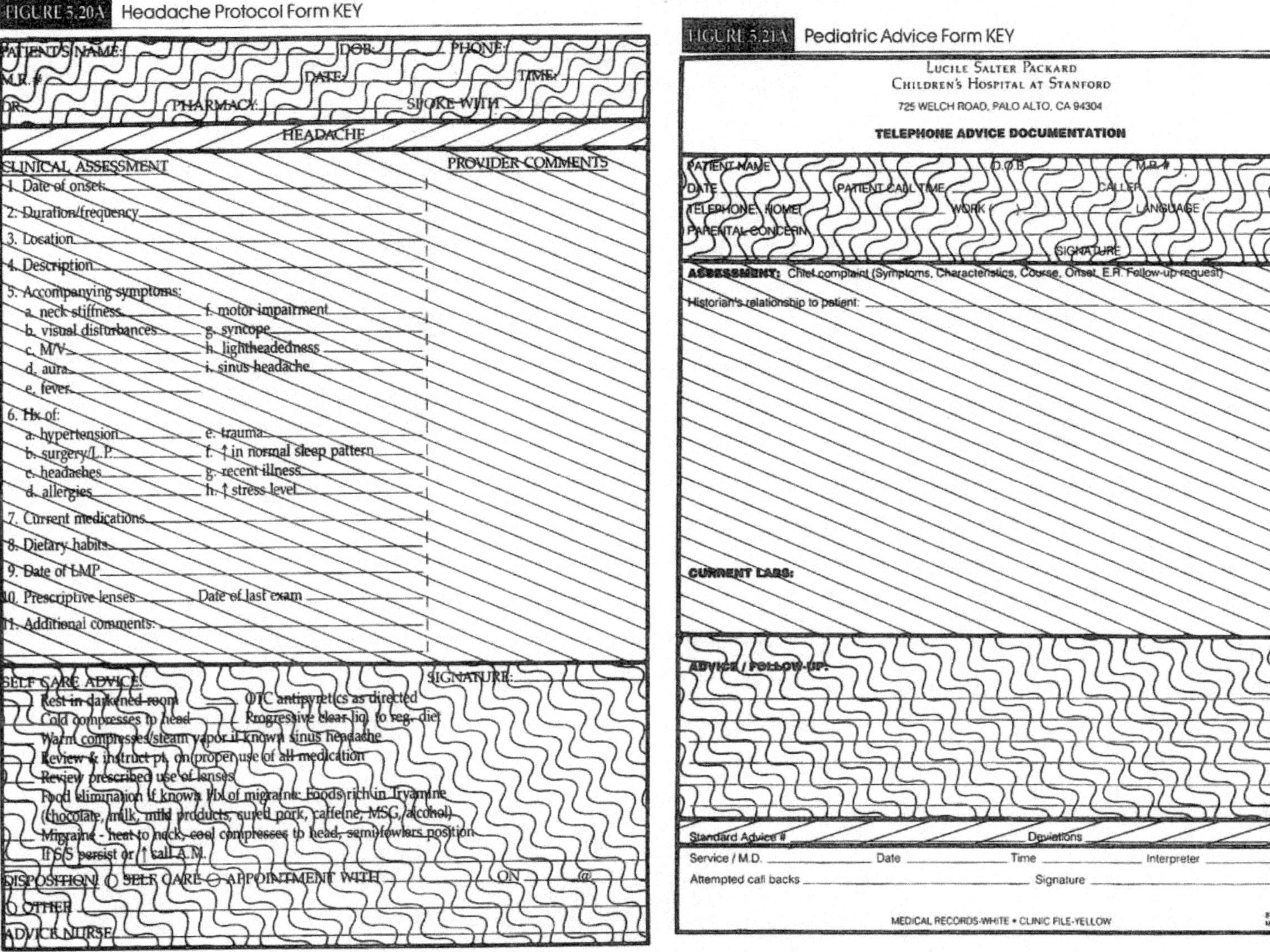

FIGURE 5.20A Headache Protocol Form KEY

PATIENT'S NAME: DOB: PHONE:
M.R. # DATE: TIME:
DR. PHARMACY: SPOKE WITH:

HEADACHE

CLINICAL ASSESSMENT | PROVIDER COMMENTS

1. Date of onset:
2. Duration/frequency
3. Location
4. Description
5. Accompanying symptoms:
   - a. neck stiffness
   - b. visual disturbances
   - c. M/V
   - d. aura
   - e. fever
   - f. motor impairment
   - g. syncope
   - h. lightheadedness
   - i. sinus headache
6. Hx of:
   - a. hypertension
   - b. surgery/L.P.
   - c. headaches
   - d. allergies
   - e. trauma
   - f. ↑ in normal sleep pattern
   - g. recent illness
   - h. ↑ stress level
7. Current medications
8. Dietary habits
9. Date of LMP
10. Prescriptive lenses Date of last exam
11. Additional comments:

SELF CARE ADVICE: SIGNATURE:
- Rest in darkened room
- OTC antipyretics as directed
- Cold compresses to head
- Progressive clear liq. to reg. diet
- Warm compresses/steam vapor if known sinus headache
- Review & instruct pt. on proper use of all medication
- Review prescribed use of lenses
- Food elimination if known Hx of migraine: Foods rich in Tryamine (chocolate, milk, milk products, cured pork, caffeine, MSG, alcohol)
- Migraine - heat to neck, cool compresses to head, semi-fowlers position
- If S/S persist or ↑ call A.M.

DISPOSITION: ○ SELF CARE ○ APPOINTMENT WITH ON @
○ OTHER
ADVICE NURSE

FIGURE 5.21A Pediatric Advice Form KEY

LUCILE SALTER PACKARD
CHILDREN'S HOSPITAL AT STANFORD
725 WELCH ROAD, PALO ALTO, CA 94304

TELEPHONE ADVICE DOCUMENTATION

PATIENT NAME D.O.B. M.R. #
DATE PATIENT CALL TIME CALLER
TELEPHONE: HOME WORK LANGUAGE
PARENTAL CONCERN
SIGNATURE

ASSESSMENT: Chief complaint (Symptoms, Characteristics, Course, Onset, E.R. Follow-up request)
Historian's relationship to patient:

CURRENT LABS:

ADVICE / FOLLOW-UP:

Standard Advice # Deviations
Service / M.D. Date Time Interpreter
Attempted call backs Signature

MEDICAL RECORDS-WHITE • CLINIC FILE-YELLOW
8700-24145(9/91) MR6003 01 90

FIGURE 5.22A Poison Control Form KEY

PCC Log Book #:
Computer Case #:

Phone line: 800 476 8058 911 5338 3182

Substance 1: Amt 1: Size: Units:
PCode 1: SF Code 1:
Substance 2: Amt 2: Size: Units:
PCode 2: SF Code 2:

Units:
1 Bite 10 Swallow/Sip
2 Grains 11 Tbls
3 Grams 12 Tsp
4 lick/taste 13 Tabs/Caps
5 μgrams 14 Vial/Ampute
6 mgrams 15 Whiff
7 mliters 16 Unknown
8 Oz. 17 Other
9 Splash/Spill

Total # Subs: 1 or

Call type: 1 Exposure 2 Drug Info. 3 Poison Info. 4 Med./Other
Victim: 1 Human 2 Animal
Exposure Type: 1 Acute 2 Chronic 3 Unknown

Reason for Exposure:
1 Acc Gen 2 Acc Occup 3 Acc Environ 4 Acc Misuse
5 Acc Unkn 6 Int Suicide 7 Int Misuse 8 Int Abuse
9 Int Unkn 10 Adv Rxn Drug 11 Adv Rxn Food 12 Adv Rxn Oth 13 Unk.

Initial Sx:
1 Asympromatic
2 Symp., Related
3 Symp., Unrelated
4 Symp., Unkn if Related
5 Unkn if Symptomatic
6 Late Symptom Develop.

Symptoms::
_ CNS-Coma _ CNS-Sz _ CNS-Major _ CNS-Minor _ CV-Hypotens. _ CV-Hypertens. _ CV-Minor _ CV-Ser. EKG _ Hyperthermia
_ Gi-Minor _ Gi-Major _ Met. Acid. _ Renal Fail. _ Rhapdo. _ Resp.-Major _ Resp-Minor _ Skin/Eye-Major _ Skin/Eye-Minor _ Other

PATIENT DATA
Name:
Phone:(
Address: ZIP:
Age: Mo Yr UNI Unkn Infant UC2 Unkn 2-5 Y UC6 Unkn 6-12 Y UAL Unkn Adolesc UAD Unkn Adult UAG Unkn Age
Sex: M F Weight: Pds Kgs Unk
Route(s): _ Ingestion _ Bite/Sting _ Inhal/Nasal _ Parenteral _ Ocular _ Unkn _ Dermal _ Other
Time since exposure: _ Min. Hr. Day or Chronic
PMHx: (mark all that apply) Pregnant?: T F Unk
_ Alcoholism _ Allergy-Drug _ Allergy-Other _ Cardiac/CHF _ Down's Synd. _ Drug Abuse _ Hepatic Dis _ Medications _ Ment. Handicap _ Psych./Schizoph _ Pulm-Asthma/COPD _ Pulm-Other _ Renal Dis _ Seizure Dis _ Other

CALLER DATA
Name:
Relation: Moth Fath Self Oth
Title: MD RN Pharm Oth
Hospital:
ZIP: Phone:(
Address:
City: State:
Country:
Site of Caller: Site of Exposure:
Residence
Workplace
Health Care Facility
School
Other
Unknown Site

Care Provided:
1 No therapy nec.
2 Observation only
3 Patient refused
IF THERAPY PROVIDED, LEAVE BLANK OR ENTER "0"
PCC #2? True False

Decontamination:
_ Ipecac _ Act. Charcoal _ Catharot
_ Lavage _ Dilute _ Irrigate/Wash
_ Fresh Air _ Other decon. _ Other ematic

Other Therapies:
_ Acidification _ Alkalinization _ Anticonvulsants _ Antiphistamines _ Antivenin _ Atropine _ BAL _ CPR _ Char Hemoper _ Cyanide Kit
_ Deferoxamine _ EDTA _ Ethanol _ Exchg. Transf. _ Fab Fragmnts _ Forced diuresis _ Glucose _ Hemodialysis _ Hyperbar Oxy _ Methylene blue
_ NAC, IV _ NAC, PO _ Naloxone _ Oxygen _ 2-Pam _ Penicillamine _ Pent. dialys _ Physostigmine _ Pyridoxine _ Resin Hemoperf. _ Other

Patient Flow:
1 Managed on site (non HCF)
2 Patient already in/enroute to HCF
3 Treated and relased
4 Admitted for medical care
5 Admitted for psych care/eval
6 Lost to follow-up/left AMA
7 Patient was referred by PCC to HCF
8 Treated and relased
9 Admitted for medical care
10 Admitted for psych care/eval
11 Refused ref/didn't arr HCF
12 Lost to follow-up/left AMA
13 Other
14 Unknown

# of F/U:

Outcome:
1 No effect
2 Minor effect
3 Moderate effect
4 Major effect
5 Unkn. nontoxic
6 Unkn. pot toxic
7 Unrelated effect
8 Death

Teaching Case?: (free area #1) Y N

HCF #2? (name)

HazMat? True False
Foreign Language? (free area #2) Y N

Signed: Reviewed:
Complete?: True False
Entered in Computer:

Notes:

FIGURE 5.23A Health Access Logsheet KEY

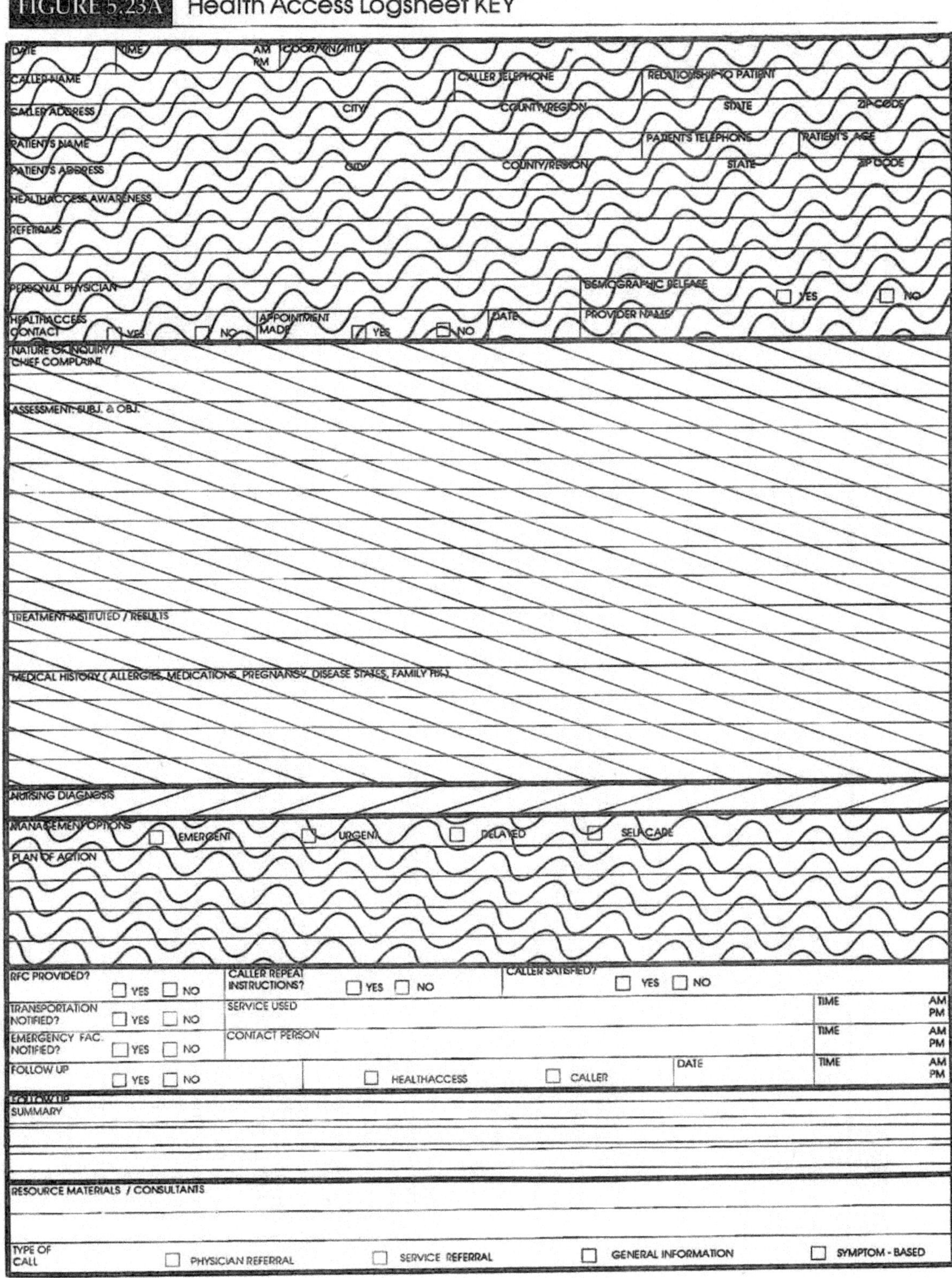

DATE | TIME | AM PM | COORD/RN/TITLE

CALLER NAME | CALLER TELEPHONE | RELATIONSHIP TO PATIENT

CALLER ADDRESS | CITY | COUNTY/REGION | STATE | ZIP CODE

PATIENT'S NAME | PATIENT'S TELEPHONE | PATIENT'S AGE

PATIENT'S ADDRESS | CITY | COUNTY/REGION | STATE | ZIP CODE

HEALTHACCESS AWARENESS

REFERRALS

PERSONAL PHYSICIAN | DEMOGRAPHIC RELEASE ☐ YES ☐ NO

HEALTHACCESS CONTACT ☐ YES ☐ NO | APPOINTMENT MADE ☑ YES ☐ NO | DATE | PROVIDER NAME

NATURE OF INQUIRY/ CHIEF COMPLAINT

ASSESSMENT: SUBJ. & OBJ.

TREATMENT INSTITUTED / RESULTS

MEDICAL HISTORY (ALLERGIES, MEDICATIONS, PREGNANCY, DISEASE STATES, FAMILY HX)

NURSING DIAGNOSIS

MANAGEMENT OPTIONS ☐ EMERGENT ☐ URGENT ☐ DELAYED ☑ SELF-CARE

PLAN OF ACTION

RFC PROVIDED? ☐ YES ☐ NO | CALLER REPEAT INSTRUCTIONS? ☐ YES ☐ NO | CALLER SATISFIED? ☐ YES ☐ NO

TRANSPORTATION NOTIFIED? ☐ YES ☐ NO | SERVICE USED | TIME AM PM

EMERGENCY FAC. NOTIFIED? ☐ YES ☐ NO | CONTACT PERSON | TIME AM PM

FOLLOW UP ☐ YES ☐ NO | ☐ HEALTHACCESS ☐ CALLER | DATE | TIME AM PM

FOLLOW UP SUMMARY

RESOURCE MATERIALS / CONSULTANTS

TYPE OF CALL ☐ PHYSICIAN REFERRAL ☐ SERVICE REFERRAL ☐ GENERAL INFORMATION ☐ SYMPTOM - BASED

FIGURE 5.24A Head Injury Protocol KEY

HEAD INJURY

Traumatic injury to the head resulting in a fall, high speed accident (car), great force (baseball) or possible child abuse

ASSESSMENT:

- Determine AVPU Scale: A-Alert, V-Responds to verbal stimuli, P-Responds to painful stimuli, U-unresponsive.
- Describe in detail the events of the accident:
  - time
  - area injured (laceration, bleeding, swelling, abrasions)
  - distance of fall or struck with what object
  - any loss of consciousness?
- Any of the following symptoms: headache, nausea, vomiting, blurred or double vision, unequal pupils (black circle in center of eyes), perfuse bleeding, confusion, unsteady gait, seizure activity, neck pain, difficulty moving arms or legs, swelling of head, change in speech or usual behavior, loss of appetite
  - Describe skin color and temperature: pin, pale, warm, cool, clammy?
- Any drainage from the ears, mouth or nose? color? amount?
- Signs and symptoms of respiratory distress? (Shortness of breath, Cyanosis, Rapid, Labored breathing? Restlessness?)
- Any difficulty arousing from sleep?
- Prior medical history of neurological deficits, surgery, seizures?
- Present list of medications taken today
- Treatment instituted? Effectiveness?

EMERGENT:

*IF PARALYZED, DO NOT MOVE PATIENT WITHOUT MEDICAL ASSISTANCE

- Head injury with subsequent loss of consciousness (immediate or delayed).
- Head injury with open laceration, active bleeding requiring sutures.
- Head injury associated with nausea, vomiting, and/or seizure.
- Head injury with severe neuro deficits (respiratory distress, decreased level of consciousness, change in pupils, pale skin color, change in gait, speech, affect).
- Drainage from ear, nose or mouth (not related to cold).
- Any muscle weakness, twitching, paralysis.
- Head injury with complaint of stiff-sore neck.
- Change in status, decreased level of consciousness, difficult to arouse, loss of nerve function as described above.

URGENT:

- Head trauma with:
  - minor swelling, controlled bleeding from laceration
  - minor swelling, controlled bleeding from laceration
  - headache unrelieved with home management
  - post trauma fever greater than 100 degrees

DELAYED:

Not applicable

SELF-CARE:

A head injury which causes confusion, loss of memory or a brief period of unconsciousness is called a concussion. Some person with concussions will also vomit one or more times. Children may sometimes vomit once even though they do not have a concussion. Nearly all persons with concussions will recover within one to three days. Occasionally, however, complications develop. Follow these instructions carefully and call your doctor promptly if you are concerned for any reason.

WHAT TO DO:

1. A responsible person should watch a person who has any sign of concussion carefully for signs of complications.
2. Have the person rest. He should be allowed to sleep if he wants to, but awakened every 1–2 hours for the first 24 hours to be checked. Ask person to identify familiar family members or objects.
3. Have the person drink only liquids if he is feeling nauseated.
4. Take Tylenol/Panadol, as directed by manufacturer, as needed for pain. Do not use any stronger pain medicine.

REASONS FOR CONCERN:

- Increasing sleepiness or inability to awaken
- Bleeding from ears, mouth or nose
- Close discharge from the nose (not associated with crying or a cold) or ear
- Blurred or double vision
- Garbled speech or any other difficulty that occurs in talking
- Unusual stumbling or inability to use arms or legs
- Unusual behavior, personality change or confusion, irritability, combative
- Muscle weakness in arms or legs
- Convulsions or seizures
- Unequal pupil size not present prior to injury
- Vomiting more than twice, loss of appetite
- Severe persistent or worsening headache unrelieved with home management
- Persistent fever over 100 degrees orally (101 degrees rectally)
- Any other symptoms that might seem unusual to you

NOTE: The single most important sign that a complication of head injury is developing is inability to arouse the person and get him to respond appropriately to questions or instructions.

CROSS-REFERENCE:

Balance Problems, Coma, Confusion, Convulsions, Dizziness, Headache, Nausea and Vomiting

FIGURE 5.25A Abdominal Pain Protocol KEY

SUBJECT Surgery Advice Protocols	NUMBER: 2	PAGE 1 OF
TITLE: Abdominal Pain	EFFECTIVE DATE: 10/75	
PERSONNEL APPLICABLE TO:	REVISION DATE: 8/80, 4/81, 6/90	

ABDOMINAL PAIN

1. Inquire from patient:
   a. Where is it?
   b. How long have you had it?
   c. Have you had recent surgery? If so, what and where and when?
   d. How severe is it?
   e. Have you vomited? If so, what?
   f. Do you have fever?
   g. Do you have headache or muscle aches?
   h. Do you have frequent or painful urination?
   i. Do you have diarrhea, bloody or black stools?
   j. Do you have gall stones, ulcers or chronic intestinal disease?
   k. Do you have yellow eyes or skin?
   l. For women: When was your last period? Do you have any vaginal bleeding or discharge?
2. If patient has had:
   a. Surgery recently (within one month)
   b. Is being followed for a specific problem by a surgeon, refer message to patient's surgeon, surgeon on-call, or clinic surgeon.
3. If patient complains of:
   a. Severe pain of recent onset.
   b. Vomiting of blood or coffee ground emesis.
   c. Bloody or tarry stools.
   d. High fever (over 101).
   e. Yellow eyes or skin or dark urine.
   f. Localized abdominal tenderness.
   g. Heavy vaginal bleeding.

DIRECT PATIENT TO THE EMERGENCY DEPARTMENT.

4. If patient complains of:
   a. Pelvic pain as in menstrual cramps, abnormal bleeding (less than heavy) vaginal discharge.

TRANSFER TO GYNECOLOGY ADVICE NURSE

5. All others transfer to Medical Advice Nurse.

FIGURE 5.26A Protocol Checklist KEY

PROTOCOL TITLE: FEVER IN CHILDREN

1. FORMAT	YES	NO
Effective, consistent hierarchy of acuity?	X	
Overlapping time frames?	X	

Comments **Time and place of treatment are both present**

2. DATA COLLECTION METHOD	YES	NO
Comprehensive?	X	
Consistent?	X	

Comments **Uses *specific* questions drawn from SCHOLAR/PAMPER/ADL method**

3. TEACHING/ADVICE SECTIONS	YES	NO
Advocacy/consumer information?	Not applicable	
Self-help and support groups?	X	
Informationally sound?	X	
Follow-up advice?	X #4 under routine disposition section	
Includes time frames for self-evaluation		X

Comments **Revise to include time frame of 2 hours in #2 under routine disposition section**

4. USER FRIENDLY	YES	NO
Lay language?	X	
Cookbook approach?		X
Lay language/symptom based titles?	X	
Well presented graphically?		X
Easily accessed?		X
Quick cross-reference system?		X

Comments **Cookbook approach: Streamline entire protocol for a more cookbook approach. Use bullets and short sentences. Graphics: Graphic presentation needs work—place hierarchy of acuity vertically instead of horizontally for best use of space. Access: Protocol size requires binder—a change in format will allow for placement in Kardex.™ Cross-reference: Too long. Reduce to six generic options—ear problem, abdominal pain, URI symptoms, rash, urinary symptoms, gastrointestinal symptoms.**

5. ENHANCEMENTS	YES	NO
Reference section?		X
Follow-up mechanism?		X
Computer adaptable?	X	

Comments **Reference section: A few current references relating to treatment for fever would add credibility and reliability. Follow-up mechanism: Add #5 "automatic follow-up call" under Routine Disposition advice. Computer adaptable: After rewriting sections to a more cookbook approach and revising format, this protocol could be easily adapted to a computer format.**

FIGURE 5.27A Documentation Form Checklist KEY

	YES	NO
1. INTEGRATED WITH PROTOCOL	x	
Comment: Incorporates SCHOLAR/PAMPER/ADL data collection methods.		
2. GENERIC	x	
Comment: Used for pediatrics, geriatrics, and ob/gyn		
3. ADEQUATE SIZE	x	
4. DUPLICATE/TRIPLICATE	x	
5. HEADING	x	
Comment: Telephone Triage Data Form is descriptive but not too long.		
6. ABBREVIATIONS	x	
7. LOGICAL SEQUENCE	x	
a. Client demographic information	x	
b. Data collection	x	
c. Working diagnosis/impression	x	
d. Advice/disposition (treat, teach, appt)	x	
e. Verbal contract/disclaimer	x	
f. Follow-up	x	
8. CHECKBOXES/SLOTS	x	
Age	x	
Pregnancy status	x	
Medication	x	
Allergies	x	
Risk management safeguards:		
Protocol number or name	x	
Disclaimer	x	
Contracts	x	
Protocol override/deviations	x	
Pertinent negatives?	x	
Working diagnosis/impression	x	
9. SUFFICIENT SPACE	x	
10. DATE OF LAST REVISION		x
Comment: Date of last revision needs to be added.		

EXERCISE 3: PROTOCOL AND FORM DESIGN

No answer key provided.

EXERCISE 4: FORM DESIGN

No answer key provided.

CHAPTER 6
High-Risk Populations

THE PEDIATRIC CALL

Children, the elderly, and women of reproductive age are heavy utilizers of telephone triage services. Pediatric calls, however, comprise the largest volume of calls (Curtis, et al, 1983). This finding should not be surprising because most new parents need frequent telephone support, especially in the early days and months. In one study, pediatricians spent about 12% of their office time and 25% of their total practice time in telephone consultation (Curtis & Talbot, 1981).

Like calls from other high-risk clients, pediatric calls fall into one of three categories: administrative, medical advice, or counseling. Administrative calls include requests for medication refills, appointments, lab results, routine forms to be filled out, immunization questions, and appointments for camp and school physicals. Advice calls revolve around care and nutrition of the newborn and children, sleeping, crying, elimination and routine illnesses such as upper respiratory infections, diarrhea, cough, fever, and minor injuries. Counseling calls usually involve behavioral problems, school fears, developmental issues, and underlying family stress. Most predictable concerns can be remedied through patient education and reassurance.

Most experts agree that telephone support enhances the adaptation to motherhood and alleviates new parents' anxiety (Gosha, 1986; Graef, et al, 1988). One study found that such factors as age, perceptions of the birthing experience, support systems, maternal and infant temperaments, maternal and child illness, and self-concept can affect adaptation to motherhood (Curry, 1983). The author found that lack of experience was a major factor in difficult adjustment to motherhood, concluding that classes, group experience, and pairing with experienced mothers would help remedy this educational and experiential gap. The author concluded that nursing interventions such as telephone support, home visits, and referral to infant play groups were beneficial.

Another study (Sumner & Fritsch, 1977) focused on the difficulties of adjustment in the first six postnatal weeks. They observed that the enormous tasks of "identifying with the infant, determining the relationship and altering lifestyle patterns" (p. 27) take place at a time when mothers are physically fatigued and emotionally dependent. They determined the type of concerns by monitoring calls and developed a specialized form to facilitate data collection. The results showed that 62% of the calls were made by primiparas and 38% by multiparas. The average length of the calls was about 6 minutes. Questions revolved around feeding and gastrointestinal, skin, sleeping, and crying problems. Interestingly, they found that *mothers of males had twice as many breastfeeding questions as mothers of females.* Call volume was highest in the third week of life when there is often the least support available. It was concluded that early calling behavior was more for reassurance and validation than for information. The authors suggest that "possibly, one of the biggest helps to a new mother is other mothers with whom she can compare her baby's behavior and validate her own mothering skills."

In their 1987 study of pediatric "warmlines," Samuels and Balter found that 41 programs were operating across the country, and that these programs filled a void. Nearly 50% of the calls concerned children under 3 years of age and 5% were about children over 13 years of age. Calls concerning boys were more numerous than those about girls. The major concerns in order of frequency were negative behaviors, sleeping, combination of problems, separation anxiety, toilet training, academic concerns, referral, social problems, and feeding problems. From these studies it could safely be said that the newer the mother and the younger the child, the greater the need for support, much of which can be supplied by telephone.

In addition to warmlines, the telephone can be used in other specialized ways for pediatric populations. An Auckland study (Hornby & Murray, 1987) described the implementation of a telephone support service for families of handicapped children. Parents of handicapped children were trained as volunteers to provide telephone support. In another study, a visual telephone was used as a self-help tool for a pediatric rehabilitation inpatient (Handler, 1989). In this study, a four-year-old patient with spinal cord injury required intensive prolonged rehabilitation far from his home. Through the use of a telephone equipped with a small screen, the patient was able to communicate with his mother, who transmitted pictures of the boy's favorite toys, room, and gifts, while he transmitted his drawings. His mother was also able to see him when he began standing. Researchers concluded that the use of the visual telephone was a key factor in the improvement of his maladaptive behaviors and in his early discharge.

For the pediatric population and both new and experienced parents, the telephone is a vital lifeline to support, information, reassurance, and advice. The growth of warmlines indicates an unmet need for information, reassurance, and support. The implications are that telephone triage nurses can either develop the counseling aspect or expand and develop their ability to refer to such agencies. Interfacing with these agencies is a tangible way to develop all telephone triage services. For example, warmline counselors could share their expertise with nurses through an inservice. By knowing what services each other offers, nurse and counselor can better cross-refer to each other. The visual telephone demonstrates a new use of communications technology, which could concievably be used in the home care setting as well. In certain instances, telephone triage could include visual data collection.

CALL PATTERNS

Experts have found that, to a certain extent, call content and volume are predictable. Brown (1980) has identified six peak call periods: early morning, late afternoon, early evening (dinnertime), late evening (bedtime), Friday, and weekends. He found that the time of the call may provide a clue to the degree and type of problem. For example, parents who have been up all night often call in the early morning and are anxious to have their child seen. Calls concerning school age children returning from school or sent home by the school nurse occur late in the afternoon. Early evening or dinnertime is the "uproar time" when everyone in the family tends to be irritable, and accidental injuries and ingestions are common. Children are bored, tired, and hungry; parents are preoccupied with dinner and fatigued from the stress of work and commuting.

Late evening calls (10 P.M. to 11:30 P.M.) are often from parents who have monitored an illness which has failed to improve as the evening progressed. They want reassurance that they "have done everything possible" before they settle down for the night. Although such "hand-holding" calls seem like a nuisance, they actually reduce middle-of-the-night phone calls and emergency department visits.

Interestingly, even the weather can influence call volume. Brown (1980) notes that in warm weather parents take children out, even with low grade illness, thus decreasing call volume. Expect a flurry of Sunday evening calls for the purpose of deciding if children are well enough to attend school the next day. Friday afternoon calls come from parents who have monitored a routine illness all week and want their child "cleared for takeoff," or given a clean bill of health before traveling to see grandparents.

Nurses in practice report increased volume and acuity of calls during flu season. There are also call flurries triggered by media reports of meningitis, Lyme disease, or reactions to vaccine. Call volume is an indicator of need, even if it is simply for information. Develop informational protocols to address knowledge deficits in an appropriate and responsible way.

Brown (1980) recommends establishing a waiting period prior to examination, stating that "the likelihood of detecting an illness that is diagnosable and treatable at the time of examination is greater when symptoms have been present for 24 hours, rather than when they first appear." (p. 5) Although waiting periods may screen out illnesses of short duration and help parents bolster their confidence, some experts consider this approach to be outside the domain of nursing.

Another major factor in telephone triage utilization is whether the family has one or two parents. Moreno (1989) found a trend toward higher utilization of telephone advice by single parent families. Although single-parent families were more likely to feel they needed appointments than two-parent families, they often failed to come in.

GENERAL RULES

In general, even healthy children have several risk factors: young age, impaired veracity, and questionable emotional status. For this reason, appointments are usually given freely to children. Because the child is highly valued in society, it seems to be a universal practice to always err on the side of caution with this population; whereas with women and the elderly, this is not usually the case.

Global Assessment with the SAVED Format

Severity and Age. Common wisdom states that infants "get sicker quicker" due to underdeveloped immune systems; those under 6 months or premature are at greater risk. With all infants under six months, determine if the the birth was premature. If the infant was premature, obtain the birth weight, gestational age at birth or number of weeks premature. With all young infants, remember to verify and document the age in days or weeks as appropriate. This is important baseline information that influences assessment of symptom severity as well as medication dosages. Young age and impaired communications place all children under eight at risk for two out of five risk factors: age, veracity, and emotional status. Because children lack verbal skills to be adequate historians, it is difficult to ascertain the severity of symptoms. Most children are unable to quantify or qualify pain. However, by gathering specific, concrete, measurable data, (numbers of wet diapers, ADL, etc.) the nurse can overcome this obstacle.

Veracity. Most calls regarding children are second- or third-party calls. For example, talking to a working parent who has only communicated with the day-care worker requires extra caution. In all cases regarding children 8 years old and over, it may be helpful to talk with both child and caretaker.

Emotional Status. Explore the child's underlying emotional style as well as the reaction to the current illness. Exercise caution with a child who is normally quiet and easygoing who suddenly becomes irritable and fussy.

Ask yourself: "Must this problem be seen before 10 P.M. tonight or can it wait until morning?" A rule of thumb recommended by Schmitt (1980), is that "night crises" can be avoided by giving day appointments when possible. Directing new parents to call before everyone retires for the evening is a good general guideline.

Frequent calls may be an indicator of anxiety as well as urgency. With children, two or more calls in an 8-hour period require automatic appointments. This requirement also applies to any parent who lacks confidence or seems uncomfortable about managing the problem at home. The diagnosis "worried parent" (Schmitt, 1980) is defensible. It is expected that inexperienced, insecure parents or parents under stress will be anxious in reaction to their child's illness. The nurse can later bolster confidence by instructing parents how to differentiate between emergencies and urgencies, either by phone or in person.

Debilitation. Examples of chronic illness in children are birth defects, diabetes, asthma, HIV, and crack exposure. Less obvious, but also relevant are *recurrent illnesses*—for example, any recurrent infection, frequent ear infections, or croup. Calls regarding children with recurrent or chronic illness are more time-consuming and require cautious assessment, extensive education, and emotional support.

Persistent failure to progress or respond to the prescribed treatment must be evaluated. An example might be the child on antibiotics for an ear infection who still seems sick after 48 hours. In general, treat all children (especially under 6 months) with caution. Their symptoms may be vague but can change rapidly.

Primary Data

It is always difficult to collect data about children. For a preverbal child who appears to be in pain, it may be impossible to ask routine questions (SCHOLAR). Likewise, with young children, pregnancy, allergies, medication, recent medical history may not apply (PAMPER). However, it is possible to describe the effects of the pain on the child's normal daily routine. Activities of daily living are a valid way to measure the effects of illness and may be the first choice used to elicit information about preverbal children.

Activities of Daily Living. For children especially, activities of daily living are among the best barometers of health. Assess the following habits and behavior and compare them to the child's norm: How is the child eating, drinking, sleeping, and playing? What is the child's color and general appearance? What is the output (bowel and bladder) and is it normal? Avoid ambiguous terms such as "lethargic" and "listless." A description such as "sleeping all day, disinterested in television, and refusing food and fluids" is more concrete. Behavioral changes—extremes of fussiness, irritability, or sleepiness—are good indicators. A child who is very ill may not care about TV, may have no interest in normally entertaining activities, and may even refuse to get up to go to the bathroom.

> *A mother called regarding her child's fever. She estimated it to be about 550 degrees. When asked how she took the temperature, the mother replied that she turned the oven on, held the child near it and took a reading when the temperature of the stove approximated the baby's.*

Teach all new parents how to take a temperature properly and then instruct them to do it before calling. If done accurately, the temperature is the most basic and easily quantified information about the child's condition. It is so fundamental that on the basis of fever alone many pediatricians require that all infants under 6 months receive automatic appointments. When documenting temperatures, include the route by which it was taken, the time of onset, and as appropriate, the duration in time frames of 8, 16, or 24 hours. Other quantifiable symptoms include numbers of wet diapers, diarrhea stools, vomiting episodes, amounts of fluids ingested, presence or absence of tears, marked behavior changes, constant crying, and marked changes in activities of daily living. Teach parents what constitutes acute dehydration, respiratory distress, and unusual sleepiness.

Many parents initiate some form of home treatment (activities, medications, or foods) prior to calling. Ask what has been tried and whether it relieved or exacerbated symptoms. Collecting this data reveals three kinds of information about the parent: level of medical expertise, ability to manage symptoms and level of parenting sophistication.

Secondary Data

> *A mother called regarding her 16-year-old daughter, who had missed a period. The nurse asked if there was possibility of pregnancy. The mother replied, "Oh no, she's always in by 9:30."*
>
> *A 17-year-old primipara called with questions about the mucus plug. The nurse gave her reassurance and teaching. At the close of the conversation the teenager thanked her, adding happily "Great, now I can go trick-or-treating tonight!"*

Pregnancy. As adolescent sexual activity increases, so do the issues of adolescent pregnancy, birth control, and sexually transmitted diseases. Much depends upon client population and sexual precocity. Nurses must determine if clients are sexually active, their birth control method, and possible sexually transmitted disease (STD) exposure.

Remedy knowledge deficits with current, complete information on STD and HIV risks. Cultivate the ability to confront inconsistencies in clients' knowledge and behavior. Encourage responsibility for oneself and "ownership" of the problem and solution. Counseling newly sexually active teenagers is time-consuming. Therefore, limit these calls to 15 minutes and then offer referrals to hot lines, classes, support groups, and physicians as appropriate.

It is dangerous to make any assumptions about sexual activity before asking teenaged clients directly. Some postulate a rule of thumb that "all women of reproductive age are pregnant unless proven otherwise." Carefully explore unexplained abdominal pain or vague symptoms of possible ectopic pregnancy. Preserve client confidentiality for sexually active teenagers by having them call in for test results and consultations, rather than contacting them at home.

Allergies. Always ask parents what they mean by "allergies" before labeling symptoms as such. "Allergies" may turn out to be sensitivities. Allergies are rare in small infants. Food and environmental allergies appear at about 1 year. Common causes of allergies in toddlers are foods, medications, soaps, lotions, detergents, fabric softeners, and scented diapers.

Medications. With infants, always elicit the weight, and instruct parents to relay this information when seeking telephone advice. Determine all the prescription and OTC medications the child has taken recently. If the child is breast-feeding, ask if the mother is taking any medications, recreational drugs, or alcohol. Ask whether the child's medication seems to be effective, determine if the dosage is correct, and whether there have been any side effects. Finally, ask about possible accidental ingestion of medications and drug or alcohol abuse.

It may be difficult to verify the accuracy of the child's weight. Gauge parent reliability by the quality of data and self-care measures attempted. Ask the parent how recently the child was weighed and where. Compare the weight to standard growth charts—if there is wide variation between them, it is possible that the weight is inaccurate and cannot be relied upon.

Emotional Status.

> *A mother called saying that her child had swallowed a pacifier. The child had gone to sleep with it in its mouth. When he awakened it was gone. (It was later found).*

Obviously, this parent overreacted, and the "worried parent" diagnosis applies. While some seem overanxious, however, others tend to react with denial, as illustrated by the following example:

A mother called about her two-year-old. He had just had a fourth seizure. The temperature was 105. The child had no previous history of seizures. She wondered if these symptoms were cause for concern. She failed to come in or contact her physician later as advised.

Recent Injury, Infection, Ingestion. When there is no apparent explanation for a child's symptoms or behavior, explore the possibility of an unwitnessed accident. Explore any recent illness or exposure to infection, recent injuries, possible child abuse, or unwitnessed ingestions.

A nurse received an early morning call from a mother about her 14-year-old daughter who had been vomiting hourly since midnight the night before. After she arrived for an appointment, it was learned that the teenager had taken an overdose of Tylenol following an argument with the mother about not being allowed to go to a school dance. OUTCOME: No major liver damage.

A mother called from a welfare hotel regarding her 13-year-old son, apparently dead from an overdose.

With adolescents, always be alert to the potential for suicidal gestures, particularly ingestions. Depression in adolescents can trigger suicidal ideation or actual attempts. Adolescents tend to be impulsive and have extreme mood swings. Some experts feel that any severely depressed adolescent, *even without suicidal ideation,* is at risk for suicide (R. Allen, personal communication, February, 1992). In California, for example, suicide is the second highest cause of death for young people between the ages of 15 and 35 (R. Allen, personal communication, February, 1992). (See Chapter 7 for suicide intervention techniques.)

INTERVIEW TECHNIQUES

"Hand-holding" or reassurance calls decrease as parents gain experience. Parents can be taught assessment and observation skills. They can be encouraged to use reference books prior to calling. Nevertheless, expect hidden agendas when dealing with pediatric clients. Ask "Do you have any further questions or worries?" Parents may overreact to media scares or worry about complications or side effects of medicines. Many simply fear appearing ignorant.

Certain questions and statements reinforce continuity and credibility. Brown (1980) recommends using similar wording each time one gives advice. Appropriate questions and comments are:

What treatments (activities, foods, approaches) have you tried so far?

Is there anything else that is bothering you?

Repeat back my instructions.

What do you mean by that?

Is this the sickest you've ever seen your child?

Do you feel comfortable managing this problem at home?

I'm only a phone call away. Please call back if you have further questions.

Self-Assessment Techniques

Some evaluation can be performed by phone using the parents as observers. To facilitate observation of respirations, instruct parents to remove the child's shirt before observing, and to direct the child to count from 1 to 10 without taking a breath. Inability to do this is a sign of respiratory distress.

Evaluate the level of consciousness by directing parents to rouse the child, turn lights on, take them outside, and offer them food or drink. A quiet but alert child is probably not seriously ill. Lack of tears or lack of drooling may be an indicator of dehydration. In toddlers, favoring of arm or leg suggests limb injury.

Some symptoms can be auscultated by parents. With training using a technique known as orophonics (Kravitz et al, 1963), respirations can be auscultated for quality and quantity.

Follow-Up Calls

As mentioned before, follow-up calls provide opportunities to receive feedback, clarify instructions, enhance risk management, and demonstrate concern. They also help to insure client compliance. Parents are very appreciative of this gesture. Some experts recommend automatic follow-up calls for febrile seizures, sickle-cell crises, fevers of unknown origin, children at risk for dehydration, croup, and *parents whose compliance is doubtful* (Jones, Clark, Bradford, & Dougherty, 1987).

Ingestion Calls

Ingestion calls are every pediatric nurse's nightmare. Contrary to popular belief, however, these incidents are usually not life threatening. For example, according to one expert, less than 1% of all poisonings result in death, 45% of the victims suffer no ill effects, and 90% of toxin exposures are accidental rather than intentional (San Francisco Poison Control, 1989).

One interesting study focused on time of day, change in physical location of the substance, and child characteristics as factors in poisoning injuries (Garrettson, Bush, Gates, & French, 1990). Researchers found that in 51% of the incidents, the substance had recently been moved from the usual place of storage, and 62 out of 85 children studied were between one and three years old. More than 2/3 of all poisonings occurred between 4 and 6 P.M. These results indicate a need for extra vigilance regarding pediatric calls at the dinner hour.

An area of controversy is the percentage of poison exposures that can be safely managed at home, in the workplace or at school with appropriate follow up. One expert, Kathy Keller, relates that *every substance is a potential toxin. It is the dose which makes it so.* (K. Keller, personal communication, March, 1988) Ingestions of a nontoxic amount of a nontoxic substance or a nontoxic amount of a toxic substances are not serious. She also relates that 65% of victims are under 6 years old and in most cases, poisoning histories tend to be wrong. Use the following guidelines to assess these calls (San Francisco Poison Control, 1989):

1. Obtain address, phone number, age, and substance ingested. When referring to poison control, place a follow-up call within a few minutes.
2. Obtain the victim's weight to assess the toxicity and prognosis.
3. Instruct the parent to bring the container to the phone and spell the name of the substance. In a panic, people often misspell or misread names of drugs. Instructing the caller to perform certain actions (counting numbers of pills left, spelling out the name) dispels panic. In addition to providing vital information, this action helps callers to focus, feel in control, and feel less guilt.
4. Determine the route of ingestion (oral, inhalation, topical, intravenous, smoking, or enema).
5. Determine the time of exposure.
6. Obtain signs and symptoms.
7. Direct the caller in first aid measures.
8. Some drugs are toxic if more than 48 hours' dosage is taken at once. Check with local poison control for this list.

Diligently check compliance to assure that parents have followed directions. They may say that they have administered the ipecac and fluids when in fact they gave too little to be effective. Be specific with instructions. For example, for an eye wash, have the parent "mummy" the child in a large bath or beach towel, lay the child over the kitchen sink, and gently drip a steady stream of tepid tap water directly into the eye for *5–10 minutes by the clock.* Encourage them if they lack confidence and assure them that their child's resistant behavior is "expected and normal" but that they must be persistent or the child may suffer severe complications.

Follow-up teaching for ingestion calls includes instructions on how to use poison control centers and to keep a bottle of syrup of ipecac for every child under 5 years old, to be used as directed by a physician or poison control center.

Keep an updated list of commonly ingested substances by the triage phone for quick reference. Poison control is the best resource in questionable cases and staff often know which substances are toxic and which are not, eliminating unnecessary treatment. They are also able to identify capsules and tablets quickly by entering the numbers and letters into the computer.

Parental Stress Calls

Telephone hot lines offer immediate, accessible, anonymous "talk therapy" for parents under stress. In any case where abuse is suspected, clients should be seen as soon as possible. Child abuse is defined as "bruises, burns, cuts, poisoning, sexual abuse, neglect, and homicidal threats inflicted by adults" (Crime Prevention Center, 1988). If the family fails to come in within 1 hour, refer the call to the police.

Office Policies

Clinics and offices each have their own way of doing things and patient education includes instructions on how to "navigate the system," whether that system is a small office, a clinic, or a large HMO. For example, most systems discourage nonurgent or administrative calls after 5 P.M. Some pediatricians prefer to see urgent situations in the office after hours rather than having parents go directly to the emergency department. In general, counseling calls should be limited to 5 minutes or less. Anything beyond that time limit requires an appointment. (See Appendices O and P for Pediatric Antipyretic Dosage Chart and Office Policy Sheet.)

THE GERIATRIC CLIENT

Old Age—A Period of Loss

Much has been written about the plight of the elderly and old age as a period of loss. This section is based heavily on two books. *Suicide and the Elderly* by Susan Osgood (1985) and *You and Your Aging Parent* (1976) by Silverstone and Hyman. Both books paint a poignant portrait of the process of aging and loss.

Loss of Social Stimulation.

> *An elderly lady called about the fact that her front door was impassable due to ice and snow. She was upset that personnel from the hospital would not come to help. The police were notified and responded.*
>
> *One ED nurse related the story of Wanda, who called the emergency department every day between 7:15 A.M. and 7:30 A.M. She lived alone and wanted to "see if everything was okay." After 4 months the nurses invited her for a visit and Wanda came and had coffee.*

For the elderly, life and the world begin to shrink. The social losses can be devastating. The greatest social losses are brought on by severe physical impairment or financial hardships. Work, communication, and socialization patterns become restricted. Spouses become widows and widowers. Personality, quality of marriage, relationship with children and to the community, and attitude toward aging and dying determine how each individual adjusts to these changes. Nurses report that some calls from frail elderly are "attention seeking." They may manufacture symptoms and even request an ambulance unnecessarily (Silverstone & Hyman, 1976).

Loss of Key Roles. Most people enjoy several different roles in their lifetimes: parent, spouse, homemaker, worker. After retirement, the worker role is lost. When spouses die, survivors are deprived of the role of partner and spouse. Many elderly sell their homes and move into retirement communities, where their homeowner role becomes diminished. Some adjust well to shedding these responsibilities and feel relief. Others maintain some roles through part-time work or maintaining an active sexual and social life. If any role relinquished is vital to the self-image of the individual, that person feels a loss of self-esteem and well-being.

Many elderly, including those at the middle income level, fear poverty in old age. Retirement drastically reduces income, and inflation erodes Social Security benefits. Many are forced to live on their life savings.

Loss of Physical Health. Aging is an inevitable, irreversible, and very individual process. Sensory losses affect overall pleasure in daily life. For example, the lens of the eye loses elasticity, hearing becomes impaired, the sense of taste is blunted. The elderly even experience pain as less acute than younger people, often injuring themselves without being aware of it. They may have "walking pneumonia" or a "silent myocardial infarct" because the nervous system failed to send the proper signals.

The elderly are at higher risk for accidents. A variety of factors can affect memory, comprehension, and reasoning ability. Osteoporosis makes the elderly, especially women, more susceptible to fracture. Slowed reaction time and impaired hearing and vision lead to higher accident and injury rates for the elderly.

The excretion ability of the kidneys diminishes, the speed with which nerve impulses are conducted slows, the heat output decreases. Muscle tissue decreases, resulting in loss of strength. Lung capacity is reduced. All functions of digestion are less efficient, leading to constipation. Simple, ordinary, daily activities of dressing and walking become more difficult. Finally, the immune system wears out, and the body's ability to fight off infection is diminished. Viral infections can be devastating and recuperation from a serious illness is more precarious (Silverstone & Hyman, 1976).

Global Assessment

The frail elderly have nearly every high risk factor: advanced age, unreliable veracity, emotional extremes, and probable debilitation. They may be poor historians due to overmedication, or faulty judgment, comprehension, and memory. Chronic disease and weakened immune systems make them more vulnerable to communicable disease. Thus the nurse may find that the very old, like the very young, often need automatic appointments.

Primary and Secondary Data

Many elderly are careful observers of their own symptoms. For example, a number frequently monitor their own blood pressure using a home monitoring device. If the call is regarding their blood pressure, document the source of the measurement.

Age and gender gaps, social taboos, and upbringing may make elderly clients reluctant to discuss openly intimate details of medical problems that involve sexual activity or genitourinary symptoms, requiring considerable finesse and utmost tact. Many elderly have active sex lives, resulting in the possibility of sexually transmitted disease.

Although pregnancy/breastfeeding status is not an issue with the elderly, all other categories of concern must be explored with special emphasis on medications, previous medical history, emotional status, and recent injury, illness, or infection. Many elderly have several chronic diseases as well as medications to treat them. This information helps to establish acuity, define confusing symptoms, and identify drug reactions or overmedication. As with the very young, injury and exposure to infection must always be explored fully. Because they are at the highest risk for suicide, intentional overdoses must always be considered.

Emotional stress. Along with the increased social isolation, financial insecurity, and physical disability come a variety of psychological problems. Alcoholism, depression, organic brain syndrome, paranoid reactions, and severe neurotic and even psychotic episodes are not uncommon (Silverstone & Hyman, 1976). The incidence of these problems is on the rise among those over 65.

The process of mourning is a normal reaction to any loss and allows new energies and interests in life to emerge. Whether the elderly person has recently lost a spouse, friend, or the ability to drive, it is normal to work through the grief. Anxiety, anger, and fear are normal reactions to failing eyesight or a recent heart attack.

Extreme reactions to loss include severe depression, hypochondriasis, psychotic reactions, and chronic organic brain syndromes. Hypochondriasis, or abnormal concern about one's health, can be a positive sign *in small doses* (Silverstone & Hyman, 1976). Carried to extremes, it can be an all-consuming activity. Some theorize that the elderly focus their attention inward as they lose interest in the world around them.

The frail elderly often need support to negotiate the health care system, making consumer information and patients' rights an important teaching component.

Activities of Daily Living. With the elderly, many symptoms are vague, clouded by previous medical problems, or the caller is a poor historian. Nurses who work with the elderly state that activities of daily living often give the most accurate baseline picture of the elderly caller.

Interview Techniques

Communicating with an elderly person who is hearing impaired, confused, forgetful, agitated, or anxious may be time-consuming. Ideally, all callers, and especially the elderly, should write down instructions. If agitation or confusion limits a caller's ability to follow instructions, give an automatic appointment rather than risk miscommunicating by phone. If the primary population of a system is made up of people over 55, it may be necessary to customize the program to this population's needs, lengthening talk time and developing support services.

Intervention. Many elderly clients neither drive nor have anyone to transport them. Develop a list of organizations, cab services, ambucabs, and non-paramedic ambulances. Implement special precautions for elderly recuperating at home alone, including routine follow-up calls and visits.

Elderly clients with nonacute symptoms can be monitored by phone if they demonstrate reliability in following home treatment measures. Conditions which may preclude home monitoring are confusion, emotional distress, inability to read a thermometer, inability to hear well, severe memory loss, or physical impairment.

Support Systems and Warmlines

As with the pediatric population, warmlines and telephone alarm systems for the elderly have proliferated in part due to technological advances. Warmlines play an important role in reassurance and support for frail elderly who are housebound. There are several reasons why nurses working in telephone triage should be aware of telemetry and warmlines. Referral is a large part of telephone triage and an elderly client's need for reassurance might be better answered by such a service rather than the telephone triage nurse. Also, warmlines counselors may have expertise in telephone communications with the elderly to share with nurses by way of an inservice. Finally, in the interest of developing a team approach, the interface between nurse, warmlines, and alarm systems should be encouraged and developed. Although telemetry and alarm systems are not part of the nurse's responsibility, in the future it may very well be routine activity.

Suicide in the Elderly. Statistically, the elderly are more prone to complete the suicide act (Osgood, 1985). White, retired widowers have a suicide rate four times the national average. Some theorize that it may be because marriage benefits men more than women. Living alone is felt to be a contributing factor to suicide, and single persons are more likely than married persons to commit suicide. Elderly whites are three times more likely to commit suicide as their black counterparts. Recent retirement and "downward mobility" results in higher risk. Elderly persons who live in lower-class, inner-city neighborhoods are more likely to commit suicide. The loss of health, social standing, occupation or marriage, financial security, relationships, emotional adaptability, and mental functioning may lead to feelings of stress, fear, and vulnerability. Finally, the coping mechanisms of the elderly may fail as they experience extreme loneliness and low self-esteem. With the elderly, suicidal ideation may be a hidden agenda, hinted at obliquely.

Suicide prevention programs are sophisticated telephone-based crisis intervention services providing 24-hour hot lines. Services include education, counseling, and consulting as well as grief counseling for survivors. Many programs provide training in grief counseling and suicide prevention for professionals and school programs to educate youth about suicide. Some perform research and postmortem psychological evaluations that investigate unexplained deaths. If these community-sponsored programs are jeopardized by cutbacks, it will leave telephone triage nurses to shoulder a heavy burden for which they are ill-prepared (R. Allen, Personal Communication, January 1992).

Alarm Systems. Studies of utilization show that women are more frequent callers than men, and calls increase with age in both men and women (Greenlick et al., 1973). One study on the effect of telephone support in reducing the use of medical care among the elderly uncovered interesting results (Infante-Rivard, Krieger, Petitclere, & Baumgarten, 1988). In this study, researchers compared elderly who received regular calls from a public health nurse with a control group who received no intervention. Although the results were not statistically significant, telephone support seemed to reduce office visits, resulting in a more cost-effective system.

Telephone support services for the elderly have grown in recent years (Moreland & Grier, 1986; Fritz & Talley, 1982; Dibner, Lowt, & Morris, 1982). This support takes three different forms: home monitoring devices, alarm systems, and "hand-holding" or reassurance lines. These programs are aimed at enhancing independence, postponing institutionalization, increasing self-reliance, and reducing anxiety and loneliness among the elderly. Two types of monitoring systems are *Buddy Systems* and *Lifeline*, both of which provide electronic devices to monitor the clients. *Lifeline* is an alarm system to trigger automatically to summon help in the case of falls or other emergencies (Dibner et al., 1982). This alarm is linked to an emergency response center, usually located in a hospital, which in turn calls a list of responders—friends, neighbors, or relatives—to check on the client. *Lifeline* is a telemetry service for the frail elderly. Telemetry can provide home monitoring, eliminating the need for hospitalization. Falls, other medical emergencies, and dangers such as fire or burglars are ever-present risks for the frail elderly living alone. *Lifeline* provides emergency physical assistance and psychological relief for clients and their families. An automatic dialing unit can be activated by a remote control trigger carried by the client. When the client triggers a call, it sends a signal to the central monitoring unit, which immediately calls the client back.

Lifeline benefits users in several ways. It cuts costs for the family and the community while allowing clients to continue to live at home. It decreases the need for home health services and allows people to return home sooner postoperatively. Family members know that help is available and thus feel some relief from anxiety and responsibility. In September of 1982, over 300 *Lifeline* programs were in use in 42 states. Similar services are available for the elderly and are used in hospitals and retirement homes. Hospitals often provide *Lifeline* services as a marketing tool.

Buddy Systems is composed of a computer console that measures and records blood pressure, weight, heart rate, EKG, and other data (Fisher, 1989). These data are then transmitted to the office or home care agency via telephone, where they can be printed out for assessment. Both of these systems will help cut costs by allowing earlier discharges. By providing services which might be performed by a visiting nurse, they also reduce the number of visits.

Warmlines. *Telecare* is an example of a reassurance or hand-holding line (Marshall, 1977). In the program, the members receive daily phone calls made at a prearranged time to check on their well-being. A follow-up visit is made if there is no response.

Telephone support is ideal for people who are geographically distant from health care facilities, housebound, or want anonymity—all of which apply to many elderly and their caregivers. For example, a study by Goodman and Pynoos (1990) focused on telephone information and support for caregivers of patients with Alzheimer's disease. They stated that because of the burden of Alzheimer's, caregivers are at increased risk for mental health problems and stress symptoms due to "increased responsibility, emotional loss, overload, and isolation" (p. 399). Participants who only listened to lectures showed greater information gain and more frequent emotional support from family and friends, whereas those who participated in the telephone support (Careline) had less frequent support from family and friends. The researchers suggested that this result might be due to support substitution. They concluded that information gained increased perceived social support and increased satisfaction with social supports overall.

Hospice. Originally, hospice meant a place of refuge where pilgrims to the Holy Land could stop and rest. Today, it has come to mean a way of helping the dying to live as fully and comfortably as possible (Sergie-Swinehart, 1985). Hospice programs address the range of medical, psychological, social, spiritual, and practical problems caused by terminal illness. The approach is interdisciplinary, and family and client are considered a unit of care. Hospice enables people to remain at home for much or all of their illness. Staff teach families how to care for the client and are available 24 hours a day to assist with ongoing problems. Much support is carried out by phone, including medical advice, teaching, referral, counseling, and coordinating. Examples are:

- Pain and symptom management
- Medical treatments
- Instruction and supervision of family members in patient care
- Arrangement for home health aides
- Arrangement for respite care
- Assistance to obtain medical equipment
- Spiritual support

Hospice nurses report that early on in the dying process, clients call to "test" the system, thereby reassuring themselves that it works and that help is indeed only a phone call away.

WOMEN OF REPRODUCTIVE AGE

In the Western world, women live longer than men. However, during their lifetimes, they suffer from more physical and mental illness than men, which results in increased use of health care services by women, including telephone triage. Women call twice as often as men, though this is partly because they call for children or husbands as well as for themselves (Curtis & Talbot, 1979; Curtis et al., 1983).

Studies of mortality and morbidity for men and women show a paradoxical relationship (Fogel & Woods, 1981): women report more illness and yet live longer. Perhaps women are more willing to report less severe symptoms, have more time to be ill, or are trained to take better care of themselves when ill. Fogel and Woods cite other studies of perception of illness that theorize that women are more sensitive to bodily discomforts as well as biologic studies that surmise that women are more resistant to degenerative processes because of estrogen. Psychosocial studies cited by Fogel and Woods theorize that women's roles are more stressful, therefore they have more illness. Although the gap between the sexes is narrowing, Fogel and Woods cite studies showing that women still smoke, drink, and drive less than men, leading to a lower death rate from these factors (Cole, 1974; Nathanson, 1975; Rivkin, 1972; Verbrugge, 1977; Verbrugge, 1976; Moriyama, Krueger, and Stamler, 1971). A recent study of telephone triage in the ob/gyn office setting (Kelley & Mashburn, 1990) produced some interesting results. Researchers found that 66% of all gynecological calls involved symptoms, counseling or medication questions, while 67% of all obstetrical calls were about test results, symptom complaints, or counseling. The authors were surprised at the high proportion of counseling calls, stating that this finding indicates a need for additional training and skill refinement in counseling. Other recommendations to streamline the system and reduce administrative calls included giving larger supplies of prenatal vitamins to eliminate callbacks for refills, implementing a formal notification process for test results to eliminate administrative calls, and educating clients more thoroughly about medications.

Global Assessment

A young husband called regarding his pregnant wife who was complaining of a backache and was one week overdue. She denied cramps in the lower abdomen or uterine area. He said "she was acting fine—kinda bitchy—but she's pregnant". The woman snapped, "Get the hell off the phone. I hurt." The nurse asked if this was her normal behavior. The man replied, "Oh no, she never uses foul language." He then added that "a lot of water came out about 3 to 4 hours ago." The nurse advised him to go to the nearest hospital as soon as possible. A baby boy was born 20 minutes later.

A woman who was 8 months pregnant called. She said that contractions had started and that the baby was crowning. She was alone.

A 38-year-old woman who was 32 weeks pregnant called. She gave a previous medical history of chronic hypertension. She complained that her right arm and face were very swollen. She was later admitted to the Critical Care Unit after an emergency C-section and was found to have pneumonia and temporary paralysis.

A postpartum client called, sounding emotionally disturbed. She was later found to have postpartum depression.

A man called about his pregnant wife, explaining that she'd had a headache for one week. He stated that she "was having difficulty seeing and has been jerking around."

Although women as a group, have no major risk factors (severity, age, veracity, emotional status, and debilitation), the reproductive years, (approximately 40 years) are a high-risk period. Thus, symptoms such as abdominal pain must be viewed as serious until proven otherwise. Symptoms of illness in a pregnant woman must also be handled with care. Headache, chest pain, and dizziness can be considered serious symptoms in the woman who is on hormonal therapy. As illustrated by these case histories, pregnancy and childbirth can lead to medical emergencies. If the number of high-risk pregnancies increases, the number of telephone triage calls about these pregnancies will also increase.

Although with new artificial insemination methods it is now possible for post-menapausal women to bear children, normally the reproductive years extend from 12 to 50 years of age. However, sexual activity may precede 12 years and extend indefinitely. STDs are not restricted to the young. Avoid the common pitfall of stereotyping teenagers or elderly women, assuming teenagers are sexually active or that the elderly are not.

Secondary Data

Pregnancy. It is not enough to simply ask, "Are you pregnant?" Elicit concrete details: "Have you been sexually active?" "Is there any chance you might be pregnant?" "What is your current method of birth control? Have you used it faithfully?" "When was your last normal menstrual period?" "Have you had any irregular or missed periods?" Always ascertain if clients are taking oral contraceptives. Document the method of birth control used. IUDs, contraceptive sponges, and birth control pills have a higher incidence of serious complications than do diaphragms, condoms, foam, or natural contraceptive methods. Don't exclude those who have had tubal ligations; they can also experience ectopic pregnancies.

It is critical to be well versed in counseling and sorting out problems related to sexual activity, birth control, and reproduction. Life experience provides invaluable firsthand knowledge of the major health and emotional issues. Hidden agendas for women of reproductive age might include spousal abuse, drug abuse, and fear of sexually transmitted disease.

Medications. Medication calls are an important concern for women of reproductive age, especially antibiotics and medication when pregnant or breastfeeding. Many women in reproductive years are either trying to prevent, postpone, or achieve pregnancy through hormonal therapy. Women of menopausal age may opt for estrogen replacement therapy.

Standards for estrogen replacement therapy (ERT) and birth control (BC) pill refill calls may include a complete physical examination (CPE) and normal Pap smear within the last 12 months. Document the date of the last CPE and Pap smear and whether the Pap smear was within normal limits. Delayed or silent menses, missed pills, variable ERT schedules, and irregular bleeding are but a few of the possible concerns relating to hormonal management, necessitating thorough knowledge and client education.

Other medication questions concern monitoring effects of antibiotic therapy for STDs. Others are strictly informational, such as which medications are allowed in pregnancy and breastfeeding. *Always document pregnancy or breastfeeding status when recommending either OTC or prescription drugs of any type.*

Recent Infection. Heterosexual women have always been at higher risk for STDs than heterosexual men. However, the HIV epidemic has reordered priorities. No longer is the worst-case scenario an unplanned pregnancy, herpes, or even syphilis. HIV infection, often asymptomatic in the carrier, is the new worst case scenario. Teaching efforts must focus on STD and HIV prevention as a priority.

Unfortunately, some nurses seem unaware of the shift in priorities, and the group at greatest risk: black women of reproductive age. Women in this group are dying of HIV infection at a rate "nine times higher than white women of the same age" (Bishop, 1990). According to the article, in 1989 AIDS was the leading cause of death in New York and New Jersey among black women aged 15 to 44. Death rates from AIDS in this group jumped from 18 in 1980 to 1,430 in 1988.

Tactfully inquire about safer-sex practices. Determine if clients are using reliable, high quality condoms consistently and properly. Do not assume that experience with one type of condom qualifies one to teach about condom use. The current range of choices is wide. Some condoms have better quality control and are therefore safer and more reliable. "Beginner's mistakes" are common. Client noncompliance can be overcome through written information, classes, and telephone support.

There are two groups who are at extreme risk for HIV and AIDS: those with histories of repeated STDs and illicit drug users. Clients with multiple episodes of STDs ("repeaters") need intensive counseling and education as well as periodic follow-up calls. Core STD populations (illicit drug users, prostitutes, and some ethnic minorities with low education and socioeconomic levels) will require extensive education and counseling. Illicit drug users also have a higher risk for STDs and HIV, making treatment more complex because the natural course of STDs is altered by the impaired immune response. If a client with diagnosed HIV presents with a STD, it indicates unprotected sexual activity has occurred and the client needs intensive counseling.

Medications for vaginal infections are available OTC and by prescriptions. Carefully question clients with a self-diagnosis of yeast infection to rule out urinary tract infection. If a UTI cannot be ruled out, the client should come in for examination and treatment. Remind clients that symptoms should abate after 24 to 48 hours on antibiotics.

Telemetry

In the past, women at risk for preterm birth spent weeks or months in the hospital prior to delivery. Advances in telemetry are making this practice obsolete. Tokos is a company which provides in-home services combining telemetry, medication, and telephone support to high-risk mothers. High-risk pregnancies may include twins or triplets, previous preterm labor or delivery, DES daughters, abnormal uterine shape, two or more second trimester abortions, incompetent cervix, hypertension, diabetes, severe kidney infections, and age of less than 18 or over 35 with unusual physical or mental stress.

Tokos nurses relate that a major challenge in caring for their clients is achieving compliance. They have discovered that counseling is a large part of their telephone practice and that certain problems tend to recur. For instance, many clients simply lack information, making teaching extremely important. Some find the telemetry machine invasive and resent it. Allowing clients to set the time of telephone contact demonstrates sensitivity to client individuality and acknowledges the client's need to feel in control and to collaborate. Many clients are grieving the loss of the "perfect pregnancy experience." Clients often use denial as a defense mechanism. Thus, high-risk mothers may have many hidden agendas that act as impediments to eliciting information. When clients fail to call as directed, they are referred to physicians for additional counseling or possible hospitalization.

Rape Crisis

Currently, rape crisis calls are infrequent in telephone triage, although this situation may change if continued lack of funds forces hot lines to close. Such calls can be both information- and counseling-intensive. If a nurse is not trained in rape crisis intervention, the best approach is to initiate a conference call with rape crisis and then pass the call on. San Francisco Rape Crisis counselors offer the following advice: address the caller by first name and give your first name; obtain the address, phone number, age, and name of the caller. Callers may exhibit extreme fear, shock, or extreme calm related to denial of the emotional impact of what has occurred. After stressing confidentiality, obtain details of the rape, address any immediate needs (serious injuries, continued physical threat), and implement paramedic transport as appropriate. Advise survivors (no longer referred to as victims) not to bathe or douche; or to smoke, drink, or eat after oral copulation. Advise the survivor to seek appropriate aid accompanied by a friend. Also advise the person to bring a change of clothing. Some articles of clothing may be kept as evidence. (San Francisco Women Against Rape, 1987)

The examination includes a pelvic for injuries, sperm analysis, combing of body hair, complete physical exam for injuries, written report of results, treatment for STDs, pregnancy test, follow-up appointment in 6 weeks, morning-after pill dispensed on request, photos as needed, and follow-up AIDS testing. Counselors advise urging survivors, even if resistant, to seek medical treatment. Finally, they stress that their role is to support, facilitate, act as a sounding board and encourage callers to "own the decision."

Most crisis lines offer a variety of programs and services, including a 24-hour hot line for counseling and referral, support groups, and medical, legal, housing, and self-defense referrals. All services are confidential.

Women: The Ultimate Marketing Target. From cradle to grave, women tend to be in high-risk groups, first, by virtue of childhood, again during reproductive years, and, later, because of old age. Sexually active women risk serious complications associated with pregnancy, birth control, and sexually transmitted disease. Traditionally high utilizers of health care services, women have become a prime marketing target and many hospitals link telephone advice to special in-house programs for women. These include classes or support groups on menopause, new parenting, PMS, stress and meshing career with child rearing. Evaluate the quality and intent of such programs before recommending them to clients. Programs must offer clients unbiased, comprehensive, and reliable information.

In summary, high-risk populations are heavy utilizers of telephone triage. This overview of issues is intended only as a framework for deeper examination of high-risk clients. As recommended by Kelley and Mashburn (1990), nurses working with high-risk populations must develop continuing education courses. These may include guest speakers from suicide prevention, rape crisis, AIDS hot lines, parental stress hot lines, and geriatric specialties to discuss the complex needs, communication styles, and health problems of these populations. See Appendices A, E, F, G and H for sample protocol lists, protocols, and support groups.

CHAPTER 6

EXERCISE—MOCK CALLS

OBJECTIVES:

1. To practice thorough, concise data collection and telephone interviewing skills.
2. To practice formulating a working diagnosis and time frame for disposition. Use time frames: emergent—0–2 hours, urgent—2–8 hours, and routine—8–24 hours.
3. To practice using a data documentation form.

METHOD: In teams of three, each nurse takes a turn role-playing nurse, client, and scorekeeper, using mock calls provided. Tape the mock calls. Play back the call and, using the forms provided, score for call proficiency.

ROLES:

THE CLIENT uses the mock call *script* to provide information about symptoms to the nurse, without offering too much information. In other the words, the nurse should have to work a little to collect data. Try to make your "call" as realistic as possible. You may use your imagination and add information if you wish, keeping in mind that a change in data may change the outcome.

THE NURSE elicits and documents information in a personable and professional manner, formulating and documenting a working diagnosis (e.g., sudden onset, abdominal pain, severe, etiology unknown), and a time frame (e.g., 0–2 hours, 2–8 hours, 8–24+ hours) in which client should be seen, as appropriate. (See example, Figure 6.1)

THE SCOREKEEPER scores the call for completeness as objectively as possible using the Telephone Triage Scoresheet. (See example, Figure 6.2)

HOW TO SCORE:

- Give 1 point for each item of interview and documentation skills performed by the nurse.
- Give 1 point if category is "not applicable." (For example, pregnancy information would be inappropriate for a client who is an infant).
- Give a 0 for any failure to document data, either with positive statements or pertinent negative or a symbol for negative—$\overline{0}$.

- Nurses must demonstrate basic interpersonal communication skills such as a helpful attitude, open-ended questioning, and eliciting client age. Therefore, give a total score of "0" for the entire exercise if there is:
  - Failure to document age of client
  - Failure to act in a helpful manner from the onset
  - Consistent or inappropriate use of leading questions

Add all points. A perfect score is 32. An acceptable score is 27 or more. Anything less than 27 indicates a need for review and practice. Scoring may seem arbitrary at times; however an approximation by general consensus is acceptable.

Recording mock calls can help to assess skills in other ways:

- Does the nurse create a warm climate and reflect a commitment to healing?
- What is the speed of conversation, inflection, intonation, warmth?
- Is the interaction conducted in a professional manner according to institutional standards?
- Did the nurse use open-ended questions?
- What was the listen-to-talk ratio? (Transaction time should be divided approximately into $\frac{2}{3}$ listening and $\frac{1}{3}$ talking)
- Did the nurse use lay language, disclaimers, and follow-up instructions?
- Was the nurse articulate, facilitative, and resourceful?
- Was the data collected complete, comprehensive, and concrete?

After completing all mock call exercises, you may continue to record actual calls *(nurse's side of conversation only)* and score them in the same manner. Actual calls provide a more accurate and valid picture of the nurse's interpersonal style and job performance. Call recording, review, and feedback can be used for skill refinement and job performance evaluation.

Example:

FIGURE 6.1 Telephone Triage Data Form with Sample Documentation (Courtesy of Wheeler and Associates)

SOON/WK

TO Jones, M.D. FROM Smith, R.N. DATE 12-12-93 TIME 3pm CHECKED BY MD

NAME Doe, Jane AGE 26 WT 0 CALLER Self PHONE HOME 454-4444 WORK —

SX. CHAR/COURSE/HX/ONSET/LOC/AG.FX/REL.FX

c/o Sudden onset headache TEMP WNL O R AX

Severe (9 on scale of 10)

Denies visual problems

Feels "weak, dizzy."

N. + V. x 6°

ADL Did not go to work today

Unable to eat or drink

x 10 hours

PREG/BRSTFDG ☐ Y ☒ N LNMP 10-93

ALLERGIES none known

MEDS none

PREVIOUS CHRONIC ILLNESS Previous history migraines

EMOTIONAL STATUS anxious

RECENT INJURY, ILLNESS OR INGESTION denies

WORKING DIAGNOSIS Severe (L) sided Headache

ADVICE/PROTOCOL per Headache Protocol

DEVIATIONS none ☒ VERBAL CONTRACT ☒ DISCLAIMER

DISPOSITION ☐ ED ☒ UCC 4PM ☐ ADVICE ONLY ☐ APPT.

FOLLOW-UP CALL TIME

Rx

PHARMACY

OUTCOME: PHONE

SIG S. Smith, RN

Telephone Triage Data Form

FIGURE 6.2 Telephone Triage Scoresheet with Scoring Sample (Courtesy of Wheeler and Associates)

ROLES	Call 1	Call 2	Call 3	Call 4	Call 5	Call 6	Call 7	Call 8	Call 9	Call 10
*Helping	1									
Teaching/Coaching	1									
Diagnostic/Monitoring	1									
Monitoring Interventions	1									
Crisis Intervention	1									
INTERVIEW SKILLS	Call 1	Call 2	Call 3	Call 4	Call 5	Call 6	Call 7	Call 8	Call 9	Call 10
*Asks open-ended questions	1									
Concrete data collection/directions	1									
Uses confrontation appropriately	1									
Speaks directly to client	1									
Uses layman's language	1									
Restates problem	1									
States working diagnosis	1									
States disclaimer	1									
Elicits hidden agendas	1									
Elicits verbal contract	1									
Uses time frames	1									
Uses proper abbreviations/terms	1									
DATA COLLECTION SKILLS	Call 1	Call 2	Call 3	Call 4	Call 5	Call 6	Call 7	Call 8	Call 9	Call 10
*Age	1									
Symptom(s)	1									
Characteristics	1									
Course/ADL	1									
History of complaint	1									
Onset of symptoms	0									
Location of symptoms	1									
Altering factors	1									
Pregnant/breastfeeding status	1									
Allergies	1									
Medications	1									
Previous chronic illness	1									
Emotional status	1									
Recent injury/illness/ingestion	1									
Pertinent negatives	1									
SCORE	31									

FIGURE 6.3 Telephone Triage Scoresheet (Courtesy of Wheeler and Associates)

ROLES	Call 1	Call 2	Call 3	Call 4	Call 5	Call 6	Call 7	Call 8	Call 9	Call 10	Call 11	Call 12
*Helping												
Teaching/Coaching												
Diagnostic/Monitoring												
Monitoring Interventions												
Crisis Intervention												
INTERVIEW SKILLS	Call 1	Call 2	Call 3	Call 4	Call 5	Call 6	Call 7	Call 8	Call 9	Call 10	Call 11	Call 12
*Asks open-ended questions												
Concrete data collection/directions												
Uses confrontation appropriately												
Speaks directly to client												
Uses layman's language												
Restates problem												
States working diagnosis												
States disclaimer												
Elicits hidden agendas												
Elicits verbal contract												
Uses time frames												
Uses proper abbreviations/terms												
DATA COLLECTION SKILLS	Call 1	Call 2	Call 3	Call 4	Call 5	Call 6	Call 7	Call 8	Call 9	Call 10	Call 11	Call 12
*Age												
Symptom(s)												
Characteristics												
Course/ADL												
History of complaint												
Onset of symptoms												
Location of symptoms												
Altering factors												
Pregnant/breastfeeding status												
Allergies												
Medications												
Previous chronic illness												
Emotional status												
Recent injury/illness/ingestion												
Pertinent negatives												
SCORE												

MOCK CALL 1

61-year-old female
Noted chest tightness when jogging
Stopping makes it better
Has had it 2 to 4 weeks, 3 to 4 times per week
Feels like she has sore throat sometimes
Denies shortness of breath, dizziness, sweating, nausea
Medical history—hypertension
Medication—Atarax
Allergies—salicylates, tomatoes, green peppers

TO	FROM	DATE		TIME	CHECKED BY MD	
NAME		AGE	WT	CALLER	PHONE HOME	WORK
SX. CHAR/COURSE/HX/ONSET/LOC/AG.FX/REL.FX				WORKING DIAGNOSIS		
		TEMP O R AX				
				ADVICE/PROTOCOL		
				DEVIATIONS		☐ VERBAL CONTRACT
						☐ DISCLAIMER
ADL				DISPOSITION ☐ ED ☐ UCC ☐ ADVICE ONLY ☐ APPT.		
				FOLLOW-UP CALL	TIME	
PREG/BRSTFDG ☐ Y ☐ N LNMP						
ALLERGIES				Rx		
MEDS						
PREVIOUS CHRONIC ILLNESS						
EMOTIONAL STATUS				PHARMACY		
RECENT INJURY, ILLNESS OR INGESTION				OUTCOME	PHONE	
				SIG		
Telephone Triage Data Form				© 1990 Shelia Quilter Wheeler		

Data Form (Courtesy of Wheeler and Associates)

MOCK CALL 2

61-year-old male
History of hypertension
Feet and ankles look like "balloons"
Fatigue for 2 days
Taking Theodur, Prednisone, Wytension, Valium
4-plus pitting edema
Seems worse today than yesterday
Ankles $11\frac{1}{2}''$ on circumference on left, $12\frac{1}{4}''$ on the right
History of emphysema, colitis
Hypertension for 3 years

TO FROM DATE	TIME CHECKED BY MD
NAME AGE WT	CALLER PHONE HOME WORK
SX. CHAR/COURSE/HX/ONSET/LOC/AG.FX/REL.FX	WORKING DIAGNOSIS
TEMP O R AX	
	ADVICE/PROTOCOL
	DEVIATIONS ☐ VERBAL CONTRACT
	☐ DISCLAIMER
ADL	DISPOSITION ☐ ED ☐ UCC ☐ ADVICE ONLY ☐ APPT.
	FOLLOW-UP CALL TIME
PREG/BRSTFDG ☐ Y ☐ N LNMP	
ALLERGIES	Rx
MEDS	
PREVIOUS CHRONIC ILLNESS	
EMOTIONAL STATUS	PHARMACY
RECENT INJURY, ILLNESS OR INGESTION	OUTCOME PHONE
	SIG
Telephone Triage Data Form	© 1990 Sheila Quilter Wheeler

Data Form (Courtesy of Wheeler and Associates)

MOCK CALL 3

21-year-old female
Abdominal pain × 3 to 4 days
Near navel, painful to touch, also sl. to left of umbilicus and above
Laying on back helps
Laying on stomach makes it worse
Slight nausea
Vomited 2 hours ago
No diarrhea or constipation
No medications
No allergies
On BC pills 5 years ago
LMP 1 month ago—4 days late
Possible parasitic infection 1 month ago
No vaginal discharge
Car accident 1 month ago—headache for 4 days following accident
Back pain

TO	FROM	DATE	TIME	CHECKED BY MD
NAME	AGE	WT	CALLER	PHONE HOME / WORK

SX. CHAR/COURSE/HX/ONSET/LOC/AG.FX/REL.FX	WORKING DIAGNOSIS
TEMP O R AX	
	ADVICE/PROTOCOL
	DEVIATIONS ☐ VERBAL CONTRACT
	☐ DISCLAIMER
ADL	DISPOSITION ☐ ED ☐ UCC ☐ ADVICE ONLY ☐ APPT.
	FOLLOW-UP CALL TIME
PREG/BRSTFDG ☐ Y ☐ N LNMP	
ALLERGIES	Rx
MEDS	
PREVIOUS CHRONIC ILLNESS	
EMOTIONAL STATUS	PHARMACY
RECENT INJURY, ILLNESS OR INGESTION	OUTCOME / PHONE
	SIG
Telephone Triage Data Form	© 1990 Sheila Quilter Wheele

Data Form (Courtesy of Wheeler and Associates)

MOCK CALL 4

44-year-old woman
Severe stomach pains
Temp 103
Became ill 28 hours ago
Sweating
No diarrhea
Bowel movement today looked like pellets
Pain is 4" below umbilicus
No history of previous pain like this
Earlier felt constipated, now has dull tender spot in left lower pelvis
Medical history—kidney stone
Allergies—none
Medications—none
No appetite, drinking poorly

TO	FROM	DATE		TIME	CHECKED BY	MD
NAME		AGE	WT	CALLER	PHONE HOME	WORK
SX. CHAR/COURSE/HX/ONSET/LOC/AG.FX/REL.FX				WORKING DIAGNOSIS		
		TEMP O R AX				
				ADVICE/PROTOCOL		
				DEVIATIONS		☐ VERBAL CONTRACT
						☐ DISCLAIMER
ADL				DISPOSITION	☐ ED ☐ UCC ☐ ADVICE ONLY	☐ APPT.
				FOLLOW-UP CALL		TIME
PREG/BRSTFDG	☐ Y ☐ N	LNMP				
ALLERGIES				Rx		
MEDS						
PREVIOUS CHRONIC ILLNESS						
EMOTIONAL STATUS				PHARMACY		
RECENT INJURY, ILLNESS OR INGESTION				OUTCOME	PHONE	
				SIG		
Telephone Triage Data Form						© 1990 Sheila Quilter Wheeler

Data Form (Courtesy of Wheeler and Associates)

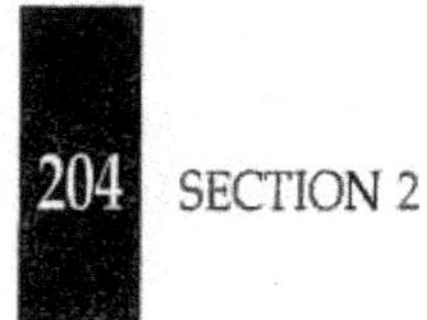

MOCK CALL 5

35-year-old unmarried woman
C/o "flu" symptoms
BC method—IUD × 2 years (Copper T)
Fever chills, muscle aches
Headache
Recent STD exposure
Menses late × 2 months
Sexually active

TO	FROM	DATE	TIME	CHECKED BY MD
NAME		AGE / WT	CALLER	PHONE HOME / WORK
SX. CHAR/COURSE/HX/ONSET/LOC/AG.FX/REL.FX			WORKING DIAGNOSIS	
		TEMP O R AX		
			ADVICE/PROTOCOL	
			DEVIATIONS	☐ VERBAL CONTRACT
				☐ DISCLAIMER
ADL			DISPOSITION	☐ ED ☐ UCC ☐ ADVICE ONLY ☐ APPT.
			FOLLOW-UP CALL	TIME
PREG/BRSTFDG ☐ Y ☐ N LNMP				
ALLERGIES			Rx	
MEDS				
PREVIOUS CHRONIC ILLNESS				
EMOTIONAL STATUS			PHARMACY	
RECENT INJURY, ILLNESS OR INGESTION			OUTCOME	PHONE
			SIG	
Telephone Triage Data Form				© 1990 Sheila Quilter Wheeler

Data Form (Courtesy of Wheeler and Associates)

MOCK CALL 6

40-year-old multipara, 8 months pregnant
Recent refugee to this country from Nicaragua, speaks little English
C/o headache, "stomach pain," dizzy

TO	FROM	DATE		TIME	CHECKED BY MD
NAME		AGE	WT	CALLER	PHONE HOME / WORK

SX. CHAR/COURSE/HX/ONSET/LOC/AG.FX/REL.FX	WORKING DIAGNOSIS
TEMP O R AX	
	ADVICE/PROTOCOL
	DEVIATIONS ☐ VERBAL CONTRACT
	☐ DISCLAIMER
ADL	DISPOSITION ☐ ED ☐ UCC ☐ ADVICE ONLY ☐ APPT.
	FOLLOW-UP CALL TIME
PREG/BRSTFDG ☐ Y ☐ N LNMP	
ALLERGIES	Rx
MEDS	
PREVIOUS CHRONIC ILLNESS	
EMOTIONAL STATUS	PHARMACY
RECENT INJURY, ILLNESS OR INGESTION	OUTCOME / PHONE
	SIG
Telephone Triage Data Form	© 1990 Sheila Quilter Wheeler

Data Form (Courtesy of Wheeler and Associates)

MOCK CALL 7

17-year-old female
History of parasites
Temp 101
History of endameoba histolitica
Has not seen MD, only NP
Sick for 1 month
Shaking chills
Severe headaches, 8 on scale of 10
Taking Vermox, Flagyl
Passing blood in stools
Abdomen grossly distended × 3 weeks
Symptoms are much worse in last few days

TO	FROM	DATE		TIME	CHECKED BY MD
NAME		AGE	WT	CALLER	PHONE HOME / WORK

SX. CHAR/COURSE/HX/ONSET/LOC/AG.FX/REL.FX	WORKING DIAGNOSIS
TEMP O R AX	
	ADVICE/PROTOCOL
	DEVIATIONS ☐ VERBAL CONTRAC
	☐ DISCLAIMER
ADL	DISPOSITION ☐ ED ☐ UCC ☐ ADVICE ONLY ☐ APPT.
	FOLLOW-UP CALL TIME
PREG/BRSTFDG ☐ Y ☐ N LNMP	
ALLERGIES	Rx
MEDS	
PREVIOUS CHRONIC ILLNESS	
EMOTIONAL STATUS	PHARMACY
RECENT INJURY, ILLNESS OR INGESTION	OUTCOME / PHONE
	SIG
Telephone Triage Data Form	© 1990 Sheila Quilter Whe

Data Form (Courtesy of Wheeler and Associates)

MOCK CALL 8

57-year-old woman
"Fainting episode" preceded by "palpitations"
Lost consciousness
Denies incontinence
Recent "flu" × 1 week
Taking Actifed, Robitussin

TO / FROM / DATE	TIME / CHECKED BY ... MD
NAME / AGE / WT	CALLER / PHONE HOME / WORK
SX. CHAR/COURSE/HX/ONSET/LOC/AG.FX/REL.FX	WORKING DIAGNOSIS
TEMP O R AX	
	ADVICE/PROTOCOL
	DEVIATIONS ☐ VERBAL CONTRACT
	☐ DISCLAIMER
ADL	DISPOSITION ☐ ED ☐ UCC ☐ ADVICE ONLY ☐ APPT.
	FOLLOW-UP CALL TIME
PREG/BRSTFDG ☐ Y ☐ N LNMP	
ALLERGIES	Rx
MEDS	
PREVIOUS CHRONIC ILLNESS	
EMOTIONAL STATUS	PHARMACY
RECENT INJURY, ILLNESS OR INGESTION	OUTCOME / PHONE
	SIG
Telephone Triage Data Form	© 1990 Sheila Quilter Wheeler

Data Form (Courtesy of Wheeler and Associates)

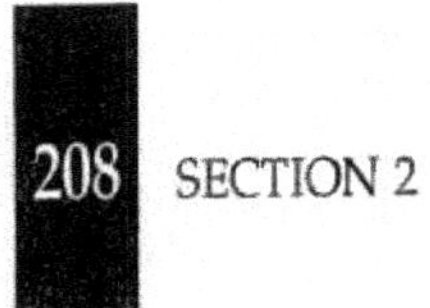

MOCK CALL 9

11-month-old infant
Temp 104
Lying around moaning
Cranky, miserable
Mother states fever is "difficult to control by normal measures"
Eating and drinking poorly—12 oz. total today
Normal amount of wet diapers
Seems much worse than last night

TO	FROM	DATE		TIME	CHECKED BY	MD
NAME		AGE	WT	CALLER	PHONE HOME	WORK

SX. CHAR/COURSE/HX/ONSET/LOC/AG.FX/REL.FX	WORKING DIAGNOSIS
TEMP O R AX	
	ADVICE/PROTOCOL
	DEVIATIONS ☐ VERBAL CONTRAC
	☐ DISCLAIMER
ADL	DISPOSITION ☐ ED ☐ UCC ☐ ADVICE ONLY ☐ APPT.
	FOLLOW-UP CALL TIME
PREG/BRSTFDG ☐ Y ☐ N LNMP	
ALLERGIES	Rx
MEDS	
PREVIOUS CHRONIC ILLNESS	
EMOTIONAL STATUS	PHARMACY
RECENT INJURY, ILLNESS OR INGESTION	OUTCOME PHONE
	SIG
Telephone Triage Data Form	© 1990 Sheila Quilter Whe

Data Form (Courtesy of Wheeler and Associates)

MOCK CALL 10

20-month-old male
Sick $1\frac{1}{2}$ days
Temp 104.6
Swollen glands under earlobes
Previously treated with Amoxicillin for otitis
Now on Gantrisin for chronic otitis $\times$ 2 months
Eating poorly, drinking fair, urine output scanty

TO	FROM	DATE		TIME	CHECKED BY MD	
NAME		AGE	WT	CALLER	PHONE HOME	WORK

SX. CHAR/COURSE/HX/ONSET/LOC/AG.FX/REL.FX	WORKING DIAGNOSIS
TEMP O R AX	
	ADVICE/PROTOCOL
	DEVIATIONS □ VERBAL CONTRACT
	□ DISCLAIMER
ADL	DISPOSITION □ ED □ UCC □ ADVICE ONLY □ APPT.
	FOLLOW-UP CALL TIME
PREG/BRSTFDG □ Y □ N LNMP	
ALLERGIES	Rx
MEDS	
PREVIOUS CHRONIC ILLNESS	
EMOTIONAL STATUS	PHARMACY
RECENT INJURY, ILLNESS OR INGESTION	OUTCOME PHONE
	SIG
Telephone Triage Data Form	© 1990 Sheila Quilter Wheeler

Data Form (Courtesy of Wheeler and Associates)

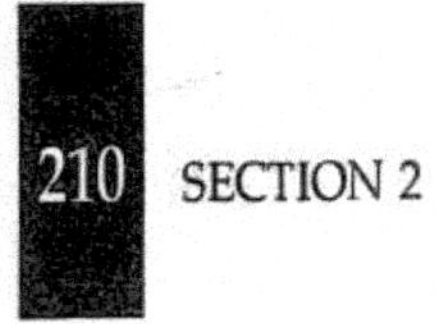

MOCK CALL 11

23-year-old male
L sided pain × 2 days
Brown urine × 2 days
Pain 6 on scale of 10
Denies chills, fever, or loss of energy
Appetite good
Sore throat × 2 weeks
No meds, allergies, health problems

TO / FROM / DATE	TIME / CHECKED BY MD
NAME / AGE / WT	CALLER / PHONE HOME / WORK
SX. CHAR/COURSE/HX/ONSET/LOC/AG.FX/REL.FX	WORKING DIAGNOSIS
TEMP O R AX	
	ADVICE/PROTOCOL
	DEVIATIONS ☐ VERBAL CONTRACT
	☐ DISCLAIMER
ADL	DISPOSITION ☐ ED ☐ UCC ☐ ADVICE ONLY ☐ APPT.
	FOLLOW-UP CALL TIME
PREG/BRSTFDG ☐ Y ☐ N LNMP	
ALLERGIES	Rx
MEDS	
PREVIOUS CHRONIC ILLNESS	
EMOTIONAL STATUS	PHARMACY
RECENT INJURY, ILLNESS OR INGESTION	OUTCOME / PHONE
	SIG
Telephone Triage Data Form	© 1990 Sheila Quilter Wheel

Data Form (Courtesy of Wheeler and Associates)

MOCK CALL 12

57-year-old pharmacist calls at 7:30 A.M. regarding his wife
Wants an appointment in a "day or two"
Wife had had a seizure during the night and is not totally alert now
No history of epilepsy
Diet for weight loss × 2 months—lost 25 pounds

TO / FROM / DATE	TIME / CHECKED BY / MD
NAME / AGE / WT	CALLER / PHONE HOME / WORK
SX. CHAR/COURSE/HX/ONSET/LOC/AG.FX/REL.FX	WORKING DIAGNOSIS
TEMP O R AX	
	ADVICE/PROTOCOL
	DEVIATIONS ☐ VERBAL CONTRACT
	☐ DISCLAIMER
ADL	DISPOSITION ☐ ED ☐ UCC ☐ ADVICE ONLY ☐ APPT.
	FOLLOW-UP CALL TIME
PREG/BRSTFDG ☐ Y ☐ N LNMP	
ALLERGIES	Rx
MEDS	
PREVIOUS CHRONIC ILLNESS	
EMOTIONAL STATUS	PHARMACY
RECENT INJURY, ILLNESS OR INGESTION	OUTCOME / PHONE
	SIG
Telephone Triage Data Form	© 1990 Sheila Quilter Wheeler

Data Form (Courtesy of Wheeler and Associates)

ANSWER KEY

MOCK CALLS: WORKING DIAGNOSIS (WD) AND TIME FRAMES (TF)

1. WD: "Poss. chest pain"
   TF: 0–2 H
2. WD: "Severe swelling of feet, hx hypertension"
   TF: 2–8 H
3. WD: "Abdominal pain, localized"
   TF: 2–8 H
4. WD: "Abdominal pain, severe"
   TF: 2–8 H
5. WD: "STD exposure with IUD"
   TF: 2–8 H
6. WD: "Abdominal pain/pregnant × 8 mo./non-English speaking"
   TF: 0–2 H
7. WD: "Severe headache, fever, shaking chills, increasing sx."
   TF: 2–8 H
8. WD: "Fainting episode, poss. palpitations"
   TF: 0–2 H
9. WD: "Fever/irritability"
   TF: 2–8 H
10. WD: "Fever/possible dehydration"
    TF: 2–8 H
11. WD: "Flank pain × 2 days"
    TF: 2–8 H
12. WD: "Seizures, decreased L.O.C."
    TF: 0–2 H

SECTION 3

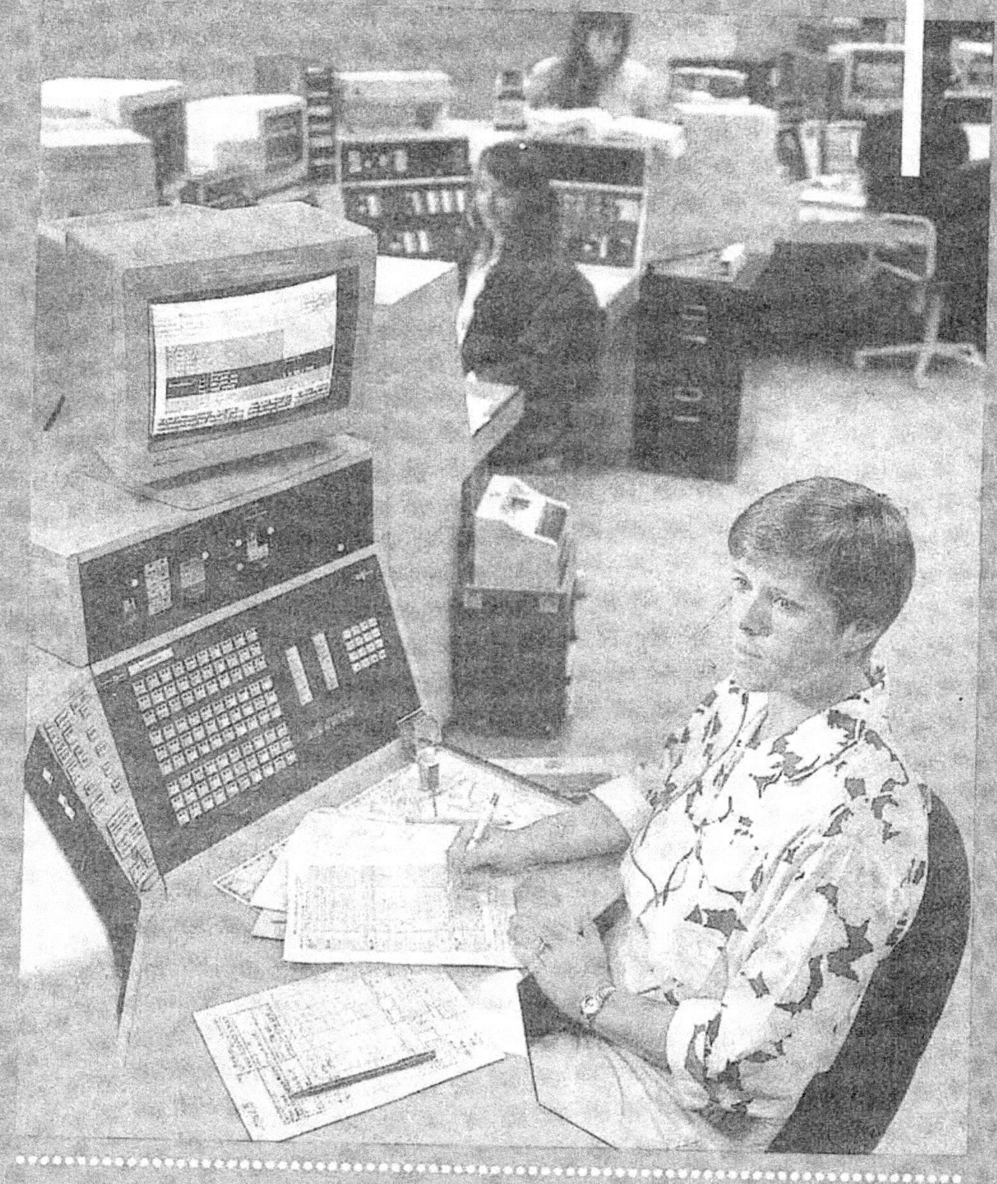

(Photo on previous page) *Marin County Communications Center features a state-of-the-art communications console for emergency medical dispatchers. (San Rafael, California. Richard Wheeler, photographer.)*

CHAPTER 7
Crisis Intervention

If there is an expert level of telephone triage, it is crisis intervention. Fortunately, the body of knowledge about crisis intervention techniques has been growing. Emergency medical dispatch (or 911), rape crisis lines, and suicide prevention have paved the way for crisis-level telephone triage. Still, nurses may be inadvertently thrust into the role of "first responder," the person receiving the call who manages the crisis initially. The first responder role may include triage, dispatch of emergency equipment, CPR coaching, or suicide prevention. With the exception of emergency equipment dispatch, most of these skills are within the scope of telephone triage nurses.

Crisis intervention is extraordinarily time-consuming and emotionally taxing. Those who administer high-volume systems view such time-consuming calls as impractical. Nonetheless, they happen, and it is irresponsible to fail to recognize and prepare for them. This chapter proposes methods for handling such calls. Because all crisis-level medical calls are psychological as well, the first part of the chapter covers psychological problems.

PSYCHOLOGICAL CRISIS INTERVENTION

This section deals almost exclusively with suicidal calls because they represent the bulk of calls about psychological crises and are often life-threatening. However, many of the techniques recommended here can be adapted to calls about chronic or acute psychosis, non-suicidal depression, severe phobias, panic attacks, and dementia.

> *A battered young college wife calls the ED. She is suicidal.*
>
> *A woman shoots herself while on the phone.*
>
> *A man overdoses on Lanoxin. He arrives at the ED after a long delay but is dead upon arrival.*
>
> *A woman calls, saying she has a loaded gun and is about to kill herself. She then hangs up without identifying herself.*

Though nurses who work in telephone triage may not encounter such problems every day, they happen eventually. Handling suicidal or homicidal calls effectively and without intense feelings of helplessness, or, in case of a bad outcome, guilt, requires resourcefulness, training, and support. This section covers the techniques nurses need for handling these extraordinary calls.

Communication Techniques for Establishing Trust

Suicide intervention calls, like all crisis calls involves five tasks: (1) engage the client, (2) identify whether or not the client is considering suicide, (3) inquire into the reasons behind the contemplated suicide, (4) assess the immediate risk, and (5) take action (California Helper's Handbook, 1992). Although the order of importance of these objectives depends on the situation, establishing trust is an important step before callers volunteer information, such as location or overdose information. Usually, if suicidal callers initially encounter a nonjudgmental, sympathetic voice on the line, they will later allow nurses to gather data.

Confront the Issue. Suicide is a taboo subject in our society. Some people worry that simply mentioning the "s" word can precipitate a suicide or plant the idea in a person's mind. This is a common misconception (Reubin, 1979). Callers are already thinking about suicide. In fact, experts say that confronting the issue allows clients to be honest, opens lines of communication, and initiates the therapeutic process (R. Allen, personal communication, February, 1992).

Asking if someone is suicidal feels strange at first. One way to overcome these feelings is through role-playing. Role-playing sessions overcome the taboo by teaching participants to ask *the question:* "Are you thinking of killing yourself/committing suicide/taking your life?" Ask the question with timeliness, directness, calmness, and composure. To be effective, use exactly these words, without evasion.

Buy Time While Establishing Trust. Occasionally, someone tries to rescue people about to jump from bridges or buildings. Often this heroic, impulsive act precipitates the actual suicide. Experts advise against using heroics without regard for the feelings of the suicidal person (R. Allen, personal communication, February, 1992). Such an act increases feelings of helplessness. Even with suicides in progress, when the caller's life is at immediate risk, try to establish trust. Recruit family, friends, emergency teams, or clergy teams. Contact 911 if callers persist in refusing help.

Likewise, premature attempts to gain vital data such as location or phone number often induce the caller to disconnect. In all but the most critical situations, nurses have time to hear callers out before attempting to obtain vital information. In the following example, the nurse attempted to elicit information prematurely:

The nurse answered the phone and a female voice very calmly stated, "I have just taken a major overdose of pills and I want to know how long it will take me to die."

Nurse: *"Miss, you need to be seen in the Emergency Department. What kind of pills did you take?"*
Caller: *"I want to die."*
Nurse: *"Where do you live? What is your name?"*
Caller: *"I don't want to tell you."*
Nurse: *"I am trying to help you! Please tell me where you live or at least your name?"*
Caller *(very angrily): "I want to die! You don't care! All of you SOBs don't care!"*
The caller then hung up the phone. (Wheeler, 1989)

The nurse's premature attempts to collect data rather than establish trust precipitated a disconnection. By contrast, talking first would probably have defused the situation and helped the crisis to pass. Experts say that crises such as suicidal impulses are time-limited (R. Allen, Personal Communication, 1992). "Talking the caller down," or letting the person "talk it out" may reduce the need to act out feelings of despair, helplessness, and hopelessness. Allow clients to express their feelings freely, no matter how angry, depressed, repellent, or manipulative callers might seem at the time. More than anything else, suicidal callers have a deep need to verbalize feelings of sadness and pain to an empathic listener. By acknowledging and validating the caller's pain, nurses provide a "psychological lifeline" (Neville & Barnes, 1985, p. 15). Similarly, it is important to listen before attempting to transfer or trace any call.

Suicide counseling calls can last as long as 30 minutes. "Buying time" and establishing rapport diminishes the likelihood of impulsive acts and makes phone tracing possible. Use your first name only and ask the caller's first name, bearing in mind that many callers may wish to remain anonymous. Using names personalizes the interaction and strengthens rapport.

Be Authentic. All crisis intervention, and suicide prevention calls especially, require congruence and authenticity. A genuine response ("Your story makes me very sad," or, "I'm overwhelmed by what you've told me,") is credible, congruent, and effective. Self-disclosure helps to convey the caregiver's feelings and fosters trust: "I remember how awful I felt when my boyfriend and I broke up. Tell me about your breakup." Do not offer platitudes or unwanted advice. "Rescuing" (taking over in a way that assumes you know best) denies the client's autonomy, fosters dependency, and aggravates feelings of helplessness.

Be Resourceful. Allen (Personal Communication, 1992) suggests that suicidal callers need "hooks" to pull them back toward life. The very fact that the client has called demonstrates an ambivalence about dying. Capitalize on this ambivalence. Use whatever works—guilt, uncertainty, religious faith, even pets—to take advantage of the client's ambivalence. For example, some Catholics believe that they will go to hell if they commit suicide. Capitalizing on this belief may dissuade the caller from suicide. Ask directly, "Do you believe that you will go to hell?" If the caller is looking forward to heaven you might say, "No one really knows what happens after death." To a client with pets you could say, "Your cats will miss you a lot. Who will take care of them if you kill yourself?"

Avoid Psychobabble. Many suicidal callers are psychologically sophisticated from having experienced psychotherapy. Using trite psychological phrases sounds artificial. Callers respond better to authenticity in speech, feeling, and manner. Reflecting feelings is another overused and superficial technique. Neville and Barnes (1985) note that if a client is distraught about losing a job and is afraid of never finding another, saying, "You sound really upset about being laid off" seems phony and even uncaring. Instead of repeating back callers' feelings, they suggest saying something like, "I don't blame you for being angry." This response validates the client's feelings. Afterwards use a more directive problem-solving approach like "Have you considered other kinds of work?"

Counseling Techniques. Rather than trying to impose a solution, facilitate problem-solving by helping callers to identify and mobilize their own strengths and resources. Explore past solutions and resources rather than preaching. Acknowledge that, though suicide may be a way out of the problem, it is only one of many choices. Even in crises, choices exist. The nurse can help the client discover what those solutions are. Ask, "Have you considered any other options besides suicide?"

Ownership of the problem and solution leads to feelings of control. One approach is to reinforce coping strategies. Acknowledge and recognize positive feelings and acts. For example: "Some part of you must want to live, because you have reached out for help." Even a simple "Uh-huh," or "Yes," or "Go on," said in an encouraging tone of voice heartens callers. Facilitative questions leading toward concrete solutions help reinforce coping: "What people (or places, or interests) help you when you're feeling this way? Would they help you now?"

Don't ask "Why?" Even though it is an open-ended question, it serves no useful purpose, and invokes exactly those universal issues that callers are struggling with. Callers will be frustrated because they probably do not have the answers.

Remain With the Caller. No matter how skillfully the nurse establishes a trusting relationship, if the caller is cut off, the chance for intervention is lost. Callers in crisis need immediate support. Asking them to hang up and redial another agency is insensitive and risky. It may evoke feelings of abandonment. Instead, if suicide prevention or poison control hot lines are available in your community, install telephone lines with conference call capability. Conference calls provide instantaneous interface and continuity with the appropriate agency, facilitate call transfer, and shunt time-consuming calls safely and effectively to appropriate agencies. When a suicidal call comes in, and if the case does not require medical intervention, you may place a conference call to a suicide prevention agency after building trust with the client. Counselor, caller, and nurse can then all talk together. The conference call provides a temporary lifeline until the nurse feels confident that the counselor has gained the caller's trust. Conference calls demonstrate sensitivity while eliminating accidental disconnection and inadvertent abandonment.

In rural communities without suicide prevention agencies, nurses may have to handle suicide calls on their own. Under these conditions, it may be necessary to devote considerable time and emotional energy to these calls. If a suicidal call comes in, stay with the caller. Write notes to co-workers so that they can take other calls and perform tasks such as contacting relatives, obtaining addresses, or arranging for a telephone trace (Neville & Barnes, 1985). Facilities that encounter suicidal calls in addition to routine telephone triage require administrative support, adequate staffing, conference call capability, and specialized crisis intervention training. Develop a protocol for tracing calls. Check with police or EMD agencies for the best way to proceed.

Data Collection: Assessing Risk of Lethal Outcome

The concept of lethality was developed in the suicide prevention field. It means the likelihood that suicide will occur. There are two measures of lethality: predictors and indicators. Predictors include lack of resources, a plan, and a history of prior attempts. Indicators include risk factors such as second-party calls, alcohol and drug abuse, age, sex, stress, symptoms of depression, lifestyle and others. Of this group of risk factors, second-party calls and alcohol/drug abuse carry the greatest risk. However, research has shown that "current suicide plan . . . prior suicidal behaviors . . . and [lack of] resources" are factors which "identify those who are at much greater risk of suicide," within the next 2 years (California Helper's Handbook, 1992, p. 27). Suicidal behavior can be further divided into three levels of lethality: suicidal thoughts, suicidal threats, and suicide attempts. Suicide risk can be classified as high, moderate, or low. For example, ideation is low, threats are moderate, and attempts are high.

All suicide calls are potentially serious. In Marin County, California, for example, 40% of all calls are truly suicidal. In the remaining 60%, callers' problems include feelings of loss and relationship problems. Many calls to suicide prevention are "maintenance calls" or repeat callers who need ongoing support (R. Allen, personal communication, February, 1992).

The nurse assesses lethality through expert *direct* questioning. After establishing trust, ask directly whether the client plans to commit suicide.

Ask about the intended method and its availability. Strive for concrete responses. The more risk factors that apply to the situation, the more likely the outcome could be lethal. The lethality scale can be used to form the basis of a protocol for suicide (ideation, plan, and in process). If the threat to life is not immediate, help the client explore feelings using more open-ended questions and counseling techniques. Explore the following risk factors:

Lack of Resources. Resources are any emotional, financial, or social strengths that give life meaning and enhance its quality. The most obvious resources are friends, family, co-workers, and professional helpers. As the number of *meaningful* relationships increase, the risk of suicide decreases. Other resources are affiliation with a religion, children, a satisfying job, interests, hobbies, or pets. The fewer the resources, the higher the lethality risk.

Method/Plan. The deadliness of the proposed method, the availability of the means, and other details provide clues about whether suicide is imminent. Highly lethal methods include shooting, hanging, drowning, carbon monoxide poisoning, crashing a car, jumping off a bridge or building, burning oneself, barbiturates, and high doses of aspirin or acetaminophen. Less lethal methods include natural gas, certain nonprescription drugs, tranquilizers, and wrist-slashing. Ask how available the method is. If the caller is holding a loaded gun, the situation is highly lethal. If the caller has made preparations such as suicide notes, changing or making out a will, or setting a time, suicide becomes extremely likely (R. Allen, personal communication, February, 1992). If, however, the caller has a plan but no gun or is only thinking about suicide, the lethality risk may be low.

History of Prior Suicide Attempts. More than half of all people making suicide attempts have a history of at least one prior attempt. Experts feel this phenomenon may be a result of callers having broken their own taboo. Any history of a previous suicide attempt increases the client's risk by a factor of 40 (R. Allen, Personal Communication, February, 1992). Suicide attempts are more likely in the first years following previous attempts. Family history, such as a parent's or sibling's suicide, is considered a self-destructive modeling pattern which increases risk.

Second-Party Calls. Second-party calls from concerned friends or family of a potential suicide victim are a serious prognosticator of a high-risk situation. Follow up on these calls, as they are early warning signs of potentially lethal conditions.

Alcohol or Drug Use. Alcohol increases lethality because it lessens inhibitions, enabling the person to "act out" more easily. It also increases feelings of helplessness and hopelessness and potentiates the lethality of other drugs.

Age and Sex. Generally, suicide rates increase with age. Although youthful suicides are on the rise, the elderly are more at risk for suicide. Women are three times more likely to *attempt* suicide than men, while men are twice as likely to *complete* suicide. Older men are at the highest risk, followed by older women, and then young men. Young women are at least risk (R. Allen, Personal Communication, 1992).

Recent Stress. Divorce, separation, being fired or retiring, impending surgery or illness, accidents, legal threats, and loss of money are sources of stress. Interestingly, even a recent promotion or increased responsibilities can lead to suicidal threats.

Symptoms of Depression. Insomnia, weight loss, anorexia, apathy, lack of interest in life, hopeless or helpless feelings, and psychological and physical exhaustion are symptoms related to depression and linked with suicide. Psychotic and agitated states—tension, anxiety, guilt, rage, hostility, restlessness, and pressured speech—may also be related to suicide. (R. Allen, Personal Communication, 1992)

Medical Status. Many suicidal callers have a history of physical complaints, real or imagined chronic disease, or pain. Chronic medical problems can cause deterioration of relationships with medical personnel, hospitals, and family, thus increasing lethality risk. (R. Allen, Personal Communication, 1992)

Life-Style. Persons who live transient existences or who frequently change jobs, relationships, and living situations are considered at risk. Homosexuals have a six times higher risk than heterosexuals, and transvestites, drug abusers, alcoholics, and loners are also at higher risk for suicide. Physician's wives, physicians, nurses, female pharmacists, dentists, and therapists are at high risk (Allen, 1989).

Season/Day/Place. Spring and fall are more likely times of suicide attempts. People often choose Mondays for attempts. Most suicides occur in the home. (R. Allen, Personal Communication, 1992)

Diagnosis

Like all protocols, the lethality scale should be used judiciously. Because each category means something different to each individual caller, it is hard to weigh each risk equally. However, remember that second party calls, alcohol and drug abuse carry greater risk among the indicator factors. Even in the absence of predictors, enough indicators may express a high risk suicide call. Thus, suicide prevention agencies have no rigid rules about lethality scores for indicators, and do not rely on a numerical score per call. They suggest using "informed intuition" plus the predictors and indicators to assess an overall risk of high, moderate, or low (L. Brown, personal communication, September 25, 1992). The lethality score then becomes part of the working diagnosis. Thus, a client who says, "Sometimes I wonder whether ending it all might not be easier all around" would be assessed as a person with "suicidal ideation and low risk," whereas someone who says she is going to jump off a bridge would be described as one who represents a "suicidal threat and high risk." Of course, this method is by no means infallible, and in every case the nurse must use good judgment and err on the side of caution.

Disposition

> *A high school teacher had counseled a student who was suicidal, securing a promise that if the student ever felt suicidal, she would call the teacher. Two years later, the same student called long distance from college, pills in hand, and was able to talk through the feelings with the counselor and overcome the urge to kill herself. (R. Allen, personal communication, February 1992)*

This story demonstrates the power of a contract. The goal in any suicide call is to have the client stop destructive behavior and adopt a new behavior. A contract, or "no-suicide pact," can facilitate compliance. It is an agreement which results from negotiation, and both nurse and client must accept it. For clients to "own" the contract, they should repeat it back out loud. Experts say that if callers refuse to make any pact or are intoxicated or high on drugs, the risk increases (R. Allen, Personal Communication, 1992). Neville and Barnes (1985) give as an example a client who says, "I will not kill myself unless my husband leaves me" (p. 16). In this case, they recommend pointing out that the client is allowing someone else to control whether she lives or dies, and to make a countersuggestion: "I will not kill myself within the next week no matter what happens" (p. 19). However, Allen (Personal Communication, 1992) points out that such a contract may not be realistic, suggesting that "Sometimes an 'incremental contract' is more realistic," e.g., "I will not do anything to harm myself until I see my therapist," or "talk to my minister," or "for the next two hours." Clients may be more amenable to a contract not to commit suicide within a certain period of time—before morning, for example. If this is the case, try to have them agree to call you again before that time. Allen also suggests making an overall contingency plan such as: "If I feel like acting on suicidal feelings I will contact Suicide Prevention." She states that some suicide prevention counselors ask callers to place follow-up calls at two-hour intervals. For example, they might ask the caller to "keep calling back until you reach a counselor with whom you feel comfortable talking." Allen stresses the importance of "client ownership" of the contract—restating it in their own words, perhaps altering it in some way that suits their needs. It is not desirable for the caller to mechanically repeat what the counselor has suggested as a contract, because it indicates client passivity and failure to participate in the contract process. Strive for the most life-enhancing contract possible.

Suicide and Homicide

A 30-year-old man called from a Holiday Inn lobby saying he had a gun and "voices were telling him to kill people." Police were notified by 911. The nurse kept him on the line until the police located him.

Like the suicidal caller, homicidal callers are ambivalent about their desperate plans. Unconsciously, they want to be stopped. In such cases, it is standard practice to have a co-worker place a call to police while the first responder remains on the phone with the caller. Such calls require resourcefulness, perseverance, and creativity to keep callers talking. Role-playing homicide calls will develop these skills.

Drug and Alcohol Crises

In communities with high drug abuse, be alert to calls that reveal a threat to life. For example, one cocaine hot line handles 1500 to 1600 calls per month relating to all drugs, including cocaine. Most callers are seeking information, but a small number (about 3 to 4 calls) are either suicidal, homicidal, medical, or psychological emergencies. Drug abusers are extremely unpredictable and may be disoriented or psychotic. Expect impaired judgment, noncompliance, and disorientation. Listen to background sounds for clues in locating clients.

Suicidal and homicidal calls impose great stress on nurses. Some report that these calls make them feel "impotent and depressed" (Wheeler, 1989). Supportive debriefing sessions help alleviate feelings of helplessness. Reviewing calls is useful for staff development as well. Additional training is often available from local suicide prevention agencies.

MEDICAL CRISIS INTERVENTION

The nurse must know how to recognize an emergency and how to respond to one calmly, quickly, and effectively. Training develops these skills.

What Is A Crisis?

Determining whether a crisis exists is much easier in person than by phone. Experts differ in their definitions of what constitutes a crisis or emergency. For example, The American College of Emergency Physicians (ACEP) defines an *emergency* as "the onset of a medical condition manifesting itself by symptoms of sufficient severity that the absence of immediate medical attention could reasonably be expected by a prudent layperson, possessing an average knowledge of health and medicine, to result in placing health in jeopardy; serious impairment to bodily functions; serious dysfunction of any bodily organ or part; or development or continuance of severe pain" (pp. 97–98). ACEP defines the following conditions as emergent:

> Any condition resulting in admission of the patient to a hospital within 24 hours.
>
> Evaluation or repair of acute (less than 72 hours) trauma.
>
> Relief of severe pain.
>
> Evaluation and/or treatment of acute infection.
>
> Obstetrical crises and/or labor.
>
> Hemorrhage or threat of hemorrhage.
>
> Shock or impending shock.
>
> Investigation and management of suspected abuse or neglect of person which, if not interrupted, could result in temporary or permanent physical or psychological harm.
>
> Decompensation or threat of decompensation of vital functions such as sensorium, respiration, circulation, excretion, mobility or sensory organs.
>
> Management of a patient suspected to be suffering from mental illness and posing an apparent danger to the safety of himself, herself, or others. (Annals of Emergency Medicine, 1988, p. 98)

While ACEP defines what an emergency is, Derlet and Nishio (1990) describe a situation in which a triage system defines which clients are not suffering from an emergency. They report that the ED at the University of California at Davis adopted a policy in 1988 of refusing treatment to walk-in clients unless triage nurses determined that the clients were experiencing a genuine emergency. The purpose of this policy was to reduce demand on the ED for treatment of minor complaints. At the triage area, nurses screened clients for vital signs, took a brief history, and examined them, concentrating on the chief complaint. If vital signs fell within acceptable parameters, and if clients had one of 50 minor complaints, they were referred to an assistance desk, where a receptionist gave them information about other treatment options, including information about insurance. All other clients were seen in the ED. The triage guidelines were conservative, excluding, for example, abdominal and chest pain from the list of minor complaints. Nearly 20% of walk-in clients were referred elsewhere. The authors note that "resources were better focused on caring for remaining patients" (p. 267) and that those referred away from the ED "appeared not to be harmed by this system" (p. 268).

Offering a psychological perspective, Stanhope and Lancaster (1988) characterize a crisis as a disequilibrium and note that "people in crisis feel helpless and often desire assistance in relieving their misery" (p. 650). They further suggest that crises offer an opportunity for growth and the development of new coping mechanisms.

In contrast to the medical, resource-sparing, and psychological definitions of emergency, Colman and Robboy (1980) report that laypersons define emergencies by the social situation surrounding the event more than by the actual symptoms presented. Social definitions are more complex than medical definitions and include such factors as social class, age, ethnicity, sex, religion, and distance from help. These factors alter perceptions and intensify responses to emergencies. Thus, the caller's perception of what constitutes an emergency may differ widely from that of the nurse.

Colman and Robboy (1980) synthesize a number of studies which found that people in different cultural, ethnic, and socioeconomic groups experience pain differently and regard symptoms of illness with differing degrees of stoicism or urgency. For example, people in lower socioeconomic groups ignored chest pain, fainting spells, and chronic cough while those in middle- and upper-income groups perceived them as urgencies requiring medical intervention. Nurses should be alert to the possibility that social or cultural factors may influence a client's response to a possible emergency, but they should also guard against stereotyping.

Not surprisingly, social standing heightens others' perceptions of emergencies. For example, if the victim is famous, wealthy, or simply beautiful, an illness or accident is more likely to be defined as an emergency. Colman and Robboy (1980) cite one study in which ambulance crews exhibited the highest competency when transporting prominent citizens.

The victim's age is also a major influence. Children's symptoms were more often perceived as emergencies when compared to adults, and sick children elicited greater first aid efforts from ambulance crews. Likewise, ED staff performed resuscitation longer and more aggressively on young victims as compared with the elderly (Colman and Robboy, 1980).

In many cases, even before the physician has confirmed their emergency status, victims are accorded the social status of being sick or injured. For example, even though they may only have minor injuries, car accident victims are perceived as emergencies. This is not an unreasonable assumption considering the possibility of internal injuries. Location affects perceptions of emergencies. The farther the distance to aid, the more likely the event is to be defined as an emergency. Although laypersons may be unaware of the "golden hour" concept, most instinctively feel vulnerable when emergency help is remote.

Develop a sensitivity to social interpretations of emergency and to the possibility of differences among individuals and cultural groups in their reaction to emergencies. Factor in the client response when making a global assessment using SAVED. Such information can foster awareness of prejudices. This awareness can be critical when overriding protocols to upgrade emergency status.

Be alert to common misconceptions. For example, a caller might minimize chest pains because she first experienced them while watching television rather than while shoveling snow. Eisenberg (1986) found that, prior to collapse, victims of cardiac arrest were sleeping 27% of the time, resting 45% of the time, and involved in heavy work or sexual relations only 1% of the time. Finally, remember that in the clinic and emergency department, true emergency-level calls are still uncommon. Even emergency medical dispatchers estimate that only about 1 in 10 calls is a true life-threatening emergency, while in the pediatric setting, 50% of callers need advice, 47% need office visits, and only 3% of all calls are true emergencies (Schmitt, 1980).

A final caution is in order in the matter of defining an emergency. Some HMOs have limited access to emergency care because of cost considerations. For example, a survey of seven HMOs in the Milwaukee area (Kerr, 1986) found that the HMOs did not include information about calling paramedics or an ambulance in their client information brochures. These HMOs permitted clients to call the nearest ED in life-threatening situations, but directed them to call their physicians first if the situation was not life-threatening. "They are warned that if they go to an ED without authorization and in a nonlife-threatening situation, their bill will not be paid by the HMO. The client thus is confronted with the nearly impossible situation of having to decide whether he is dying" (p. 727) and thus may lose valuable time by calling the physician to get permission for ED treatment.

In response, one HMO system has instituted a cooperative agreement with another institution and has developed a 24-hour emergency triage system for clients to help alleviate the confusion about where to turn in a crisis (Daley, Leaning, & Braen, 1988). The American College of Emergency Physicians (1988) has recognized the problem and issued a document stating that the ACEP "believes that access to emergency care must be readily available to every person without regard to ability to pay or the nature of insurance coverage" (pp. 97-98). ACEP issued a set of recommendations to help implement this position, including one which states: "Claims analyses should be based upon the prospective definition of a bona fide emergency rather than the discharge diagnosis" (p. 97).

Telephone triage nurses, especially those in HMOs, must educate themselves about a possibly complex list of emergency providers, including 911, paramedics, and various EDs, in order to make the safest choice for the client without being constrained by cost considerations. In any case, speedy dispatch may be cost-saving as well as lifesaving in the long run. One study (Valenzuela et al., 1990) points out that effective prehospital care for cardiopulmonary arrest can reduce the need for costly heart transplants.

General Rules

To a certain extent, in handling crisis calls, nurses can act as intermediaries between clients and emergency medical systems such as 911, poison control, suicide prevention, and rape crisis lines. Remember that community standards vary widely and not all EMDs are highly trained. In such cases, learning crisis intervention principles can be lifesaving.

Stay with the Caller. This approach is based on years of experience in the field. Clawson maintains that "when someone calls in a crisis, that call becomes our responsibility" ("60 Minutes," December 25, 1988). Most medical dispatchers feel that it is dangerous to ask panic-stricken callers to hang up and redial another agency. They fear the outcome may result in further catastrophe. According to Bill MacMurray of the Marin County Emergency Dispatch Center (Personal Communication, 1992):

- Some callers might simply "load up" the victim and drive in, creating potential for further injury.
- Suicidal callers might feel that they are getting the runaround or feel abandoned, possibly leading to a suicide attempt.
- Callers who are alone in a life-threatening situation may hang up to redial, lose consciousness, and be unreachable by medical aid.

Community standards and resources will determine the course of action for such calls. Three possible options are:

1. Direct ring-through. This procedure allows the transfer of callers to the correct agencies without redialing by the caller.
2. Conference call. By this method, the telephone triage nurse places a call to the appropriate agency (poison control, suicide prevention, or 911) and then acts as intermediary between agency and caller.
3. Acting as first responder in the absence of any agency or more highly trained personnel.

Direct ring-through and conference calls allow immediate, direct access. Conference calls allow caller, nurse, and staff to communicate simultaneously;

nurses can remain with callers until the agency has taken over the call. They also allow for feedback to nurses, who often do not know call outcomes. Before such procedures can be implemented, telephones must be equipped for conference call or ring-through capability, and guidelines for jurisdiction for out-of-area calls must be in place so that calls are expedited rather than misdirected.

At facilities which lack direct ring-through or conference call capability, nurses may be forced to act as intermediaries between callers and dispatchers who are sending aid, relaying information back and forth between two parties, and giving pre-arrival instructions to callers. Be aware that this approach introduces risks of misinterpretation and errors, especially if callers are emotionally upset, very young, elderly, or not proficient in English. Also be aware that callers may call from areas which are not part of your 911 jurisdiction. Work out contingency plans for such eventualities with the medical dispatch agency to avoid bureaucratic snags.

Consider Distance and Traffic Flow. Where distance or traffic present an obstacle, upgrade the urgency rating. In rural areas, where distances to emergency departments are greater, urgencies are upgraded to emergencies and emergencies to life-threatening emergencies. This rule applies to inner-city hospitals as well, when rush hour traffic creates gridlock. *Thus, the farther from medical intervention the victim, the more urgent the situation, and the shorter the acceptable time frame for arrival (Clauson & Dernocoeur, 1988).*

Second-Party Calls as an Indicator of High Acuity. The fact that someone is making the call for the victim may itself be an indicator of urgency, as illustrated by the following case histories:

> *The wife of a 40-year-old man called, stating that he had been diagnosed that morning with pneumonia. She said he was having difficulty breathing. He was on antibiotics and had no fever. The man suffered a cardiac arrest and died within 3 hours of his arrival in the emergency department. (Wheeler, 1989)*
>
> *The wife of a 30-year-old man called stating that he had collapsed during sexual intercourse and wasn't breathing. The man died of a dissecting aortic aneurysm. (Wheeler, 1989)*
>
> *A 74-year-old man called about his wife, saying that she had vomited blood, was sweating profusely, and complaining of mild chest pain and shortness of breath. (Wheeler, 1989)*

First Responder Skills Development

A recent survey (Wheeler, 1989) demonstrated that on rare occasions, ED nurses receive calls in which the caller's life is at risk, possibly because the caller found the 911 lines busy, as they often are in large cities (see "Curse of 911," 1990). HMO advice nurses frequently relate that some members contact them prior to calling 911, to be sure that ambulance expenses will be paid for.

Crisis intervention requires expert-level knowledge, sophistication, resourcefulness, and what Benner (1984, p. 109) characterizes as the "effective management of rapidly changing situations." Nurses must respond quickly and effectively in the face of emotional extremes: shock, hysteria, panic, even hostility. Because clients are fearful, *the manner of communication is as important as the information communicated*. Clear, simple directives, and concrete, congruent, and contractual communications enable clients to act, and action is the antidote to fear.

Data Collection. In a crisis, the address and phone number are more important than a name. This information enables the nurse to relocate callers in case of disconnection. Always determine *the address from which the call is made*. Never assume that the call is being made from home. In emergencies, people sometimes panic and give their home address even though they are calling from a restaurant or phone booth. Clawson and Dernocoeur (1988) recommend collecting the following essential data: chief complaint, age, and breathing and consciousness status—in that order. These "Four Commandments" can be built into special logs or flow charts as checkboxes or key words to expedite documentation and promote quality assurance.

After collecting the Four Commandments, obtain additional information about the victim's condition, and landmarks and cross streets. Ask callers to turn on house lights, collect medications, and lock up animals which might attack the paramedics. Determine the type of equipment and personnel to send. For example, the "jaws of life" (used to extricate accident victims from cars) are not standard equipment on all paramedic rigs and must be specifically requested (Clawson and Dernocoeur, 1988).

Coaching. Although callers in crisis seem unlikely candidates for coaching over the telephone, excellent outcomes are possible (Kellerman, Hackman, & Somes, 1989). Clawson feels the key lies in the ability to focus the client's attention by *anticipating predictable periods of panic and repeating certain calming and directive phrases.* This technique is grounded in actions which people unconsciously and instinctively perform in crises. (See Clawson and Dernocoeur, 1988, for a complete description of pre-arrival instructions and techniques.) Most trained medical dispatchers read verbatim from pre-arrival instructions.

As with any unfamiliar procedure, explain actions to alleviate anxiety and increase collaboration. For example: "I must leave the line to contact the ambulance. *Don't hang up.* I'll be back in a moment." Remind the caller frequently that help is on the way and you will stay on the line until help arrives.

Not all callers are willing or able to perform measures such as CPR or the Heimlich maneuver. Some frail elderly may be unwilling or unable physically to perform CPR (Eisenberg, 1985a). If they do not wish to aid the victim, perhaps they can quickly find someone who will. Clawson and Dernocoeur (1988) discourage asking the caller if they wish to help, as this approach invites inaction.

Anticipating Panic and Hysteria. Clawson and Dernocoeur (1988) have found that in a crisis, callers have predictable responses and patterns. They tend to experience panic and hysteria at three predictable points:

1. When the victim is brought to the phone and the caller again visually confronts the seriousness of the situation.
2. When the caller finds that vital signs (breathing and pulse) are absent.
3. When the treatment measures seem ineffective.

In the case of a near drowning, for example, the mother may leave the child to call for help. She feels renewed panic and terror when she returns to the child who is now blue and lifeless. Her behavior is predictable and normal under the circumstances. Learn to anticipate panic reactions before they happen to maintain control of the call.

Repetitive Persistence. When anticipating panic is insufficient to forestall it and asking open-ended questions to build trust would waste valuable time, repetitive persistence will usually bring clients around (Clawson & Dernocoeur, 1988). This technique is designed to calm hysterical clients, forge the trust necessary for effective coaching, and facilitate quick action. It consists of frequent word-for-word repetition of instructions in a calm, confident manner. The repetition helps to center and focus the caller, and the calm, authoritative manner engenders trust. Now focused and in control, the caller is receptive to coaching. Repetitive persistence works quickly, an advantage in crisis intervention, when speed is crucial. This technique is part of the standard, concrete, first aid coaching that dispatchers call "pre-arrival instructions" and analogous to "crash cards," the quick directions given prior to paramedics' arrival.

Benefits of CPR Coaching. Medical dispatchers relate that CPR coaching benefits staff and callers as well as victims. Even if attempts to revive victims are unsuccessful, the act of performing CPR helps callers to feel a sense of control and to come to terms with a death later on. In the case of children, and especially babies who have died of sudden infant death syndrome, parents are comforted by the fact that they did everything possible. Dispatchers report that despite initial resistance, training has raised staff self-esteem and morale. (B. MacMurray, Personal Communication, 1992)

Crisis intervention requires instant, high-level response. Telephone triage nurses should have frequent CPR drills and an ongoing program to refine skills in medical and psychological crisis intervention. Role-playing is an excellent practice to strengthen these skills. This discussion of crisis intervention techniques, however, is not intended as a substitute for in-depth, well-developed training programs.

Disposition

The two interventions for emergent or urgent level calls are (1) paramedic or ambulance transport and (2) immediate transport by car to the nearest emergency department. Basic life support or advanced life support is reserved for the most urgent of calls. Transport by car is an option only if the caller can safely drive or be driven the distance within the appropriate time frame. Callers require ambulance transport if they appear too panic-stricken or distracted to drive or are not within 20 minutes of the hospital.

Poison Control Calls

Studies of poison hot lines report obstacles that plague many who practice in telephone triage—such as hearing-impaired callers, difficulty in visualizing the situation, being required to work through intermediaries, and directing laypersons in emergency procedures (Broadhead, 1986). One interesting finding is that callers to poison control are likely to have hidden agendas. Callers may withhold information because of embarrassment or guilt. Some people mask the fact that they are calling about a pet; parents may feel that they have been irresponsible.

Approximately 15% of all calls are from physicians and other health care providers who hide their identities. They are embarrassed about not knowing how to manage a poisoning or a situation that they caused. In one instance, an office nurse called for a dentist regarding a severe reaction to lidocaine (Broadhead, 1986). Physicians, pharmacists, nurses, and dentists, motivated by the desire to protect client confidentiality or themselves, may be reluctant to volunteer information.

It is estimated that about 8% of all poison control calls involve suicide attempts (Broadhead, 1986). Suicidal callers may call seeking information about lethal dosages. Suspect callers who ask about hypothetical situations or who conceal the reasons for the call. These may be clues to suicidal intent. Broadhead tells of a caller who asked what would happen if someone took "a bottle of Compose or Sominex." Assuming that they were calling in good faith, and failing to sense the danger, the nurse answered the question rather than confronting the issue of suicide. The caller hung up when the nurse left the line momentarily to answer another call.

Another communications barrier is the use of colloquialisms or slang. For example, one caller to poison control said that her house had been "bombed" by the landlord. A lengthy, confusing conversation ensued, until the nurse realized that the house had been fumigated (Broadhead, 1986). Another caller to an ED asked whether "gas could kill you." The nurse, thinking the caller was referring to flatus, gave a routine response, realizing too late that the caller was referring to lethal gases.

Poison-related calls require expert questioning techniques. If the call sounds suspect, do not hesitate to ask, "Are you thinking of committing suicide?" Other key questions or directives include:

> "What is your relationship to the victim?"
>
> "Exactly what is the situation?"
>
> "Where are you calling from?"
>
> "Exactly how many pills are missing?"
>
> "How long ago did you notice a change in behavior?"
>
> "Get the bottle and spell out the name of the ingredients for me."

Most poison control hot lines screen out nonurgent calls and refer only about 10% of callers to the emergency department (Broadhead, 1986). Callers receive instruction in administering emergency self-treatment, an effective approach. Poison control staff have found that sometimes a directive and forceful manner must be employed to insure caller compliance. For example, parents may panic and become uncooperative when told to give ipecac to their fearful, uncooperative child to induce vomiting. Brief, concrete explanations help ensure compliance. For example, you might say, "By giving the ipecac immediately, you will reduce the chance of life-threatening complications."

The timing of the call may be an important indicator of acuity. From a study (Amitai, Mitchell, Carrel, Luciw, & Lovejoy, 1987) a rule of thumb might be: calls received within 10 minutes of ingestion are most likely accidental ingestions by children; whereas, calls received 30 minutes or more after ingestion may indicate intentional poisonings in adults. Most calls, however, came within the first 10 minutes after exposure. Researchers also found that ipecac was available in 59% of the homes of callers with children younger than 5 years, and that among children whose households had ipecac, significantly fewer had to be referred to the hospital. The study concluded that poison exposures can be managed effectively at home if treated promptly.

With poisoning calls, use direct ring-through or conference calls to the poison control center when possible. Because relaying information from the caller to poison control is cumbersome, time-consuming and ineffective, poison control staff prefer to have direct contact with callers. The final disposition rests with poison control, but always document the call and disposition.

EXPECTED DEATH CALLS

Although studies have not been performed, some feel that the number of home deaths has increased in the last 10 years. This phenomenon may be due to cost containment efforts, to the hospice movement, and to increased home health care. Expected death calls—those involving clients who are expected to die at home—may range from cardiac invalids to people with AIDS.

After collecting the Four Commandments, ask if the death was expected. If death was anticipated, ask the client's diagnosis. Instruct callers in how to discern the signs of death: blank stare, no breathing, no pulse, no movement, no response upon being shaken, loss of bowel or bladder contents, relaxed jaw. Depending on local standards, a nurse, a paramedic, or a physician must pronounce the client dead. Some hospice nurses will come when death has occurred and are available on a 24-hour basis. They will notify the doctor and the funeral home so there is no hurry or need to panic.

As appropriate, inform medical dispatchers of the expected death status and diagnosis, especially in cases of AIDS. Include the circumstances of the death, signs of death, diagnosis, and length of illness. Such information can aid dispatchers in setting priorities. For example, trained EMDs have a protocol for "obvious death" which limits the number of responding vehicles. To send paramedics on each call is wasteful and dangerous. It is wasteful, because every paramedic intervention is very costly. Overuse of paramedics may deplete resources at a critical moment. Prudence is especially important in urban areas where medical dispatchers are forced to allot limited numbers of vehicles and personnel carefully.

Crisis intervention requires exceptional skill in communication, leadership, and setting priorities to insure the safe, effective disposition of problems and to prevent inadvertent abandonment of clients. In this area of greatest challenge, as nowhere else, telephone triage is an art and a lifesaving tool. See Appendices for Emergency Department protocol lists and a crisis-level protocol.

CHAPTER 7

EXERCISE 1: EFFECTIVE AND INEFFECTIVE CRISIS INTERVENTION TECHNIQUES

OBJECTIVE: To distinguish between effective and ineffective intervention techniques.

METHOD: Label each of the following approaches as ineffective (I) or effective (E).

______ 1. Offer platitudes
______ 2. Identify self
______ 3. Lie
______ 4. Act judgmental
______ 5. Express a desire to help
______ 6. Give advice
______ 7. Use stock phrases
______ 8. Use lay terms
______ 9. Criticize
______ 10. Listen intently
______ 11. Act interested and warm

EXERCISE 2: STATEMENT MATCHING

The following techniques are not meant to be followed verbatim or in any specific order. The more natural and spontaneous communications are, the better.

OBJECTIVE: To apply more effective interview techniques.

METHOD: Match the categories in Column A with the examples in Column B.

COLUMN A	COLUMN B
CATEGORIES	EXAMPLES
1. LETHALITY ASSESSMENT	_____ A I hear you. It's been hard. You've been through a lot. Uh-huh. Tell me about it. What (How) are you feeling?
2. SELF-DISCLOSURE	_____ B Many people feel suicidal when . . . It's normal to feel suicidal when . . .
3. SELF-EXPRESSION	_____ C One time I felt suicidal. I once considered committing suicide.
4. IMMEDIACY/SPECIFICITY	_____ D Your story makes me feel very sad. What a sad story.
5. NORMALIZING	_____ E Are you thinking of suicide? Do you want to kill yourself? How do you plan to do it? How many pills do you have? Is your gun loaded?
6. ATTENDING	_____ F How are you feeling right now? What do you want from me right now? What things have worked for you in the past?

EXERCISE 3: LETHALITY ASSESSMENT

OBJECTIVE: To assess levels of lethality.

METHOD: Using the lethality scale, assess the suicide risk for the following callers. Give a plus (+) for each risk factor on the lethality scale that applies to the caller, and a minus (−) for each risk factor that does not apply. If case description does not address a certain factor (i.e., season, date, place), assign a minus.

The overall lethality assessment is reached by combining the presence of predictors with indicators. In general, the more indicators present—even without predictors—the higher the risk.

This exercise is not intended as a substitute for in-depth training, which is available through suicide prevention agencies.

EXAMPLE:

A 65-year-old male calls stating he is depressed over his wife's death last week. He states he is employed and currently seeing a therapist. He wants help and denies that he has a suicide plan. History of previous suicide attempts. He sounds inebriated and admits to heavy drinking.

Predictors:

LACK OF RESOURCES	−
PLAN	−
PRIOR ATTEMPTS	+

Indicators:

ALCOHOL/DRUGS	+
2ND PARTY CALL	−
SYMPTOMS	+
STRESS	+
SEX	+
AGE	+
MEDICAL PROBLEMS	−
LIFE-STYLE	−
SEASON/DAY/PLACE	−
LETHALITY	High

CASE STUDY 1

A mother calls regarding her 19-year-old daughter who has suicidal ideation with a history of two previous attempts—one wrist slashing and one barbiturate overdose within the last two years. Possibly other attempts. Daughter is single, employed and is close to her brother, who is 20. Parents are involved and concerned. The daughter smokes marijuana often, is a skydiver and recently almost died in a sky diving accident. The mother reports her daughter is very depressed, crying a lot.

Predictors:

LACK OF RESOURCES

PLAN

PRIOR ATTEMPTS

Indicators:

ALCOHOL/DRUGS

2ND PARTY CALL

SYMPTOMS

STRESS

SEX

AGE

MEDICAL PROBLEMS

LIFE-STYLE

SEASON/DAY/PLACE

LETHALITY

CASE STUDY 2

A 55-year-old woman calls regarding symptoms of depression. She states she is eating and sleeping normally, but she feels extremely depressed. She says she and her husband have history of marital discord. She has few relatives but one close friend. Her mother-in-law is a source of stress and is due to visit. She denies thinking about suicide and is seeking marriage counseling.

Predictors:

LACK OF RESOURCES

PLAN

PRIOR ATTEMPTS

Indicators:

ALCOHOL/DRUGS

2ND PARTY CALL

SYMPTOMS

STRESS

SEX

AGE

MEDICAL PROBLEMS

LIFE-STYLE

SEASON/DAY/PLACE

LETHALITY

CASE STUDY 3

A 60-year-old woman calls stating she is having weird feelings just like the last time she attempted suicide. She has a large number of barbiturates. She feels she will not live through the day. Five weeks ago she took a large number and variety of pills and ended up in the hospital. She states she has no friends or relatives, her money is running out, and she is currently living on her savings. She can no longer work due to health problems.

Predictors:

LACK OF RESOURCES

PLAN

PRIOR ATTEMPTS

Indicators:

ALCOHOL/DRUGS

2ND PARTY CALL

SYMPTOMS

STRESS

SEX

AGE

MEDICAL PROBLEMS

LIFE-STYLE

SEASON/DAY/PLACE

LETHALITY

CASE STUDY 4

A 30-year-old male calls, sounding inebriated. He states he wants to kill himself. He was recently diagnosed with AIDS. He is estranged from his family and has lost his job. He has been drinking and has a bottle of Seconal pills.

Predictors:

LACK OF RESOURCES

PLAN

PRIOR ATTEMPTS

Indicators:

ALCOHOL/DRUGS

2ND PARTY CALL

SYMPTOMS

STRESS

SEX

AGE

MEDICAL PROBLEMS

LIFE-STYLE

SEASON/DAY/PLACE

LETHALITY

CASE STUDY 5

A 28-year-old-male calls regarding suicidal ideation. He states he is depressed and has not slept or eaten for several days. He is separating from his wife and unemployed. He has two children. He has lost his job and car, and his wife just left him last night.

Predictors:

LACK OF RESOURCES

PLAN

PRIOR ATTEMPTS

Indicators:

ALCOHOL/DRUGS

2ND PARTY CALL

SYMPTOMS

STRESS

SEX

AGE

MEDICAL PROBLEMS

LIFE-STYLE

SEASON/DAY/PLACE

LETHALITY

CASE STUDY 6

A 30-year-old white woman is despondent over a pending divorce. She has two children and works as a teacher. She states she has had suicidal thoughts in the past when things went wrong. She is Catholic and has a circle of friends. She sounds inebriated. She is healthy, and eating and sleeping well.

Predictors:

LACK OF RESOURCES

PLAN

PRIOR ATTEMPTS

Indicators:

ALCOHOL/DRUGS

2ND PARTY CALL

SYMPTOMS

STRESS

SEX

AGE

MEDICAL PROBLEMS

LIFE-STYLE

SEASON/DAY/PLACE

LETHALITY

CASE STUDY 7

A 13-year-old girl calls saying she is very depressed. She has congenital multiple facial deformities and has been told that she is going blind. She has one close school friend but feels alienated. She says her parents deny her physical problems. She has a prescription for Tylenol with Codeine™ which she states she intends to take. She states she has thought about suicide and talked with friend about it in the last year. She has written a suicide note to her best friend.

Predictors:

LACK OF RESOURCES

PLAN

PRIOR ATTEMPTS

Indicators:

ALCOHOL/DRUGS

2ND PARTY CALLS

SYMPTOMS

STRESS

SEX

AGE

MEDICAL PROBLEMS

LIFE-STYLE

SEASON/DAY/PLACE

LETHALITY

EXERCISE 4: MULTIPLE CHOICE

OBJECTIVE: To assess overall understanding of telephone triage.

Method: Choose the phrase(s) that best completes each sentence.

_____ 1. The correct order of information needed for medical crisis intervention calls is:
   a. address, age, complaint, phone number
   b. complaint, age, phone number, address
   c. address, phone number, complaint, age

_____ 2. When interviewing the client in a crisis situation the nurse must:
   a. never ask leading questions
   b. ask some leading questions
   c. always ask leading questions

_____ 3. Giving clients a time frame within which they must arrive in the emergency department:
   a. helps insure that they will not arrive too late and that they comprehend the urgency of the situation.
   b. makes little difference in insuring safe, effective, appropriate disposition
   c. fulfills current legal requirements in the state of California

_____ 4. Currently, all emergency nurses are:
   a. trained and qualified to coach callers in CPR, Heimlich maneuvers, and first aid by telephone
   b. able to coach in CPR, Heimlich and first aid from their intuitive knowledge and medical experience in the ED
   c. not trained to coach in CPR, Heimlich, or first aid by telephone

_____ 5. Clients in a crisis situation can be expected to:
   a. always act overly calm (denial)
   b. be responsive to calming techniques and instructions by trained personnel
   c. be irrational and unreasonable

_____ 6. A predictable point when callers tend to panic is:
   a. when the treatment measures fail to revive the victim
   b. when callers realize that they are responsible for the situation
   c. when the caller realizes they should have learned CPR in the past

_____ 7. Denial can be commonly experienced by the:
   a. nurse, caller, and victim
   b. caller and victim
   c. victim

_____ 8. Fifty percent of medical dispatchers are usually:
   a. college-trained personnel with paramedic training
   b. medical personnel who respond to calls for ambulance, fire or police
   c. High school graduates with no medical background

_____ 9. The California training program for medical dispatchers is
   a. 16 hours long and includes CPR coaching
   b. 40 hours long and includes CPR coaching
   c. 90 hours long and does not include CPR coaching

_____ 10. Helpful instructions to callers to facilitate paramedic intervention in crisis calls are:
   a. to hang up the phone immediately after getting instructions
   b. to unlock the front door, turn on porch lights, remove pets, and describe landmarks
   c. to honk the horn loudly to attract a crowd

_____ 11. The group most at risk for completed suicide is:
   a. teenagers
   b. elderly, retired, white male widowers
   c. black, unemployed men between the ages of 15 and 45

_____ 12. Medical dispatchers should:
   a. routinely hang up after giving instructions to the caller so the dispatcher can be ready for the next call
   b. remain with the caller until help arrives
   c. tell the caller to call back if problems arise and then hang up

_____ 13. If there is a suicide in progress, the best approach is for the nurse to:
   a. tell the client to dial 911
   b. stay with caller, try to establish rapport, and then elicit information
   c. refer the caller to suicide prevention and disconnect

_____ 14. Child abuse hot lines, rape hot lines and drug abuse hot lines
   a. do not receive life-threatening calls level
   b. occasionally receive life-threatening calls level
   c. are not set up to deal with life-threatening emergencies

_____ 15. Psychological intervention by telephone is usually:
   a. brief and not emotionally taxing
   b. is not an important function of hot lines
   c. draining emotionally and may be time consuming

_____ 16. Trained medical dispatchers with a high school education are:
   a. not as well-trained or qualified as RNs to coach in first aid
   b. better trained and qualified than RNs in first aid coaching by telephone
   c. risking legal liabilities by coaching in first aid

______ 17. Of the following, the highest indicators of suicide lethality are:
  a. suicide plan, prior suicide attempts, lack of resources
  b. unstable personality, frequent job loss
  c. PMS, recent abortion, job loss

______ 18. The "no-suicide pact" is:
  a. a contract to establish trust and support the client's decision not to commit suicide within a certain time period
  b. a contract with doubtful value to all parties, including the client, nurse, and the health care institution
  c. a paper signed "in house" by suicidal clients

______ 19. Nurses may be placed in the role of first responder in the following circumstances:
  a. when 911 lines are busy
  b. if they work in the HMO setting
  c. when poison control is unavailable

______ 20. The best approach to interviewing the suicidal caller is to:
  a. be sensitive but direct, using concrete and confrontational questioning
  b. talk about the weather or other non-threatening subjects
  c. immediately talk about your brother-in-law's suicide attempt.

ANSWER KEY

EXERCISE 1: EFFECTIVE AND INEFFECTIVE CRISIS INTERVENTION TECHNIQUES

1. I
2. E
3. I
4. I
5. E
6. I
7. I
8. E
9. I
10. E
11. E

EXERCISE 2: STATEMENT MATCHING

1. E
2. C
3. D
4. F
5. B
6. A

EXERCISE 3: LETHALITY ASSESSMENT

CASE STUDY 1

LACK OF RESOURCES	–
PLAN	–
PRIOR ATTEMPTS (two prior attempts)	+
ALCOHOL/DRUGS	+
2ND PARTY CALL	+
SYMPTOMS	+
STRESS	+
SEX	+
AGE	+
MEDICAL PROBLEMS	–
LIFE-STYLE	+
SEASON/DAY/PLACE	–
LETHALITY	HIGH

CASE STUDY 2

LACK OF RESOURCES	–
PLAN	–
PRIOR ATTEMPTS	–
ALCOHOL/DRUGS	–
2ND PARTY CALL	–
SYMPTOMS	+
STRESS	+
SEX	+
AGE	+
MEDICAL PROBLEMS	–
LIFE-STYLE	–
SEASON/DAY/PLACE	–
LETHALITY	MODERATE

CASE STUDY 3

LACK OF RESOURCES	+
PLAN	+
PRIOR ATTEMPTS	+
ALCOHOL/DRUGS	+
2ND PARTY CALL	–
SYMPTOMS	+
STRESS	+
SEX	+
AGE	+
MEDICAL PROBLEMS	+
LIFE-STYLE	+
SEASON/DAY/PLACE	–
LETHALITY	HIGH

CASE STUDY 4

LACK OF RESOURCES	+
PLAN	+
PRIOR ATTEMPTS	–
ALCOHOL/DRUGS	+
2ND PARTY CALL	–
SYMPTOMS	+
STRESS	+
SEX	+
AGE	+
MEDICAL PROBLEMS	+
LIFE-STYLE	+
SEASON/DAY/PLACE	–
LETHALITY	HIGH

CASE STUDY 5

LACK OF RESOURCES	+
PLAN	–
PRIOR ATTEMPTS	–
ALCOHOL/DRUGS	–
2ND PARTY CALL	–
SYMPTOMS	+
STRESS	+
SEX	+
AGE	+
MEDICAL PROBLEMS	–
LIFE-STYLE	–
SEASON/DAY/PLACE	–
LETHALITY	MODERATE

CASE STUDY 6

LACK OF RESOURCES	–
PLAN	–
PRIOR ATTEMPTS	–
ALCOHOL/DRUGS	+
2ND PARTY CALL	–
SYMPTOMS	–
STRESS	+
SEX	+
AGE	+
MEDICAL PROBLEMS	–
LIFE-STYLE	–
SEASON/DAY/PLACE	–
LETHALITY	MODERATE

CASE STUDY 7

LACK OF RESOURCES	+
PLAN	+
PRIOR ATTEMPTS	+
ALCOHOL/DRUGS	–
2ND PARTY CALL	–
SYMPTOMS	+
STRESS	+
SEX	+
AGE	+
MEDICAL PROBLEMS	+
LIFE-STYLE	–
SEASON/DAY/PLACE	–
LETHALITY	HIGH

EXERCISE 4: Multiple Choice

1. C
2. B
3. A
4. C
5. B, C
6. A
7. A
8. C
9. B
10. B
11. B
12. B
13. B
14. B
15. C
16. B
17. A
18. A
19. A, B, C
20. A

APPENDICES

PART I

PROTOCOL BUILDING COMPONENTS: LISTS, SAMPLES, AND PROTOTYPES

APPENDIX A

COMMONLY CALLED PHONE NUMBERS

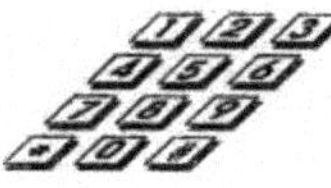

The following is a list of agencies frequently called by telephone triage nurses. Guard against referring someone to the wrong number by updating it every 6 to 12 months, as you would a protocol, adding new programs and correcting changed phone numbers. Ask about mailing lists—some agencies use them to inform clients about changes in services and phone numbers. The list can be developed further by adding days and business hours of services as well as any emergency numbers. Finally, for ease of access, post the list by the telephones.

MEDICAL EMERGENCIES—OUTSIDE LINE

MEDICAL EMERGENCIES—DIRECT LINE

SUICIDE PREVENTION

LOCAL HOSPITALS

PHARMACIES

IN-HOUSE PROGRAMS

NATIONAL AIDS INFORMATION CLEARINGHOUSE **1-800-458-5231**

LOCAL AIDS SUPPORT

ALCOHOLISM

ALATEEN

ALANON

ACOA

ANIMAL CONTROL

BATTERED WOMEN

BLOOD BANK

CHILD ABUSE

DRUG ABUSE

ELDER ABUSE

HOME HEALTH SERVICES

HOSPICE

POISON CONTROL

RAPE CRISIS

SENIOR INFORMATION

APPENDIX B

SUICIDE INTERVENTION (Post near phones)

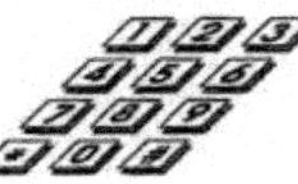

This is a summary of material in *The California Helper's Handbook for Suicide Intervention* (1990). The reader is encouraged to refer to the text for a more complete presentation.

SUMMARY OF KEY INTERVENTION TASKS
Following are the key tasks to perform to lessen the risk of immediate suicide.

ENGAGE the person in a conversation that focuses on his or her feelings. Ask the at-risk individual: "How are you feeling about all of this?"

IDENTIFY if the person is thinking about suicide. Ask the at-risk individual: "Are you thinking about suicide? Are you thinking about killing yourself?"

INQUIRE about the reasons for and against suicide at this point in time. Ask the at-risk individual: "Part of you feels suicide is the only answer, but another part wants to find some other answer. Is that correct?"

ASSESS the degree of risk for suicide at this point in time. Ask the at-risk individual: "I am seeing the risk of you harming yourself as (high, medium, or low) right now. Does that fit with what you are feeling?"

PREVENT the immediate risk by agreeing to a plan with the person. Ask the at-risk individual: "Are we agreed then that you will do a, b, and c, and I will do x and y to prevent the immediate danger?"

SUMMARY OF COMPONENTS OF PREVENTION PLANS
This is a summary of material in *The California Helper's Handbook for Suicide Intervention* (1990). The reader is encouraged to refer to that text for a more detailed discussion. Every good prevention plan should have the following components.

SPECIFICITY
Details about the things to be done must be clearly understood.

LIMITED OBJECTIVES
Your job is to intervene until the immediate danger or threat of suicide has passed or until additional assistance and resources can be accessed.

MUTUALITY
Both you and the person at risk have some things to do.

COMMITMENT

The person at risk agrees not to engage in any self-harming behavior for an agreed upon time period. Ask the person to repeat the agreement.

CRISIS CONTACT

Confirm some arrangement for emergency support if the steps of your plan for action cannot be carried out or if the commitment cannot be maintained until follow-up.

FOLLOW UP

Set the date and time for another meeting between you and the person at risk, or between the person at risk and whatever follow-up resources you have agreed to as part of the prevention plan.

APPENDIX C

MASTER PROTOCOL COLLECTION LIST

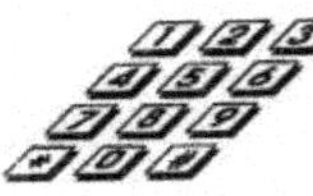

Protocol headings should be arranged alphabetically, use lay language, and have appropriate subheadings. Please note that in certain cases an appropriate protocol may not exist. In these cases, after using SCHOLAR, PAMPER, or ADL, the nurse should refer to the blank protocol containing standing triage policies which can serve as a general guide for questionable cases.

Blank Protocol (use Master Format, Figure 5.7, when no appropriate protocol exists)

Abdominal Pain
- Appendicitis symptoms
- Ectopic pregnancy symptoms
- Hemorrhage symptoms
- Peritonitis symptoms
- Pelvic inflammatory disease symptoms
- Trauma symptoms

Allergy Symptoms
- Mild/moderate
- Anaphylactic shock symptoms

Back Pain
- Upper
- Lower
- Trauma

Bites
- Animal (dog, cat, wild animal)
- Bee sting
- Jellyfish
- Human
- Snake
- Spider
- Sting ray
- Tick

Bowel Problem
- Black or bloody stools
- Constipation
- Diarrhea
- Incontinence
- Pain
- Pin worms

Breast Problem (non-lactating)
- Lump
- Discharge
- Trauma

Breastfeeding Problems
- Approved drugs for lactating mothers
- General concerns
- Infection—clogged or infected milk duct symptoms
- Mastitis symptoms

Breathing Problem
- CPR crash card
- Asthma symptoms
- Croup symptoms
- Difficult breathing
- Epiglottitis symptoms

Burns—Chemical

Burns—Thermal
- First degree
- Second degree
- Third degree

Calf Pain

Chest Pain—Adult (13 and older)
- MI or angina symptoms
- Pneumonia symptoms
- Costochondritis symptoms

Chest Pain—under 13 years old

Chest Trauma

CPR Crash Card
- Adult
- Child

Childbirth Crash Card

Choking—Heimlich Crash Card
- Adult
- Child

Cold Exposure
- Hypothermia symptoms

Confusion/Consciousness Problems
- Diabetes symptoms
- Stroke symptoms

Convulsions Adult/Child
- Diagnosed epileptic
- Unknown diagnosis
- Convulsions—Child

Coping, Ineffective Family
- Child/Elder/Wife abuse

Diarrhea
- Adult
- Child

Dizziness
Drowning—See CPR
Drug/Alcohol Problems
- Intoxication/confusion/delirium
- Support group referral, hot lines

Ear Problems
- Chemical in
- Discharge
- Foreign body
- Loss of hearing
- Pain
- Plugged
- Ringing
- Swimmer's ear symptoms
- Trauma

Electrocution
Extremities—arms, legs, hands, feet, fingers, toes
- Infection symptoms
- Trauma
- Swelling

Eye Problems
- Pain
- Foreign body
- Chemical in
- Discharge
- Trauma
- Visual problems chart
- Double or blurred vision, loss of vision, halos, floaters

Fainting—See Unconsciousness
Fall
Fever/Chills/Dehydration Symptoms
- Adult
- Child

Flu Symptoms
Glands
- Pain/swelling

Gunshot Wound
Head
- Pain
- Trauma

Heat Exposure
- Heat prostration symptoms
- Sunstroke symptoms

Infection
- General signs/symptoms
- Sepsis
- Toxic shock syndrome

Ingestion—Pediatric
- Dangerous, mild, harmless

Jaw Pain

Joint Problems
- Trauma
- Pain

Lacerations
- Abrasions
- Puncture
- Tetanus guidelines

Lice
- Adult—pubic/body
- Child—head/body

Menstrual Problems
- BCP problems
- Estrogen replacement therapy problems
- Painful periods
- Bleeding—irregular, excessive, amenorrhea
- Menopause

Nausea/vomiting
- Adult/child

Neck Problem
- Pain
- Trauma
- Stiffness

Newborn Concerns
- Crying
- Feeding
- Circumcision

Nose Problem
- Bleeding
- Foreign body
- Discharge
- Sinusitis symptoms
- Trauma

Ob/Gyn Office Procedures
- Colposcopy
- Cryosurgery
- Conception
- Cervical biopsy
- Endometrial biopsy
- Bartholin cysts

Penile Problems
- Discharge
- Lesion

Postpartum Problems
- Postpartum emergencies
- Postpartum concerns and discomforts

Pregnancy Problems and Emergencies
- Approved drugs
- Emergencies of pregnancy—Eclampsia
- Placenta previa
- Abruptio
- Preterm labor
- Labor symptoms
- Premature rupture of membranes

Reye's Syndrome Symptoms

Skin Problems
- Athlete's foot symptoms
- Boil symptoms
- Cellulitis symptoms
- Discoloration of skin—bruises, yellowing, petechiae
- Hives
- Jock itch symptoms
- Herpes symptoms
- Childhood rashes chart: diaper rash, eczema, chicken pox, poison oak, impetigo, ringworm, roseola
- Swelling/edema

Throat Problems
- Cough
- Foreign body
- Pain
- Trauma

Tooth
- Infection
- Pain
- Trauma

Shock Symptoms

Stab Wound

Suicide or Homicide
- Ideation
- Threats
- In-progress

Rape Trauma Syndrome

Rectal Problems
- Bleeding
- Fissures
- Hemorrhoid symptoms
- Itching
- Trauma

Vaginal Problems
- Pain
- Bartholin cyst symptoms
- Infections: Non-STD/STD chart: herpes, chlamydia, gonorrhea, syphilis, gardnerella, monilia, AIDS, trichomonas, hepatitis, warts

Unconsciousness

Upper Respiratory Infection Symptoms

Urinary Problems
- Blood in urine
- Decreased output
- Dark
- Excessive output
- Pain
- UTI symptoms

APPENDIX D

EMERGENCY DEPARTMENT PROTOCOL LIST

A "bare bones" set of ED protocols may be modeled after the pre-arrival instructions formulated for the Emergency Medical Dispatcher. This list is adapted from *Principles of Emergency Medical Dispatch* (Clawson & Dernocoeur, 1988). It focuses on 25 emergent presenting symptoms about which clients might call. For purposes of illustration only, the list shown here is limited to main headings only (it does not show subheadings). However, each heading should be fleshed out (i.e. Abdominal pain—appendicitis, ectopic pregnancy, hemorrhage symptoms, etc).

Abdominal pain
Allergic symptoms/hives/stings
Bites—animal, insect, human
Breathing problems
Burns—chemical, thermal, electrical
Chest pain
Choking—Heimlich maneuver
Childbirth
Convulsions
CPR—cardiac or respiratory arrest
Drowning
Electrocution
Eye problems—trauma, chemical, foreign body
Falls
Headache/head injury
Heat or cold exposure
Hemorrhage
Lacerations
Overdose/ingestion symptoms
Poisoning—carbon monoxide inhalation, hazardous materials exposure
Pregnancy complications
Psychiatric/behavioral problems, suicidal calls
Rape
Stab/gunshot wound
Unconsciousness

POLICIES

Call transfer
Call tracing
Suicide in progress
Home death/hospice/expected deaths
AIDS crisis intervention
Drug/alcohol calls

APPENDIX E

INFORMATION PROTOCOL LIST

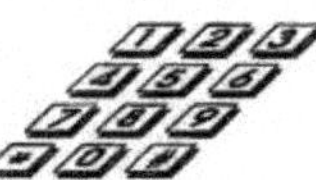

TelMed™ is a program of computerized audiotapes on hundreds of health topics accessed by telephone. Health information services such as this demonstrate clients' need for access to health information by telephone. However, callers often seek in-depth information as well as a human response—aspects that audiotapes lack. The list below is a small sample of topics about which clients frequently call, and is by no means exhaustive. After this is developed and modified, obtain administration and nursing approval and place it in the appendix of the standards manual.

AIDS
Alcoholism
Allergies
Blood donation
Blood tests (cholesterol, etc.)
Chemical dependency
Childhood communicable diseases
Childhood immunizations
Consumer
- Second opinion
- Patient rights
- Informed consent

Libraries and bookstores, medical information sources
Medication questions (generic information, common uses, side effects, contraindications, cautions)
- Analgesics
- Antipyretics
- Antibiotics
- Cardiac
- Chemotherapy
- Contraception
- Psychotropics
- Poison control

Mental health questions
Organ donation/transplants
Osteoporosis
Pregnancy
Toxic shock syndrome
Travel shots
Treatment alternatives
Sexually transmitted diseases

APPENDIX F
SUPPORT GROUP LIST

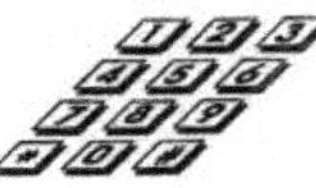

Support group referral can and should be an integral component of telephone triage. This resource is especially useful to those with limited financial resources who are undergoing life crises or have chronic emotional or health problems. The list below shows frequently used self-help groups. After it is developed and modified, obtain administration and nursing approval and place it in the appendix of the standards manual. The list can be further developed using Appendix H.

ADOPTION SUPPORT
AIDS
ALCOHOL ABUSE
ANOREXIA/BULEMIA
BEREAVEMENT FOR CHILDREN
CANCER
CAREER PLANNING
CHILDREN WITH LEARNING DISABILITIES
C-SECTION
DES
DOWN'S SYNDROME LEAGUE
DRUG ABUSE
ENDOMETRIOSIS
HAND (HELP AFTER NEONATAL DEATH)
HERPES
INCEST SURVIVOR
INFERTILITY
LA LECHE LEAGUE
MASTECTOMY
NEW MOTHER
PARENTS ANONYMOUS (CHILD ABUSE)
PARENT SUPPORT/PARENTAL STRESS
PHYSICAL ABUSE (ELDER, SPOUSE, CHILD)
RAPE
SHELTERS
SIDS DEATH
SINGLE PARENTS
WIDOWS SUPPORT

APPENDIX G

COMMUNITY RESOURCE LIST

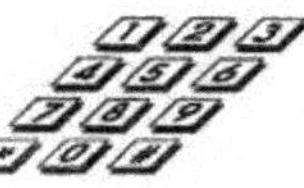

This is a list of 20 representative community resources. See Appendix H for sample community resource file card, including description, scope, fees, and purpose.

Abused women
Adoption
Advocacy
Alcoholism
Child abuse
Consumer group (healthcare-specific)
Counseling
Crisis intervention
Day care—children
Day care—elders
Drug abuse
Emergency assistance (meals, housing)
Employment services
Ethnic services
Family planning
Handicapped
Home health
Legal counsel
Pregnancy
Transportation
Volunteer opportunities

APPENDIX H

COMMUNITY RESOURCE FILE CARD SAMPLE

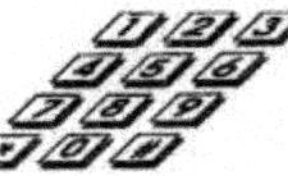

GROUP NAME:

CONTACT PERSON:

PHONE NUMBER:

ADDRESS:

OFFICE HOURS:

PURPOSE:

PROGRAM DESCRIPTION:

SUCCESS RATE:

GROUP LONGEVITY:

RESTRICTIONS/LIMITATIONS:

COST:

OTHER SERVICES:

CRISIS LINE:

APPENDIX I

MICROTEACHING SECTION SAMPLES

These suggested rules and techniques can be incorporated into assessment, treatment, or advice sections of protocol body. This list is by no means exhaustive, and users are encouraged to develop it further.

RULES OF THUMB

- Symptoms should improve after 24 to 48 hours on antibiotics
- Two calls in 4 hours or less = appt. today (diagnosis = "worried parent")
- Less than 1 wet diaper in 8 hours = appt. today
- Rectal temperature of 100 in infant of 6 months or less = appt. today
- Beware of afebrile PID (possible ectopic or ovarian cyst)
- Once an ectopic, always an ectopic
- Beware of shoulder pain associated with abdominal pain
- Diarrhea stools: more than 10 stools in 24 hours = appt. today

SELF-ASSESSMENT TECHNIQUES

BLANCHING RASH—Press area for 2 seconds and describe results.

CIRCULATION—Squeeze finger between finger and thumb for 2 seconds. Release and describe color change.

COSTOCHONDRITIS PAIN—Press on area of chest that hurts with one finger. Describe results.

DEHYDRATION—Pinch skin over top of hand for 5 seconds and release. Describe results.

FETAL ACTIVITY—5-20 kicks in 30 minutes at time that baby is normally active.

LEVEL OF CONSCIOUSNESS—Press down firmly on nailbed with thumb. Describe reaction.

PITTING EDEMA—Press firmly on the bony area of the ankle for 1-2 seconds. Describe results.

POINT TENDERNESS—Gently press along length of bone to locate injury (Hafen & Karren, 1986, p. 236)

POSTURAL HYPOTENSION—Rise quickly from sitting to standing. Describe results. (Perform only with another adult present)

PULSE—Gently place four fingers in groove along side of "Adam's apple," or place finger on thumb side of wrist. Count pulse.

RESPIRATIONS—Remove shirt and observe chest movement. Count each time chest rises. (Nurse times by the clock).

TENDERNESS TO TOUCH—Touch area. Describe results.

WEIGHT BEARING ABILITY—Attempt to walk on affected limb. Describe results.

APPENDIX J

TREATMENT MICROTEACHING SAMPLES

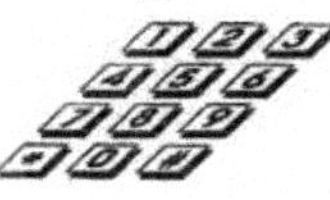

As mentioned in Chapter 4, teaching about treatments must be concrete, concise, and "cookbook" format—microteaching. These components can be added to advice and teaching sections of protocols. Some sections of these instructions are left blank for modification by the user institution.

SYMPTOM	TREATMENT MICROTEACHING
AVULSED TOOTH	TOOTH TRANSPORT: Hold in mouth between gum during transport. (Buttaravoli & Stair, 1985).
BEE STING/ INSECT BITES/ CHICKEN POX LESIONS	BAKING SODA PASTE: Apply a smooth paste of baking soda and water.
CROUP SYMPTOMS	STEAMY BATHROOM: Run hot shower with doors and windows closed for 20 minutes. (Pantell, Vickery, Fries, 1977)
CUT LIP	POPSICLE™: Give child Popsicle™ to cut down on bleeding, pain and to act as a distraction.
EYE IRRITATION	EYEWASH: "Mummy" child in large beach towel. Place on kitchen counter. Hold child down with one arm and open eye with other hand. *Gently* flood eye with water for 5 minutes by the clock. (San Francisco Poison Control, 1989)
FEVER	TEPID BATH: Shallow, warm, tub bath that does not cause shivering. Get child's head and upper body wet. Supervise child playing in tub as water cools.
GI UPSET/DIARRHEA	BRAT DIET: *Ripe* bananas, white rice, applesauce, white toast. (Refined foods that are easily digested) CLEAR LIQUIDS: Fluids you can see through: water, soda, clear fruit juice, Gatorade™, herb tea, jello, and broth.

NOSE BLEED	Pinch soft part of nose x _____ minutes by clock.
SKIN ITCHING/ IRRITATIONS	BAKING SODA BATH: Add _____ baking soda to tub of warm water.
SWELLING DISCOMFORT	COOL COMPRESS: Cold, damp cloths. Change every 10 minutes.
SWELLING—INJURY "RIP"	**R**est, **I**ce, **P**osition of Comfort (elevated to level of heart).
SWELLING/ MUSCLE SPASM	HOT PACKS: Place cloths soaked in hot water wrung out in plastic bag at _____ intervals. ICE PACK: Fill a zip-lock bag with crushed ice covered with thin cloth. Place on swelling at _____ minute intervals. *Avoid direct contact with skin.*
TEETHING	TEETHING COMFORT: Wrap ice cube in washcloth. Secure with a rubber band.
TOOTH ACHE	CLOVE REMEDY: Place whole clove between gum and painful tooth.
VAGINAL/RECTAL IRRITATIONS/ LESIONS	SITZ BATH: A _____ minute warm tub bath _____ times per day.

APPENDIX K

ABBREVIATIONS

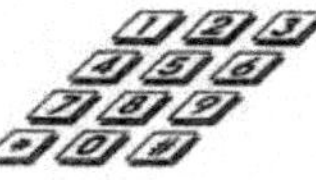

This list of common abbreviations can be used for telephone triage documentation. After it is developed and modified, obtain administration and nursing approval and place it in the appendix of the standards manual.

Abd.—Abdominal
Ac—Acute
ADL—Activities of Daily Living
Adv.—Advised
Alt.—Altered
ASWB—Altered State of Well Being
Ca.—Caller
Chr.—Chronic
Cl.—Client
c/o—Complaining Of
ED—Emergency Dept.
EMD—Emergency Medical Dispatcher
Emerg—Emergent
Et. Ukn.—Etiology Unknown
LOC—Level of Consciousness
MD—Medical Doctor
Mod—Moderate
OR—Operating room
OV—Office Visit
$\bar{o}$—no, none
$\bar{p}$—after
Poss.—Possible
Pot.—Potential for, Potential
Re:—Regarding
RN—Registered Nurse
R/T:—Related to
$\bar{s}$—without
St—States
Sev.—Severe
Sib—sibling
Surg—surgery
Urg.—Urgent
x—times
/—per

APPENDIX L

DIAGNOSTIC, CLASSIFYING, AND PRESUMPTIVE TERMS

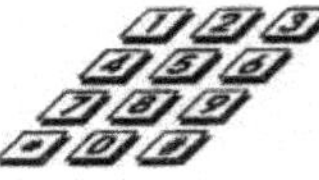

A working diagnosis necessitates developing lists of diagnostic, classifying, and presumptive terms. This sample list can be modified and developed further. After obtaining administration and nursing approval, place the list in the appendix of the standards manual.

DIAGNOSTIC
- Emotional distress
- Impaired verbal communication
- Knowledge deficit
- Noncompliance
- Pain
- Self-care deficit
- Spiritual distress

CLASSIFYING
- Acute
- Altered
- Chronic
- Diffuse
- Gradual onset
- Impaired
- Ineffective
- Localized
- Moderate
- New
- Nonacute
- Potential for
- Radiating
- Severe
- Sudden onset

PRESUMPTIVE
- Apparent
- Etiology unknown
- Possible

APPENDIX M

SAMPLE LAB TESTS FORM

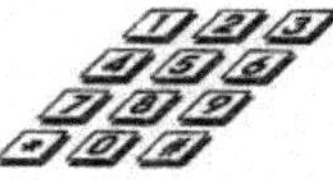

Depending on your state's Nurse Practice Act, the following tests may be ordered by nurses following protocol directives. This list may be placed in the appendix of the standards manual after obtaining nursing, physician, and administration approval.

Blood Sugar
CBC
Cholesterol
Dilantin level
Electrolyte levels
Lead level
Lithium level
Liver function
Pregnancy test
PTT/PT
Stool culture (O&P)
Stool for occult blood
Throat culture
Urine analysis
Urine culture

(Used with permission of Kaiser Permanente, Cleveland Heights, OH)

APPENDIX N

SAMPLE LIST: OVER-THE-COUNTER AND TRANSITION MEDICATIONS

The following OTC medications may be incorporated into the protocol advice sections. However, this role should not be taken lightly and the ability to recommend OTC medication does not imply that there is no risk.

As with prescription medications, allergies can develop at any time to any drug or substance, and during pregnancy and lactation, some OTC drugs can have serious effects on the fetus or nursing infant. However, there are other ways in which OTC medications can be a danger to the client: drug/disease and drug/drug interactions. Recommending aspirin to someone with ulcers or a bleeding disorder could result in a serious drug/disease interaction, whereas recommending aspirin to someone taking Coumadin could produce a drug/drug interaction. Although it is not an OTC medication, MAO inhibiters (antidepressants) combined with certain foods (aged cheeses, wine) may produce a drug/food interaction, and when combined with OTC decongestants may produce a serious drug/drug interaction. Nurses can consult texts such as *The Complete Guide to Prescription and Non-prescription Drugs* (Griffith, 1990) for interaction information, and if there is any question about an OTC drug, consult with a reliable pharmacist.

OTC:

A and D™ ointment
Acnaveen
Actifed™
Advil™
Alternagel
Aminophylline
Anacin™
Anbesol™
Anusol™
Aspergum™
Aspirin
Bacitracin
Baking Soda
Benadryl™
Benalyn
Benoxyl
Betadine
Calamine™
Caladryl™
Cheracol™
Chlor-Trimeton™
Cimetidine
Clearasil™
Colace
Cortisone Cream
Cruex™
Debrox™
Desitin™
Desenex™
Digel™
Dimetapp™
Dramamine™
Emtrol
Excedrin™
Excedrin PM™
Fostex™
Gatorade™
Gelusil
Glycerin suppository
Glyoxide
Gyne-Lotrimin™
Hydrogen peroxide
Imodium
Insulin
Iodine
Iron pills
Isopropyl alcohol
Ivy-Dry™
Kaopectate™
Lanacaine™
Maalox™
Metamucil™
Milk of Magnesia™
Monistat™
Motrin™
Murine™
Mylanta™
Neosporin™
Neosynephrine™

Nix
Novahistine™
Nuprin™
Nystatin
Oxy 5, Oxy 10™
Pedialyte™
Pepto-Bismol™
Preparation H™
Promethazine HCL
RID
Robitussin™ (except AC)
Rolaids™
Sebulex
Selsun Blue™
St. Joseph's Aspirin™
Sudafed™
Sulindac
Syrup of Ipecac
Tinactin™
Triaminic™
Tylenol™
Tums™
Tucks™
Visine™
Vagisil™
Vitamin E oil or capsules
Whitfield's™ Ointment
Zinc oxide

TRANSITION (Proposed)

Naprosyn
Seldane
Tagamet
Alupent, metaprel
Phenylpropanolamine (PPA)
Feldene
Robaxin

APPENDIX O

SAMPLE PEDIATRIC ANTIPYRETIC DOSAGE CHART

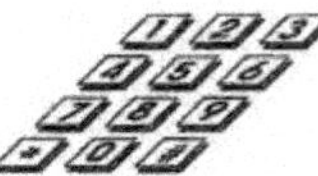

When parents call about their child's fever, they may or may not have the proper antipyretic on hand at home. Sometimes they call because they have run out of pediatric Tylenol and the pharmacy has closed. In such cases it may mean advising them to use a half or third of an adult Tylenol. In addition, antipyretics come in a confusing array of different brand names, drops, elixirs, and chewable tablets. Dosages depend on the weight and age of the child. Thus, nurses must be knowledgeable and accurate when advising antipyretics.

To prevent confusion, clarify the brand name (to be sure that the parent is not using aspirin, for example), determine the form and exact dosage. Remember that, if they don't use an accurate measuring device, for example, parents may under- or over-medicate the child—possibly leading to either an ineffective response or an overdose. A dosage chart such as the one shown here can be posted near the phone to expedite the advising process while preventing confusion. It is difficult to remember dosages for 7 different drugs and 9 different weight categories. It may be helpful to create a similar chart for OTC pediatric cough medicines and decongestants. This chart has been left blank for individual modification per institutional policy and should be revised and updated as new drugs appear on the market. After obtaining administration and nursing approval, place the list in the appendix of the standards manual, and post a copy near phone.

WEIGHT	6-11#	12-17#	18-23#	24-35#	36-47#	48-59#	60-71#	72-95#	96# & Up
TYLENOL DROPS™									
TEMPRA DROPS™									
FEVERNOL™									
TYLENOL ELIXIR™									
TYLENOL CHEWABLE™									
ADULT TYLENOL™									
EXTRA STRENGTH TYLENOL™									

APPENDIX P

TELEPHONE POLICY: PARENT INFORMATION SHEET

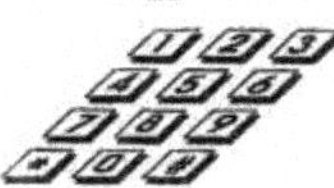

1. *Emergency calls: day and night coverage*
   a. Our practice is always covered for emergencies. Emergency calls go directly through to a physician.
   b. *Always* call in first rather than drive to an emergency room. Often your physician will be able to provide you with critical first aid instructions by phone (for example, for burns, choking, or fractures). Your physician can help you make the decision whether or not a rescue squad should be sent out or whether it is safe for you to drive in. Your physician can also tell you where to take your child for the best emergency care.
   c. When you call in, always state assertively, "This is an emergency." Do not let the clinic answering service or receptionist put you on hold. If you are put on hold, hang up and call back immediately.
   d. If for any reason you have difficulty reaching your physician, call the nearest emergency room (telephone number:__________) and ask to talk to the physician on call there for advice.
   e. Call 911 only for emergencies where your child may need resuscitation (for example, your child is not breathing). If rescue squads are not available in your community, call your physician and drive quickly to the nearest emergency room. Be sure to find out where the closest one is and the fastest route to it before an emergency strikes. In these situations, have a neighbor call ahead that you are coming.
   f. *Poisoning*. The Poison Control Center can be reached by calling______________.
2. *Calls during office hours*
   Office hours are: weekdays 8:00 to 5:30, Saturdays 8:00 to 12:00. During office hours, all medical calls are screened by our office nurse, who has been specially trained to make decisions on which patients need to be seen and how to treat the children who don't need to be seen at home. If she can't help you, she will have your physician call you back. During office hours you can call her regarding any problems or questions about your child's health. If possible, place calls about a non-sick child between 1:00 and 3:00 P.M., when our switchboard is least busy.
3. *Calling for an appointment*
   We see children by appointment only. If your child is sick and you want him or her seen, call ahead for an appointment so you won't have to wait. It is usually better to talk with the office nurse before requesting an appointment for a sick child because we may be able to treat your child easily at home, saving you travel time and the cost of an office visit.

4. *Prescription refills*
   We refill prescriptions only during office hours. Usually, we need your child's chart handy to check on dosages and the need for a revisit. Plan ahead so you don't run out of important medicines. Always have the phone number of your pharmacy available before you call the office.

5. *Nighttime calls*
   After office hours, calls should be made only for emergencies or urgent problems that can't wait until morning. At night, your physician's line must be kept open for these purposes. Calls about mild illnesses can usually wait until the next day. Our office closes at 5:30 P.M. and opens again at 8:00 A.M. During these hours your calls will be taken by an answering service. Your physician (or the one who is covering) is on a paging unit. The answering service can reach this person immediately and he or she will usually return your call within 15 minutes (immediately for emergencies).

   Don't call your physician at home. The physician may not be there or may not be on call. Always call the office number first (which is the same one as the answering service). During off hours, you must call in first if you want a physician from our group to see your child.

6. *Information that may be needed*
   Before calling us, know the following (except in emergencies):
   a. Your child's approximate weight.
   b. Your child's temperature if he or she is sick.
   c. Your pharmacy's telephone number.

(Reprinted with permission from *Pediatric Telephone Advice*. ©1980, Little, Brown and Company.)

APPENDIX Q

PROTOTYPE PROTOCOL: DIARRHEA (Pediatric)

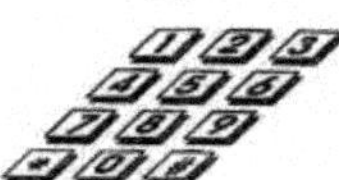

(Fill in the blanks in accordance with institutional policy.)

SPECIFIC QUESTIONS	DISPOSITION/ADVICE
EMERGENT/URGENT SYMPTOMS	**ED/MD IN 0–2 HOURS**
• Under 6 months with ______+ stools/24 hrs? • Bloody stools? • Apparent severe abdominal pain (intense crying and drawing up legs)? • Dry lips, tongue, sunken eyes, extremely sleepy, lack of tears, sunken fontanelle?	
SEMI-URGENT SYMPTOMS	**MD/APPT IN 2–24 HOURS**
• Fever × 3 days with diarrhea? • Dark or scantily wet diapers (1 or less per 8 hrs)?	• Home treatment until appt. • Call if sx. become markedly worse before appt. time • BREAST FED—Continue, offer water between fdgs. • FORMULA—Dilute to half strength. If persists, stop formula, switch to clear liq. (Pedialyte) • SOLID FOODS—BRAT DIET (see below) • Avoid milk, yogurt, cheese—irritates bowel • Substitute soy products • Avoid OTC diarrhea preparations • Observe for sx. of dehydration (see below)
ROUTINE SYMPTOMS	**MD/APPT IN 24 HOURS–2 WEEK**
• Diarrhea unresponsive to treatment × 48 hours? • MEDS—antibiotics? • Well water drinking supply? • RECENT TRAVEL to foreign country? • RECENT CAMPING trip, possible Giardia? • Mild to moderate chronic diarrhea? • *Transient, Homeless, Parental Hx. of Drug Abuse?* • *Worried parent?* • *Self limiting symptoms existing × 1 week—not becoming markedly worse?*	• *Remain at home and begin treatment* • *Call if sx becomes markedly worse, fail to improve with treatment or Rx. × 24-48 hours.* • *See home treatment above*
CROSS-REFERENCE	**BASIC TEACHING**
	DEHYDRATION—Dry lips, tongue, sunken fontanelle, lack of tears, unusual sleepiness, dark urine and/or 1 or less wet diaper or voiding per 8 hours DIARRHEA—______or more large watery stools/8 hrs BRAT DIET—Ripe bananas, white rice, applesauce, and white toast. Easily digested, nonirritating diet.

(Courtesy Wheeler and Associates)

APPENDIX R

Prototype Protocol: VAGINAL BLEEDING (Non-pregnant)

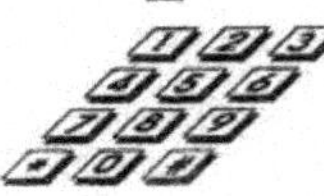

(Fill in the blanks in accordance with institutional policy.)

SPECIFIC QUESTIONS	DISPOSITION/ADVICE
EMERGENT/URGENT SYMPTOMS	**ED/MD IN 0–2 HOURS**
• More than 1 pad (2 tampons)/hour? • Pale, sweaty, thirsty, weak, dizzy, faint? • Post TAB? • Postpartum? • Recent IUD insertion? • Recent hysterectomy?	• Lie down • Have someone drive patient in
SEMI-URGENT SYMPTOMS	**MD/APPT IN 2–24 HOURS**
• Accompanied by severe abdominal pain? • Any infectious process requiring antibiotics? • Painful conditions requiring prescription drugs? • Failure to improve after 48 hours on medication? • Fever, chills? • Foul smelling discharge? • Diffuse rash, fever, muscle aches, weakness, or profound diarrhea assoc. with contraceptive sponge, cervical cap, or tampon use? • Related to IUD? • ______pads per 8 hour?	• Begin home treatment until appt. • Call or come in if sx. become markedly worse before appt. time • Rest, put feet up • Monitor number of saturated pads per hour • Increase fluid intake • Expect initial "gush" upon arising in A.M. or after lying down. Call if persistent. • Avoid aspirin or fish oils which may prolong bleeding • Tylenol™ for discomfort • Observe for sx of shock, infection (below)
ROUTINE SYMPTOMS	**MD/APPT IN 24 HOURS–2 WEEK**
• Self-limiting symptoms existing over 1 week but not becoming markedly worse? • ______pads × 8 hours? • Normal but excessively long period? • Bleeding between periods? • Late period following by heavy flow? • Last period 1 year ago? • MEDS—drug abuse, excess aspirin, blood thinners, thyroid, steroids, chemotherapy, fish oils? • Birth control pills (SEE BCP PROTOCOL)? • MED HX—thyroid disease, diabetes, bleeding disorder, Von Willebrand's disease? • Emotional distress/stress?	• SEE ABOVE HOME TREATMENT • Remain at home and begin treatment • Call back if symptoms become markedly worse or fail to improve with treatment within 48 hours.
CROSS REFERENCE	**BASIC TEACHING**
• BLEEDING POST MENOPAUSE • BLEEDING IN PREGNANCY • BLEEDING and BCP & ERT **BASIC TEACHING** • STRESS can affect bleeding patterns, leading to missed periods or excessive bleeding. • POST MENOPAUSAL BLEEDING—1 year or more after last period	• BLEEDING (SEVERE) SX: Saturation of 1 pad/hr or more. May be due to tumors or infection. • COMPLICATIONS. Shock: Pale, sweaty, faint, thirsty • INFECTION SX: Chills, fever, fatigue, foul vaginal discharge, abdominal pain • IUD may cause excess bleeding leading to anemia. Get appt. if severe × 3 months

(Courtesy Wheeler and Associates)

APPENDICES

PART II

INSTRUCTIONAL, EQUIPMENT, INFORMATIONAL, AND QUALITY ASSURANCE RESOURCES

APPENDIX S

TRAINING PROGRAMS

EMD training, consulting, and computerized pre-arrival instructions
Jeff Clawson, M.D.
Medical Priority Consultants, Inc.
139 E. S. Temple, Suite 600
Salt Lake City, UT 84111
(801) 363-9127

Telephone triage seminars and consulting
Sheila Quilter Wheeler, RN, MA, Director
Wheeler and Associates
44 Madrone Ave.
San Anselmo, CA 94960
(415) 453-8382

Nursing management, standards development, and quality assurance
Carolyn Smith-Marker, RN, MSN
Marker Systems
P.O. Box 309
Severna Park, MD 21146
(301) 544-0251

APPENDIX T

SPECIALIZED AND INFORMATIONAL PROGRAMS

(This listing does not constitute an endorsement.)

SPECIALIZED PROGRAM

TELEMETRY: Home telemetry for high-risk mothers
TOKOS Medical Corporation
1390 Willow Pass Road, Suite 300
Concord, CA 94520
(800) 682-3961

INFORMATIONAL PROGRAMS

Informational services can enhance existing telephone triage systems. For example, if an institution has subscribed to an audiotape library (e.g. Health-Line™), clients can be referred to access these libraries by telephone if they seek additional information on a medical topic or problem. There are also computerized systems (e.g. InfoTrac™, and Pediatric Advisor™), available through local public, medical, or hospital libraries. Nurses can simply refer a client to go to the library to research their question.

Telephone Accessed Audiotape Library
Health-Line™ is a library of taped messages used for community outreach, as a public relations gesture, or as a supplement to an existing telephone triage program. The library provides 300 messages covering the most commonly asked questions regarding general health issues, parenting, women, children, the elderly, diet, recreation, arthritis, cancer, dental, hospital procedures, drugs and other topics. This university-based program began in 1970 and may be the first such service of its kind. The University of Wisconsin—Madison, a major research institution, is responsible for the development of Health-Line™. The tapes are updated every 3 years. For additional information, call or write to:

Ann Whitaker, BSN, RN, Health-Line™ Coordinator
Health-Line™
University of Wisconsin—Madison
Health and Human Services
610 Langdon Street
Madison, WI 52703
(608) 262-4509

Computerized Reference Systems

Computerized systems provide databases on selected health-related subjects. Institutions can subscribe to systems like InfoTrac™ health index and/or the Pediatric Advisor™ in lieu of or to supplement in-house informational protocols. The advantage to computerized systems is that they enable nurses to find topics by phone, print out the information, and mail it to the client to reinforce instructions.

InfoTrac™ workstations, found in most public and academic libraries, provides users with direct, unlimited, and easy-access to current medical citations. Nurses should call local public, medical and hospital libraries to determine if they already have any of these systems to which the nurse can refer clients. If they are not locally available, the institution may wish to look into subscribing to such services.

Information Access Company, founded in 1976, is the world's leading supplier of periodical reference products. Their InfoTrac™ Health Reference Center is a computerized index to over 130 core publications on health, fitness, nutrition, and medicine. It provides full text summaries of professional medical journals written in lay language. For more information, call or write to:

Information Access Company
362 Lakeside Drive
Foster City, CA 94404
(800) 227-8431

The Pediatric Advisor™ computerized system is an educational aid designed for medical professionals, staff, patients, and parents. It provides information in lay language on over 500 topics related to medical and behavioral problems, newborn care, and parenting. For more information, call or write to:

Clinical Reference Systems, Ltd.
5613 DTC Parkway, Suite 350
Englewood, CO 80111-3031
(800) 237-8401

APPENDIX U

STANDARDS AND QUALITY ASSURANCE

(Adapted from Marker 1987 and 1988—see references. Used with permission.)

Standards and quality assurance (QA) are critical to the safe practice of telephone triage. Standards facilitate change and lay the groundwork for quality assurance (see Figure U.1). Implementing new units requires structure, process, and outcome standards. New forms such as telephone triage documentation forms and logs require new guidelines. New equipment such as telephones, headsets, and computers requires training. New expectations require new performance standards. To that end, nurses must work with physicians and administrators to determine what controversial measures they will perform (e.g., prescribing OTC medications, advising treatments), what high-risk measures telephone triage staff will implement (e.g., CPR, Heimlich, childbirth coaching, and suicide intervention), and which confusing aspects of the practice must be clarified (Marker, 1988, p. 13).

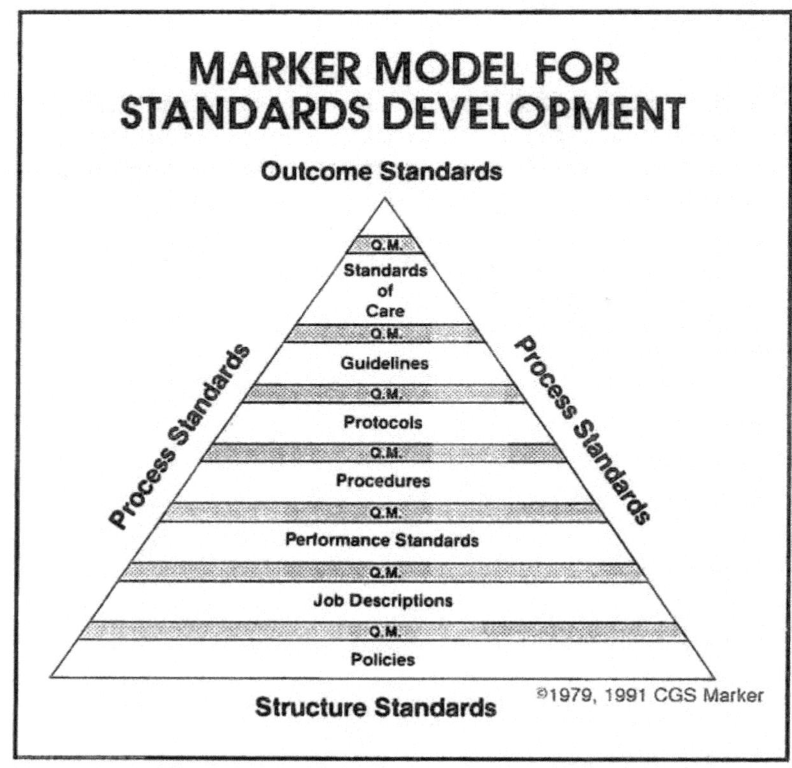

Figure U.1 (Reprinted with permission from CGS Marker)

Standards for nursing responsibilities must address certain Joint Commission on Accreditation of Healthcare Organization (JCAHO) requirements in the areas of:

1. Using the nursing process (communications, documentation and protocol use)
2. Informing the physician of significant changes (communication)
3. Crisis intervention (CPR, Heimlich, childbirth, suicidal, homicidal callers)
4. Risky procedures
5. The use of standing orders (protocols) (Marker, 1988, p. 72)

Quality assurance is a process "in which standards are set and action is taken to ensure compliance to the standards; predefined activities that are designated, implemented and documented to demonstrate compliance to establish standards." (Marker, 1988, p. 155) As illustrated by Figure U.2 quality management encompasses the monitoring and evaluating all aspects of professional practice. Practice is made up of nine different activities: standards development, credentialing, continuing education, performance appraisal, audit, concurrent monitoring, problem identification utilization review and risk management.

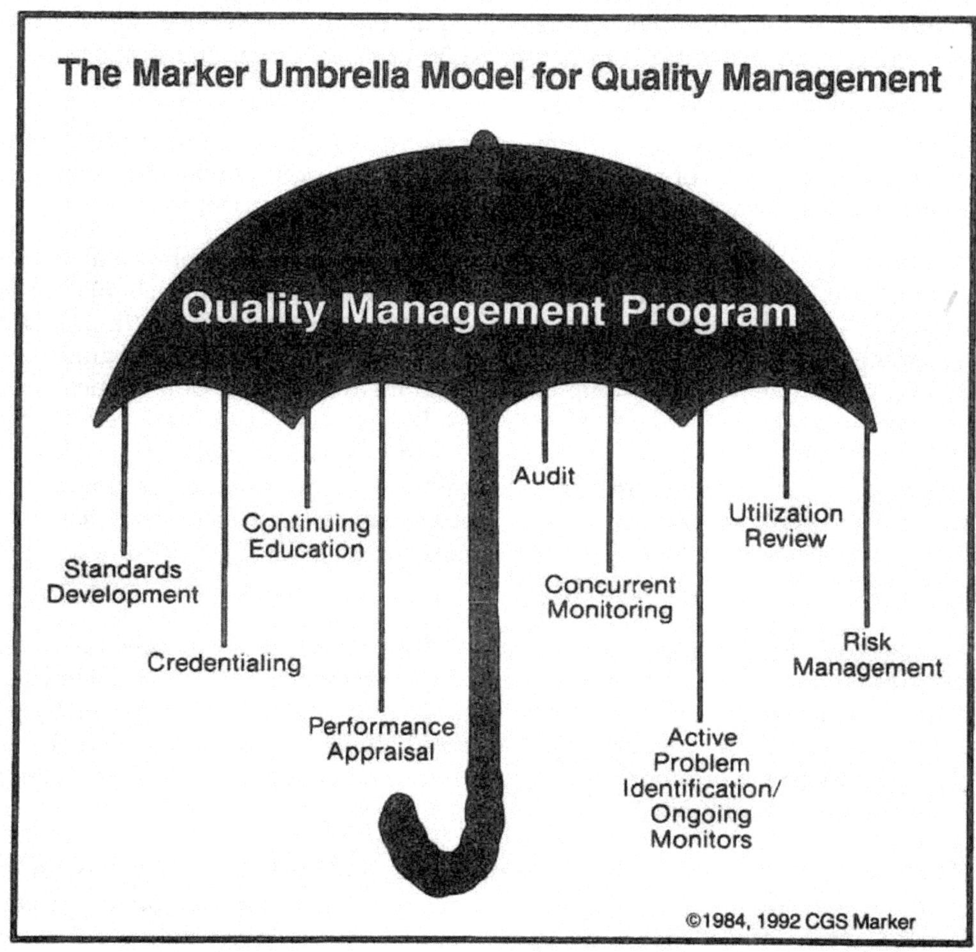

Figure U.2 (Reprinted with permission from CGS Marker)

1. *Standards* are "written statements defining the level of practice in the staff or a set of conditions in the patient or staff determined to be acceptable by some authority." (Marker, 1988, p. 116) An example of a telephone triage standard might be the standard talk time of an average of 6 minutes per call.

2. *Credentialing* means "validating competency either through testing of cognitive knowledge or psychomotor skill." (Marker, 1987, p. 52) Legal requirements are included here. Like all nurses, telephone triage nurses must possess a current license. Secondly, an annual unit-based test for knowledge and skills necessary to achieve performance standards should be given. For telephone triage nurses, this might include testing of skills in using a computer, transferring a crisis call, Heimlich maneuver and CPR coaching, as well as a written test.

3. *Continuing education* includes "all professional development events conducted on a nursing unit, including inservices, in-house and off-site staff development, covering existing standards, new competencies in new standards, and QA results (corrective actions)" (Marker, 1987, p. 58). In telephone triage, this could include in-service training on new phone or computer equipment, pharmacy or AIDS updates, or communications training.

4. *Performance appraisals* are based on employee job descriptions, which might include such tasks as "performing client assessment within an average of six minutes using the appropriate protocol and documentation form," or "evaluate the client's ability to carry out self care measures at home safely" (Marker, 1987, p. 59).

5. *Auditing* is a "formal process of data collection from a representative sample including chart reviews, direct observation and interviews of staff and clients" (Marker, 1987, p. 60). Common examples of auditing include documentation review (in this case the telephone triage form rather than the chart) and directly observing staff. Auditing is done in three areas: compliance, noncompliance, and miscellaneous. Compliance auditing might be done to test for safety and effectiveness. For example, is the new documentation form safe and effective enough for general use? Noncompliance audits are used to check staff performance. For example, are nurses actually using the protocols as directed? Miscellaneous audits examine documentation, patient satisfaction, and staff satisfaction. Thus, like other specialties, telephone triage nurses can be audited for documentation and caller satisfaction with a follow-up call.

6. *Concurrent monitoring* is data collection regarding three to four clients on five or six criteria (Marker, 1987, p. 60). An example in telephone triage might include direct observation by a supervisor, who monitors three to four calls to determine six aspects of a nurse's performance. For example, did the nurse follow the protocols? Did the nurse collect the age and phone number? Did the nurse use lay language, give a working diagnosis, and state the disclaimer?

7. *Risk management* focuses on "preventing loss and includes unit safety, infection control and incident reporting" (Marker, 1987, p. 61). Environmental safety checks are included here, for example, checks on proper use of VDT screens to prevent excessive exposure to radiation.

8. *Utilization review* is the "tracking of resources" in regard to adequacy and proper use (Marker, 1987, p. 61). Resources include staff, funds, equipment, and supplies. In telephone triage, this could mean creating a telephone log to collect and track trend data, such as numbers of calls, the level of acuity of those calls (urgent, emergent, routine), which protocols were used, and the outcome of the calls.

9. *Active problem identification* refers to "tools created by the manager to use as a data source for tracking problems" (Marker, 1987, p. 62). Examples might include problem identification sheets and problem log, care conference report sheets, supervisory report forms and shift report sheets, all of which are applicable to telephone triage.

APPENDIX V

SAMPLE REFERENCE LIBRARY

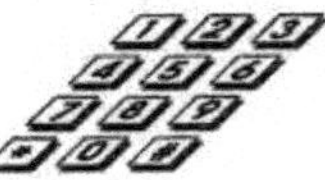

A good telephone triage library requires a minimum of 10 to 15 reference books tailored to the needs of the population served. When possible, choose books that are written in lay language, include monthly or annual supplements (such as the *USP Drug Information for the Patient*), and are less than 5 years old. After obtaining administration approval, update this list on a biannual basis. The list below is based on suggestions from managers and practitioners in the field. Asterisks indicate titles that are most recommended.

STANDARDS/QUALITY ASSURANCE/EXPERTISE

* Benner, P. (1984). *From novice to expert.* Menlo Park, CA: Addison-Wesley.
* Smith-Marker, C.G. (1988). *Setting standards for professional nursing: The Marker model.* Baltimore: C.V. Mosby.

PROTOCOL DEVELOPMENT

* Bates, B. (1991). *A guide to physical examination and history taking.* (5th ed.) New York: Lippincott.
* Berkow, R. (Ed.). (1982). *The Merck manual.* Rahway, NJ: Merck.
* California Department of Mental Health. (1991). *The California helper's handbook for suicide intervention.* San Francisco: Author.
* Clawson, J. J., & Dernocoeur, K. B. (1988). *Principles of emergency dispatch.* Englewood Cliffs, NJ: Brady.
* Doak, C. C., Doak, L. G., & Root, J. H. (1985). *Teaching patients with low literacy skills.* Philadelphia: Lippincott.
* Krupp, M., & Chatton, M. (1985). *Current medical diagnosis and treatment.* Los Altos, CA: Lange.

McGear, R., & Simms, J. (1988). *Telephone triage and management.* Philadelphia: W. B. Saunders.

McVan, B. (1988). *Signs and symptoms handbook.* Springhouse, PA: Springhouse.

* Pantell, R. H., Fries, J. F., & Vickery, D. M. (1978). *Taking care of your child.* Palo Alto, CA: Addison-Wesley.
* Schmitt, B. D. (1980). *Pediatric telephone advice.* Boston: Little, Brown.

Scott, M., & Packard, K. (1990). *Telephone assessment.* Philadelphia: W. B. Saunders.

* Seller, R. H. (1986). *Differential diagnosis of common complaints.* Philadelphia: W. B. Saunders.

* Vickery, D. M., & Fries, J. F. (1978). *Take care of yourself.* Palo Alto, CA: Addison-Wesley.

* Wasson, J., Walsh, B. T., Tompkins, R., Sox, H., & Pantell, R. (1984). *The common symptom guide.* New York: McGraw Hill.

LAY MEDICAL DICTIONARY

* Martin, EA. & Guidos, B. (Eds.). *Bantam Medical Dictionary.* (1981). Toronto: Bantam.

PHARMACOLOGY

American Pharmaceutical Association. (1982). *Handbook of nonprescription drugs,* (7th ed.). Washington, DC: Author.

Boyd, J. (1983). *Facts and comparisons.* St. Louis: Lippincott.

* Griffith, H., & Winter, M. D. (1990). *Complete guide to prescription and non-prescription drugs.* Los Angeles: Price, Stern, Sloan.

Shirkey, J. (1980). *Pediatric dosage handbook.* Washington, DC: American Pharmaceutical Association.

* *United States Pharmacopeial Convention Dispensing Information: Advice for the patient* (6th ed.) (1985). Rockville, MD: Author.

POISON CONTROL

* Olson, K., Becker, C., Benowitz, N. L., Buchanan, J. F., Mycroft. F.J., Osterloh, J., & Woo, O.F. (1990). *Poisoning and drug overdose* (1st ed.). San Mateo, CA: Appleton & Lange.

MATERNAL/CHILD AND BREASTFEEDING

* Briggs, G., Freeman, R. K., & Yaffe, S. (1986). *Drugs in pregnancy and lactation* (2nd ed.). Baltimore, MD: Williams & Wilkins.

* Huggins, K. (1986). *Nursing mother's companion.* Boston: Harvard Common Press.

CONTRACEPTION

* Hatcher, R. A., Guest, F., Stewart, F., Stewart, G. K., Trussell, J., & Frank, E. (1984). *Contraceptive technology* (12th ed.). New York: Irvington.

OTHER

Any local Medical Society Register.
* Beneson, A. S. (Ed.) (1984). *Control of communicable diseases in man* (15th ed.). Washington, D.C.: American Public Health Association.
French, R. M. (1981). *Guide to diagnostic procedures.* New York: McGraw Hill.

INFORMATIONAL AND REFERRAL SERVICES DEVELOPMENT

For informational questions not covered by protocols on medical advances and written in lay language, consult any local medical school health letter (e.g. Harvard, Tufts).

CONSUMERISM, SELF-HELP, AND SELF-CARE

Asmus-Weaver, T. (ED.) (1990). *Resources for Self-Help Groups.* Los Angeles, CA: California Self Help Center.
* American Hospital Association and Illinois Self-Help Center. (1987). *Directory of National Self-Help/Mutual Aid Resources.* Evanston, Ill: Illinois Self-Help Center.
* Baer, L. (1978). *Let the patient decide: A doctor's advice to older persons.* PA: Westminster Press.
* Carper, J. (1987). *Health Care USA.* New York: Prentice Hall.
* Denney, M. K., (1978). *Second opinion.* New York: Grosset and Dunlap
Ferguson, T. (1980). *Medical self-care.* New York: Summit Books.
Graedon, J. (1980). *The people's pharmacy.* New York: Avon.
* Huttman, B. (1981). *The patient's advocate.* New York: Penguin.
Illich, I. (1978). *Medical nemesis.* New York: Bantam Books.
LeMaitre, G. D. (1979). *How to choose a good doctor.* Andover, MA: Andover.
Lipp, M. R. (1980). *The bitter pill: Doctors, patients and failed expectations.* New York: Harper and Row.
* Madara, E. J., & Meese, A. (Eds). (1986). *The self-help sourcebook.* New Denville, NJ: St. Claire's Riverside Medical Center.
Miller, L. (1979). *The life you save.* New York: William Morrow.
Rees, A., & James, J. (1984). *The consumer health information source book.* (2nd ed.). New York: R. R. Bowker.
Rosenfeld, I. (1981). *Second opinion.* New York: Linden Press.
* San Francisco Self-Help Clearinghouse. (1989). *The whole self-help directory.* San Francisco, CA: Author.
Sehnert, K. (1975). *How to be your own doctor (sometimes).* New York: Grosset and Dunlap.

GLOSSARY

ACTIVITIES OF DAILY LIVING (ADL): A useful measure of health status, especially in children and frail elderly. How a person is eating, drinking, sleeping, working playing and eliminating waste.

ACUTE: Disease of rapid onset, severe symptoms, and brief duration (Webster's New Collegiate Dictionary, 1975).

ALGORITHM: "A step-by-step procedure for solving a problem or accomplishing some end" (Webster's New Collegiate Dictionary, 1975, p. 28).

ARTIFICIAL INTELLIGENCE (AI): A machine or computer based analytical process which parallels the thought processes, logic steps, rules, and intuition used in problem solving. AI can be used in "computer diagnostics" to help physicians think through diagnostic and treatment decisions.

CALL VOLUME: The number of calls per hour to be handled by trained professionals. May range from 2 (low volume) to 10 or more (high volume) per hour.

CALLER: The person speaking to the nurse by phone; may also be the client.

CHRONIC: Medical or psychological disease of long duration involving recurrent symptoms and very slow changes. Gradual onset. Does not imply severity.

CLIENT OR VICTIM: The person with the problem. The caller is not necessarily the client.

COMPUTER ASSISTED DIAGNOSIS: A field which utilizes computers to assist in the diagnostic process. An example is "PUFF," a computerized diagnostic tool for pulmonary problems.

CRASH CARD: A set of specific instructions for coaching callers by phone in CPR, Heimlich, and childbirth techniques.

CRISIS INTERVENTION: Action taken to aid the client in a medical or psychological emergency such as cardiac arrest or threatened suicide.

CRISIS INTERVENTION TEAM: This group consists of trained medical dispatchers, counselors from suicide prevention, poison control and rape crisis as well as telephone triage nurses.

DECISION TREE: A diagram of decision criteria.

DISCLAIMER: A final step in the telephone triage process to insure informed consent. Nurses define the working diagnosis status and remind callers that the final responsibility rests with the caller. Disclaimers apply only to routine calls, not crisis intervention.

EMERGENCY: "Any medical or psychological situation that must be attended to within 20 to 30 minutes to prevent loss of life, limb, hearing, or sight" (American College of Emergency Physicians, 1990).

EMERGENCY MEDICAL DISPATCHER (EMD): Trained medical dispatchers who respond to calls to 911. They are a certified subspecialty of emergency medical services personnel along with paramedics and Emergency Medical Technicians (EMT).

EFFICIENCY: In telephone triage, the speed with which a call is handled.

FEEDBACK: A mechanism or procedure which insures that staff receives results (positive or negative) of telephone triage dispositions.

FIRST RESPONDER: A term coined by the Emergency Medical Services System. An individual who has successfully completed a 40-hour First Responder Course, usually an EMD who responds to calls on 911.

GATEKEEPER: A person who processes or directs information flow or patients. In telephone triage, *gatekeeper* refers to an entire system or institutional approach to calls.

HIDDEN AGENDA: An unspoken, underlying emotional or psychological motivation for the client's call. Hidden agendas may also relate to anxiety or misinformation.

HOT LINE: A telephone service which delivers information, referral, or counseling by telephone, often using an 800 number.

INFORMATIONAL TEAM: This team consists of the pharmacist, medical librarian, and telephone triage nurse.

LIFE-THREATENING EMERGENCY: "Any medical or psychological situation that must be attended to within 4 minutes or less to prevent death" (American College of Emergency Physicians, 1990).

MASS CASUALTY INCIDENT (MCI): "A catastrophic accident resulting in loss of many lives or endangerment to many lives, for example, plane crash, explosion, or accidental release of toxic gases" (Clawson, 1990 p. 313).

MICROTEACHING: Short descriptions of common medical terms, assessment methods, and treatments in lay language, and "cookbook format." Microteaching sections may be included in the data collection, advice, and teaching sections of protocols.

MISTRIAGE: To give advice or disposition instructions to client that may result in inappropriate appointments, injury, or further deterioration.

NON-ACUTE: Symptom(s) which present no immediate threat or minimal threat to life, limb, or any major organ; pain of 4 or below on scale of 10.

OVER-THE-COUNTER (OTC): Considered safe if label warnings are followed. RN's may advise use as appropriate if protocols dictate and no contraindications exist.

OROPHONICS: A listening technique to evaluate client respiratory distress by telephone.

POPULATION: The clients or potential clients served by a health care facility, or a category of clients, such as "the elderly population."

PRE-ARRIVAL INSTRUCTIONS: Protocols used by trained emergency medical dispatchers to direct callers in actions that prevent further deterioration or harm to the client (Clawson, 1990).

PRESCRIPTION: Drugs prescribed only by physician (includes drugs which are habit forming, highly toxic or with serious side effects).

PRODUCT LINE: A hospital-sponsored service designed to market services or programs, thereby increasing hospital revenue. Telephone advice or health information services for new parents, the elderly, or women are examples of product lines.

PROFICIENCY: In telephone triage, proficiency relates to the safety, effectiveness, and appropriateness with which a call is handled.

PROTOCOL: Guidelines used in telephone triage for assessment, advice, teaching, crisis intervention, and referral for a range of symptoms. They may be dependent, independent, or interdependent in scope. Protocols are composed of five sections: questions, treatment advice, teaching, referral, and cross-reference.

QUALITY ASSURANCE: "A process in which standards are set and action is taken to insure compliance to the standards; predefined activities that are designed, implemented and documented to demonstrate compliance to established standards" (Smith-Marker, 1988 p. 115).

RULE OF THUMB: "Any method or procedure based upon experience and common sense. A general principle regarded as roughly correct but not intended to be scientifically accurate" (Webster's, 1975 p. 1012).

SELF-ASSESSMENT TECHNIQUES: Methods for quickly, effectively instructing clients in the assessment of their own physical condition or symptoms.

SHOPPING: A method of assessing employee and service effectiveness by hiring actors to act as patients, pretending they have a problem.

STABLE: Characterizing an overall client condition which is not becoming markedly worse, and in which the client is maintaining normal activities of daily living (eating, sleeping, elimination, drinking, work, play).

STANDARD: "Written statements defining a level of practice in the staff or a set of conditions in the patient or staff determined to be acceptable by some authority" (Smith-Marker, 1988 p. 116).

STEREOTYPING: Arriving at an uncritical judgment or oversimplified picture of the client or presenting problem, jumping to conclusions instead of hearing out the client's symptoms, thus blocking useful information that might further clarify the picture.

TALK TIME: The amount of time devoted to telephone triage interactions. In general, a standard of 5 to 7 minutes per call assures safe, effective, and appropriate disposition of client problems.

TELEMARKETING: Promotion of goods or services by telephone solicitation.

TELEMETRY: The process of "measuring a physical variable (for example, heart rate), transmitting the result to a distant station, and there indicating or recording the variable measured" (Webster's, 1975, p. 1198).

TELEPHONE CHARISMA: Warmth, magnetism, or personal charm as well as expert levels of authenticity, congruence, concreteness, and confrontation.

TELEPHONE MEDICINE, TELEPHONE MANAGEMENT: This term usually refers to telephone evaluation and advice given by physicians. Most studies of "telephone medicine" involve pediatrics.

TELEPHONE TRIAGE: The process of evaluating, advising, educating, referring and assuring safe, effective appropriate disposition of client health problems by telephone.

TIME FRAME: Refers to the length of time that symptoms have existed, or within which treatment directives should be followed to achieve a safe, effective, and appropriate disposition.

TRANSITION DRUG (PROPOSED): Drug available only from pharmacist while side effects are monitored. If safety profile is satisfactory, the drug will be approved as OTC.

TRIAGE: The sorting of client health problems into categories. Originally used under wartime conditions to divide patients into three categories of acuity.

TRICK OF THE TRADE: A quick or artful way to achieve a result (Webster's, 1975).

TOCODYNAMOMETER: A monitoring device that senses, records, transmits, and graphs uterine activity by means of telephone transmission for prompt clinical assessment. Used to monitor high risk obstetrical clients at home (Tokos, 1990).

UNSTABLE: Characterized by an overall condition that is becoming markedly worse; symptoms of shock may be present.

URGENCY: Any medical or psychological situation which must be attended to within 20 minutes to 2 hours to prevent loss of life or severe damage to limb, hearing, or sight.

VIDEO WINDOW: A television screen which allows callers to see each other when speaking by phone.

REFERENCES

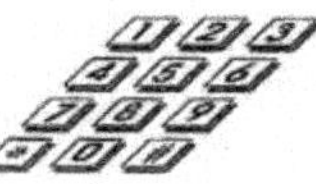

Acker, D. B., Corwin, M., Sachs, B. P., & Schulman, E. (1989). The nonstress test: Transmission from the home. *Journal of Reproductive Medicine, 34*, 971–974.

American College of Emergency Physicians. (1988). Managed health care plans and emergency care. *Annals of Emergency Medicine, 17*, 97–98.

American College of Emergency Physicians. (1990). Providing advice from the emergency department. *Annals of Emergency Medicine, 19*, 600.

Amitai, Y., Mitchell, A., Carrel, J.C., Luciw, H., & Lovejoy, F. H. (1987). Patterns of calling. *American Journal of Disease in Children, 45*, 622–625.

Bates, B. (1991). *A guide to physical examination and history taking*. (5th ed.) New York: Lippincott.

Benner, P. (1984). *From novice to expert*. Menlo Park, CA: Addison-Wesley.

Bernstein, L., & Bernstein, R. S. (1985). *Interviewing: A guide for professionals*. Norwalk, CT: Appleton-Century-Crofts.

Bishop, J. E. (1990, August 11). AIDS set to be a leading killer of women in '91. *The Wall Street Journal*, p. B4.

Broadhead, R. (1986). Directing intervention from afar: The telephone dynamics of managing acute poisonings. *Journal of Health and Social Behavior, 27*, 303–319.

Brown, J. L. (1980). *Telephone medicine*. St. Louis: Mosby.

Buttaravoli, P. M. & Stair, T. O. (1985). *Common simple emergencies*. Bowie, MD: Brady.

California Department of Mental Health. (1992). *The California helper's handbook*. San Francisco: Author.

California Nurses Association. (1989). *Nursing practice in California: Rights, responsibilities and regulations*. San Francisco: Author.

Caplan, S. E., & Straus, J. H. (1988). Strategies for reducing inappropriate after-hours telephone calls. *Clinical Pediatrics, 27*, 236–239.

Carper, J. (1987). *Health Care USA*. New York: Prentice Hall.

Cave, L. A. (1989). Follow-up phone calls after discharge. *American Journal of Nursing, 89*, 942–943.

Christensen, P. J. & Kenney, J. W. (1990). *Nursing process: Application of conceptual models*. (3rd ed). St. Louis: Mosby.

Clawson, J. J. & Dernocoeur, K. B. (1988). *Principles of emergency dispatch*. New Jersey: Brady.

Clawson, J. J. (1988, December 25). Interview, *"60 Minutes"*, CBS.

Colman, C. V., & Robboy, H. (1980). The social construction of a medical emergency. in *TEM: The prehospital care system*. Richmond, VA: Aspen.

Corcoran, S., Narayan, S., & Moreland, H. (1988). Thinking aloud as a strategy to improve clinical decision making. *Heart and Lung, 17*, 463–468.

Crime Prevention Center. (1988). *Child abuse prevention handbook*. Sacramento, CA: Author.

Curry, M. A. (1983). Variables related to adaption to motherhood in "normal" primiparous women. *Journal of Obstetric, Gynecologic, and Neonatal Nursing, 12 (2),* 115–121.

Curse of 911. *Newsweek,* November 5, 1990.

Curtis, P., & Evens, S. (1983). Using patient simulators to teach telephone communications skills to health professionals. *Journal of Medical Education, 58,* 894–898.

Curtis, P., Evens, S., Berolzheimer, N., & Beery, M. (1983). *Telephone medicine.* Chapel Hill, NC: University of North Carolina.

Curtis, P., Evens, S., Talbot, A., Baer, C. & Smart, A. (1985). Characteristics and perceptions of after hours callers. *Family Practice, 2*(1), 10–16.

Curtis, P., & Talbot, A. (1979). The after-hours call in family practice. *Journal of Family Practice, 9,* 901–909.

Curtis, P., & Talbot, A. (1980). After hours call: An aspect of primary care education. *Journal of Medical Education, 55,* 55–57.

Curtis, P., & Talbot, A. (1981). The telephone in primary care. *Journal of Community Health, 6,* 194–203.

Curtis, P., Talbot, A., & Liebeseller, V. (1979). The after-hours call: a survey of United States family practice residency programs. *Journal of Family Practice, 8,* 117–122.

Daley, W. R., Leaning, J., & Braen, R. (1988). Prehospital emergency services and health maintenance organizations: An HMO perspective. *Journal of Emergency Medicine, 6,* 333–338.

Dalton, K. J., Manning, K., Robarts, P. J., Dripps, J. H., & Currie, J. R. (1987). Computerized home telemetry of maternal blood pressure in hypertensive pregnancy. *International Journal of Bio-Medical Computing, 21* (3–4), 175–187.

Daugird, A. J., & Spencer, D. C. (1988). Patient telephone call documentation. Quality implications and attempted intervention. *Journal of Family Practice, 27,* 420–421.

Daugird, A. J. and Spencer, D. C. (1989). Characteristics of patients who highly utilize telephone medical care in a private practice. *The Journal of Family Practice, 29,* 59–64.

Derlet, R. W., & Nishio, D. A. (1990). Refusing care to patients who present to an emergency department. *Annals of Emergency Medicine, 19,* 262–267.

Dibner, A. S., Lowt, L., & Morris, J. N. (1982). Usage and acceptance of an emergency alarm system by the frail elderly. *Gerontologist, 22*(6), 538–539.

Dunn, J. (1985). Warning: Giving telephone advice is hazardous to your professional health. *Nursing, 85, 15*(8), 40–41.

Egger, R. L. (May 26, 1986). What every practice needs is more phone calls. *Medical Economics,* p. 106, 108, 111.

Eisenberg, M. (1986). Identification of cardiac arrest by emergency dispatchers. *American Journal of Emergency Medicine, 4,* 299–301.

Emergency Nurses Association. (April 27, 1991). Emergency nurses association position statement: Telephone advice. Chicago: Author.

Emery, J. L. (1959). Epidemiology of "sudden, unexpected or rapid" death in children. *Proceedings of the Royal Society of Medicine, 52,* 890–892.

Evens, S., & Curtis, P. (1983). Using patient simulators to teach telephone communications skills to health professionals. *Journal of Medical Education, 58,* 894–898.

Evens, S., Curtis, P., Talbot, A., Baer, C., & Smart, A. (1985). Characteristics and perceptions of after-hours callers. *Family Practice, 2,* 10–26.

Finley, J. P., Human, D. G., Nanton, M. A., Roy, D. L., Macdonald, J., Marr, D. R., & Chiasson, H. (1989). Echocardiography by telephone—evaluation of pediatric heart disease at a distance. *American Journal of Cardiology, 63*, 1475–1477.

Fischer, P. M., & Smith, S. R. (1979). The nature and management of telephone utilization in a family practice setting. *Journal of Family Practice, 8*, 321–327.

Fisher, A. B. (1989, July). House calls. *Inc.* pp. 72–79.

Fogel, C. I., & Woods, N. F. (1981). *Health care of women*. St. Louis: Mosby.

Ford, R. D. (Ed.) (1985). *Nurse's legal handbook*. Springhouse, PA: Springhouse.

Fosarelli, P. D., & Schmitt, B. (1987). Telephone dissatisfaction in pediatric practice: Denver and Baltimore. *Pediatrics, 80*, 28–31.

Fritz, M. S., & Talley, J. (1982). Bloomington hospital's experience with Lifeline. *Hospital Topics, 60*(5), 15–18.

Garrettson, L. K., Bush, J. P., Gates, R. S., & French, A. L. (1990). Physical change, time of day and child characteristics as factors in poison injury. *Veterinary and Human Toxicology, 32*, 139–141.

Geller, R. J., Fisher, J. G., Leeper, J. D., & Ranganathan, S. (1988). American poison control centers: Still not all the same? *Annals of Emergency Medicine, 17*, 599–603.

Ghitelman, D. (1988). Put together the right phone system for your office. *Medical Economics*, pp. 157, 160, 161, 163.

Glass cable has big potential. (November 11, 1990). *Marin Independent Journal*. p. C 1.

Gonen, R., Braithwaite, N., & Milligan, J. E. (1990). Fetal heart rate monitoring at home and transmission by telephone. *Obstetrics and Gynecology, 75*, 464–468.

Goodman, C. C., & Pynoos, J. (1990). A model telephone information and support program for caregivers of Alzheimer's patients. *The Gerontologist, 30*, 399–403.

Gosha, J. (1986). A self-help group for new mothers: An evaluation. *Maternal Child Nursing, 11*, 20–23.

Graef, P., McGhee, K., Rozychi, J., Fescina-Jones, D., Clark, J. A., Thompson, J., & Brooten, D. (1988). Postpartum concerns of breastfeeding mothers. *Journal of Nurse Midwifery, 33*, 62–66.

Gray, B. B. (1991, August 19). When drugs shift from RX to OTC. *Nurseweek*, p. 1.

Green, L. W., & Kreuter, M. W. (1991). *Health Promotion Planning*. London: Mayfield.

Greenlick, M. R., Freeborn, D. K., Gambill, G. L., & Pope, C. R. (1973). Determinants of medical care utilization: The role of the telephone in total medical care. *Medical Care, 11*, 121–134.

Greitzer, L., Stapleton, B., Wright, L., & Wedgwood, R. J. (1976). Telephone assessment of illness by practicing pediatricians. *The Journal of Pediatrics, 88*, 880–882.

Grumet, G. W. (1979). Telephone therapy: A review and case study. *Amer. J. Orthopsychiatry, 49*, 574–584.

Halberstam, M. J. (1977). Medicine by telephone: Is it brave, foolhardy, or just inescapable? *Modern Medicine, 15*, 11–12.

Hamadeh, G. (1989). Documentation of after hours telephone contacts by family medicine resident. *Family Medicine, 21*, 305–306.

Handler, E. G. (1989). Visual telephone for pediatric rehabilitation inpatients. *Archives of Physical Medicine and Rehabilitation, 70*, 854–855.

Harsham, P. (1982). Medicine by telephone rings some new numbers. *Medical Economics, 4*, 93.

Haston, L. (Ed.). (1984). *Nurse's legal handbook*. Springhouse, PA: Springhouse.

Higgs, Z., & Gustafson, D. (1985). *Community as client.* Philadelphia: Davis.

Hornby, G., Murray, R., & Jones, R. (1987). Establishing a parent to parent service. *Child: Care, Health and Development, 13,* 277–288.

Hornsby, L., & Payne, F. (1979). A model for communications skills development for family practice residents. *Journal of Family Practice, 8,* 71–76.

Huff, B. (Ed.). (1981). *Physicians' Desk Reference.* Oradell, NJ: Medical Economics.

Infante-Rivard, C., Krieger, M., Petitclerc, M., & Baumgarten, M. (1988). A telephone support service to reduce medical care use among the elderly. *JAGS, 36,* 306–311.

Isaacman, D. J., Verdile, V. P., Kohen, F. P., & Verdile, L. A. (1992). Pediatric telephone advice in the emergency department: Results of a mock scenario. *Pediatrics, 89,* 35–39.

Johnson, B. E., & Johnson, C. A. (1990). Telephone medicine: A general internal medicine experience. *Journal of General Internal Medicine, 5,* 234–239.

Jones, J., Clark, W., Bradford, J., & Dougherty, J. (1987). Efficacy of a telephone follow-up system in the emergency department. *Journal of Emergency Medicine, 6,* 249–254.

Kasche, C., & Knutson, K. (1985). Patient compliance and interpersonal style: Implications for practice and research. *Nurse Practitioner, 10*(3), 52–54, 56.

Katz, H. P. (1990). *Telephone medicine: Triage and training.* Thorofare, NJ: Slack.

Katz, H. P., Pozen, J., & Mushlin, A. I. (1978). Quality assessment of a telephone care system utilizing non-physician personnel. *American Journal of Public Health, 68,* 31–37.

Kellerman, A. L., Hackman, B. B., & Somes, G. (1989). Dispatcher-assisted cardiopulmonary resuscitation: Validation of efficacy. *Circulation, 80,* 1231–1239.

Kelley, M., & Mashburn, J. (1990). Telephone triage in the office setting. *Journal of Nurse-Midwifery, 35,* 245–251.

Kerr, H. D. (1986). Prehospital emergency services and health maintenance organizations. *Annals of Emergency Medicine, 15,* 727–729.

Kerr, H. (1989). Access to emergency departments: A survey of HMO policies. *Annals of Emergency Medicine, 18,* 274–277.

Knowles, P., & Cummins, R. (1984). ED medical advice telephone calls: Who calls and why? *Journal of Emergency Nursing, 10,* 283–286.

Korcok, M. (1983). Computer diagnostics: Technology of the future. *Canadian Medical Assoc, 133,* 231–235.

Kravitz, H., Korach, A., Murphy, J. B., Luce, H., & Kite, M. (1963). Telephone diagnosis of pediatric respiratory diseases. *American Journal of Diseases of Children, 106,* 471–472.

Kulikowski, C. A. (1985). Artificial intelligence methods for expert medical consultant systems. *The Mount Sinai Journal of Medicine, 52,* 87–93.

Leerhsen, C., Lewis, S. D., Pomper, S., Davenport, L., & Nelson, M. (1990, February 5). Unite and conquer. *Newsweek,* pp. 50–55.

Levy, J. C., Strasser, P. H., Lang, G. A., Rosekrans, J., Friedman, M., Kaplan, D., & Sanofsky, P. (1980). Survey of telephone encounters in three pediatric practice sites. *Public Health Reports, 95,* 324–328.

Lindsay, P. C., Beveridge, R., Tayob, Y., Irvine, L. M., Vellacott, I. D., Giles, J. A., Hussain, S. Y., & O'Brien, P. M. S. (1990). Patient-recorded domiciliary fetal monitoring. *American Journal of Obstetrics and Gynecology, 162,* 466–470.

Margolis, C. F., Harrigan, J. A., Franko, A. P., Gramata, J., Margolis, J., & Ebersold, D. K. (1987). The telephone management of gastroenteritis by family medicine residents. *Family Practice Research Journal, 6,* 148–149.

Marker, C. S. (1987). The Marker umbrella model for quality assurance: Monitoring and evaluating professional practice. *Journal of Nursing Quality Assurance, 1,* (3), 52–63.

Marker, C. S. (1988). *Setting standards for professional nursing: The Marker model.* Baltimore, MD: Mosby.

Marshall, D. (1977). Telecare. *Hospital Forum, 19,* 6–8.

Matherly, S. & Hodges, S. (1990). *Telephone nursing: The process.* Englewood, CO: Center for Research in Ambulatory Health Care.

McGear, R., & Simms, J. (1988). *Telephone triage and management.* Philadelphia: Saunders.

McMahon, M. M. (1986). Providing telephone advice. In J. B. Johnston (Ed.). *Emergency Nurse Reports, 1,* 8.

Moreland, H., & Grier, M. (1986). Telephone consultation in the care of older adults. *Geriatric Nursing, 7* (6), 28–30.

Moreno, C. A. (1989). Utilization of medical services by single-parent and two-parent families. *Journal of Family Practice, 28,* 194–199.

Neville, D., & Barnes, S. (1985). The suicidal phone call. *Journal of Psychosocial Nursing, 23,* 14–18.

Nicklin, W. M. (1981). The telephone—a viable medium for health education. *Dimensions in Health Service, 58* (8), 9–11.

Nurses on call reduce emergency room visits. (1991, July 8). *The Wall Street Journal,* p. B1.

O'Brien, R. P., & Miller, T. L. (1990). Urgent care center pediatric telephone advice. *American Journal of Emergency Medicine, 8,* 496–497.

Osgood, N. J. (1985). *Suicide in the elderly.* Richmond, VA: Aspen.

Ott, J., Bellaire, J., & Machakota, P. E. (1974). Patient management by telephone by child health associates and pediatric house officers. *Journal of Medical Education, 49,* 596.

Pantell, R. H., Fries, J. F., & Vickery, D. M. (1978). *Taking care of your child.* Palo Alto, CA: Addison-Wesley.

Perrin, E., & Goodman, H. C. (1978). Telephone management of acute pediatric illness. *New England Journal of Medicine, 298,* 130–135.

Physicians referral services: Boom or bust? (May 20, 1987). *Hospitals,* p. 40.

Pitts, J., & Whitby, M. (1990). Out-of-hours workload of a suburban general practice: Deprivation or expectation. *British Medical Journal, 300,* 1113–1115.

Politis, E. K. (1988). Medicolegal aspects of telephone triage. In S. Q. Wheeler, *The fine art of telephone triage* (pp. 23–28). San Anselmo, CA: Wheeler and Associates.

Radecki, S. E., Neville, R. E., & Girard, R. A. (1989). Telephone patient management by primary care physicians. *Medical Care, 27,* 817–822.

Reubin, R. (1979). Spotting and stopping the suicidal patient. *Nursing 79, 9,* 83–85.

Riley, J. (1989). Telephone call-backs: Final patient care evaluation. *Nursing Management, 20,* 64–66.

Rowland, H. (1987). *Nursing forms manual: Checklists and guidelines.* Rockville, MD: Aspen.

Roy, C. (1982). Theoretical framework for classification of nursing diagnosis. In Kim, M. J. and Moritz, D. A. (Eds). *Classification of nursing diagnosis: Proceedings of the third and fourth national conferences.* New York: McGraw-Hill.

Samuels, J., & Balter, L. (1987, May-June). An evaluation of a warmline: How useful are telephone consultation services for parents? *Children Today,* pp. 27–29.

San Francisco Women Against Rape. (1987). *Guidelines for counselors.* San Francisco: Author.

Schmitt, B. (1980). *Pediatric telephone advice*. Boston: Little, Brown.

Scott, M., & Packard, K. (1990). *Telephone assessment*. Philadelphia: W. B. Saunders.

Silverstone, B., & Hyman, H. K. (1976). *You and your aging parent*. New York: Pantheon.

Skillicorn, S. A. (1980). *Quality and accountability: A new era in America's hospitals*. San Francisco: Editorial Consultants.

Sloane, P. D., Egelhoff, C., Curtis, P., McGaghie, W., & Evens, S. (1985). Physician decision-making over the telephone. *The Journal of Family Practice, 21*, 279–284.

Smith, K. S. (1990). Telephone triage offers help and advice for patients in need. *American Medical Writers Association, 5*, 18–21.

Smith, S. R., & Fisher, R. (1980). Patient management by telephone: A training exercise for medical students. *The Journal of Family Practice, 10*, 463–466.

Spencer, D. C. and Daugird, A. J. (1988). The nature and content of physician telephone calls in a private practice. *The Journal of Family Practice, 27*, 201–205.

Spitz, L., & Bloch, E. (1981). Denial and minimization in telephone contacts with patients. *Journal of Family Practice, 12*, 93–98.

Stanhope, M., & Lancaster, J. (1988). *Community Health Nursing*. St. Louis: Mosby.

Stirewalt, C. F., Linn, M. W., Godoy, G., Knopka, F., & Linn, L. S. (1981). Characteristics of callers and noncallers to an ambulatory care hotline. *Journal of Ambulatory Care Management, 4*, 39–45.

Strain, J. E., & Miller, J. D. (1971). The preparation, utilization and evaluation of a registered nurse trained to give telephone advice in a private pediatric office. *Pediatrics, 47*, 1051–1055.

Sumner, G., & Fritsch, J. (1977). Postnatal parental concerns: The first six weeks of life. *Journal of Obstetric, Gynecologic, and Neonatal Nursing, 6*, 27–32.

Taber, C. W. (1962). *Taber's Cyclopedic Medical Dictionary* (9th ed.). Philadelphia: Davis.

Tennenhouse, D. J. (1988, September 24). Legal aspects of telephone triage. In *Future Trends in Nursing*. Seminar conducted at San Francisco General Hospital.

Tennenhouse, D. J. (1991, March-April). Minimizing liability for telephone advice. *California Nursing Review*, pp. 24–27.

Thayer, M. B. (1984). Telephone management. *Pediatric Nursing, 10*, 121–122.

Thompson, C. E., Jones, J. M., Cox, L. R., & Levy, L. E. (1983) *Adult health management*. Reston, VA: Reston.

Thompson, D. F., Trammel, H. L., Robertson, N. J., & Reigart, J. R. (1983). Evaluation of regional and nonregional poison centers. *New England Journal of Medicine, 308*, 191–194.

Trautlein, J. J., Lambert, R. L., & Miller, J. (1984). Malpractice in the emergency department—review of 200 cases. *Annals of Emergency Medicine, 13*, 709–711.

Turner, S. R. (1981). Golden rules for accurate triage. *Journal of Emergency Nursing, 7*, 153–156.

U.S. Department of Health and Human Services. (1991). *Health: United States 1990*. Hyattsville, MD: Author.

USP Dispensing Information—Advice for the patient. (1985). Easton, PA: Mack Printing.

Verdile, V., Paris, P. M., Stewart, R. D., & Verdile, L. A. (1989). Emergency department telephone advice. *Annals of Emergency Medicine, 18*, 279–282.

Vickery, D. M., & Fries, J. F. (1978). *Take care of yourself*. Palo Alto, CA: Addison-Wesley.

Wasson, J., Walsh, B. T., Tompkins, R., Sox, H., & Pantell, R. (1984). *The common symptom guide*. New York: McGraw Hill.

Wasson, J., Gaudette, C., Whaley, F., Sauvigne, A., Baribeau, R., & Welch, H. G. (1992). Telephone care as a substitute for routine clinic follow-up. *Journal of the American Medical Association, 267*, 1788–1793.

Wheeler, S. Q. (1988). *The fine art of telephone triage*. San Anselmo, CA: Wheeler and Associates.

Wheeler, S. Q. (1989). ED telephone triage: Lessons learned from unusual calls. *Journal of Emergency Nursing, 15*, 481–487.

Will, G. (1990, March 12). The trauma in trauma care. *Newsweek*, p. 98.

Willett, D. (1977). Medicine by telephone, a legal opinion. *Modern Medicine, 45*, 73–74.

Wood, P. R. (1986). Pediatric resident training in telephone management: A survey of training programs in the United States. *Pediatrics, 77*, 822–825.

Woolf, H. B., Artin, E., Crawford, F. S., Gilman, E. W., Kay, M. W., & Pease, R. W. (Eds.) (1975). *Webster's New Collegiate Dictionary.* (pp. 313, 373, 1351). Springfield, MA: Merriam.

Yanovski, S. Z., Yanovski, J. A., Malley, J. D., Brown, R. L., & Balaban, D. J. (1992). Telephone triage by primary care physicians. *Pediatrics, 89*, 701–706.

Yura, H., & Walsh, M. B. (1978). *The nursing process: Assessing, planning, implementing, evaluating*. New York: Appleton-Century-Crofts.

Zelus, P. R., & Hughes, S. (1988). Dialing for health: Electrocardiogram analysis program. *Geriatric Nursing, 9*, 230–231.

Zola, I. (1966). Culture and symptoms—An analysis of patients' presenting complaints. *American Sociological Review, 31*, 5.

ADDITIONAL READING

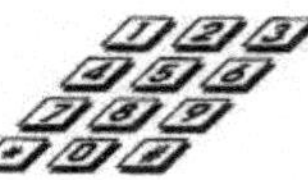

Albin, S., Wassertheil-Smoller, S., Jacobson, S., & Bell, B. (1975). Evaluation of emergency room triage performed by nurses. *American Journal of Public Health, 65,* 1063–1065.

American College of Emergency Medicine. (1990). Measures to deal with emergency department overcrowding. *Annals of Emergency Medicine, 19,* 944.

American Nurses Association. (1980). *Nursing: A social policy statement.* Kansas City: Author.

Arnold, R. G. (1973). How does a pediatrician spend his time? *Clinical Pediatrics, 12,* 611–616.

Benner, P. & Tanner, C. (1987). How expert nurses use intuition. *American Journal of Nursing,* 23–31.

Benner, P. & Wrubel, J. (1982). Skilled clinical knowledge: The value of perceptual awareness. *Journal of Nursing Administration, 7,* 28–33.

Bonovitz, A. (1990, May 14). The jury is out on safety of computers. *Nurseweek,* p 1, 4.

Broome, M. E. (1986). Telephone protocols for pediatric assessment and advice. *Journal of Emergency Nursing, 12,* 141–146.

Brown, S. B., & Eberle, B. J. (1974). Use of the telephone of pediatric house staff: A technique for pediatric care not taught. *Journal of Pediatrics, 84,* 117–119.

Brunnette, D. D., Kominsky, J. H., & Ruiz, E. (1991). Correlations of emergency health care use, 911 volume, and jail activity with welfare check distribution. *Annals of Emergency Medicine, 20,* 739–742.

Buckles, E. & Carew-McColl, M. (1991). Communication: Triage by telephone. *Nursing Times, 87* (6), 26–28.

Burda, D. (1987). Referral services can link hospitals with lawsuit. *Hospitals, 61* (10), 36.

Carlova, J. (1984). How treating by telephone rang a malpractice bell. *Medical Economics, 19,* 82–84.

Casey, R., Rosen, B., Glowasky, A., & Ludwig, S. (1985, March). An intervention to improve follow-up of patients with otitis media. *Clinical Pediatrics,* 140–152.

Ceccio, J. F., & Ceccio, C. M. (1982). *Effective communication in nursing: Theory and practice.* New York: Wiley.

Conrath, D. W., Dunn, E. V., Bloor, W. G., & Tranquada, L. B. (1977). A clinical evaluation of four alternative telemedicine systems. *Behavioral Science, 22,* 12–21.

Copeland, D. (1979, July 23). Why (and how) I charge for telephone advice. *Medical Economics,* 77–79.

Curry, T. A., & Schwartz, M. (1978). Telephone assessment of illness: What is being taught and learned? *Pediatrics, 62,* 603–605.

da Silva, V. L., & Steinberg, B. (1991). A force field evaluation tool for telephone service in ambulatory health care. *Journal of Ambulatory Care Management, 14* (4), 68–76.

Davidhizar, R. E., & Wehlage, D. F. (1987). Telephone "emergencies." *Postgraduate Medicine, 81*, 164–168.

Davis, A. J. (1984). *Listening and responding*. St Louis: Mosby.

Dial 1-900 for doctor. (1991, October 28). *Newsweek*. p. 48.

Doak, C. C., Doak, L. G., & Root, J. H. (1985). Teaching patients with low literacy skills. Philadelphia: Lippincott.

DRGs of emergency alert units. (1986). *Hospitals, 20*, 97–98.

Duggan, H. A. (1984). *Crisis intervention*. Lexington, VA: Lexington.

Eisenberg, J. M. (1979). Sociologic influences on decision-making by clinicians. *Annals of Internal Medicine, 90*, 957–964.

Eisenberg, M. (1985). Dispatcher cardiopulmonary resuscitation instruction via telephone. *Critical Care Medicine, 13*, 923–924.

Eisenberg, M. (1985). Emergency CPR instruction via telephone. *American Journal of Public Health, 75*, (1), 47–50.

Ennis, M. & Vincent, C. A. (1990). Obstetric accidents: A review of 64 cases. *British Medical Journal 300*, 1365–1367.

Fitzgerald, J. L., & Mulford, M. (1984). An experimental test of telephone aftercare contacts with alcoholics. *Journal of Studies on Alcohol, 46*, 418–424.

Fleming, M. F., Skochelak, S. E., Curtis, P., & Evens, S. (1988). Evaluating the effectiveness of a telephone medicine curriculum. *Medical Care, 26*, 211–216.

Fosarelli, P. D. (1983). The telephone in pediatric medicine. *Clinical Pediatrics, 22*, 293–296.

Fosarelli, P. D. (1985). The emphasis of telephone medicine in pediatric training programs. *American Journal of Diseases of Children, 139*, 555–557.

Freeman, T. R., (1980). A study of telephone prescriptions in family practice. *Journal of Family Practice, 10*, 857–862.

George, J. (1976). The legal problem of the telephone. *Journal of Emergency Nursing, 2* (4), 51.

Glatt, K. M., Sherwood, D. W., & Amisson T. J. (1986). Telephone helplines at suicide site. *Hospital and Community Psychiatry, 37*, 178–180.

Hafen, B. Q. & Karren, K. J. (1983). *Prehospital emergency care and crisis intervention*. Englewood, CO: Morton.

Haight, J. (1977). Steadying parents as they go—by phone. *Maternal-Child Nursing, 2* (5), 311–312.

Hallam, L. (1991). Organization of telephone services and patients' access to doctors by telephone in general practice. *British Medical Journal, 302*, 629–632.

Haynes, B. E., & Bedard, L. A. (1989). HMOs and the use of 911. *Annals of Emergency Medicine, 18*, 422.

Health Care Advisory Board. (1988). *Frontier marketing: 32 of the best/worst hospital marketing tactics*. Washington, D.C.: Author.

Hoff, L. A. (1984). *People in crisis: Understanding and helping*. Menlo Park, CA: Addison-Wesley.

Holden, G. L., & Klinger, A. M. (1988). Learning from experience: Differences in how novice versus expert nurses diagnose why an infant is crying. *Journal of Nursing Education, 27*, 123–129.

Hornblow, A. R. (1986). The evolution of effectiveness of telephone consulting services. *Hospital and Community Pyschiatry, 37*, 731–733.

Hossfield, G. & Ryan, M. (1989). HMOs and utilization of emergency medical services: A metropolitan survey. *Annals of Emergency Medicine, 18*, 374–377.

Houts, P. S., Whitney, L. C. W., Mortel, R., & Bartholomew, M. J. (1986). Former cancer patients as counselors of newly diagnosed cancer patients. *JNC, 76*, 793–796.

Hribersek, E., Van De Voorde, H., Poppe, H., & Casselman, J. (1987). Influence of the day of the week and weather on people using a telephone support system. *British Journal of Psychiatry, 150*, 189–193.

Krupp, M., & Chatton, M. (1985). *Current medical diagnosis and treatment.* Los Altos, CA: Lange.

Lancaster, J. & Lancaster, W. (1982). *The nurse as change agent.* St. Louis: Mosby.

Leikin, J. B., Frateschi, L. J., Boston, D. A., Eckenrode, P. J., Morris, R. J., Konczyk, L. J., & Hryhorczuk, D. O. (1990). Effects of nonparticipation in trauma center system on emergency department utilization. *Journal of Emergency Medicine, 8*, 545–550.

Marklund, B., Silverhelm, B., & Bengtsson, C. (1989). Evaluation of an educational programme for telephone advisors in primary health care. *Family Practice, 6*, 263–267.

Martin, B. A., Ornstein, S. M., Johnson, A. H., Jenkins, R. G., & Rust, P. E. (1990). Factors associated with frequency of after hours in person consultations. *Family Medicine, 22*, 443–446.

Mayer, T. R., Solberg, L., Seifert, M., & Cole, P. (1983). Family practice after-hours telephone use. *Journal of Ambulatory Care Management*, 14–19.

McBean, B. J., & Balckburn, J. L. (1982). An evaluation of four methods of pharmacist conducted patient education. *Canadian Pharmaceutical Journal, 115*(5), 167–172.

McCarthy, M., & Bollam, M. (1990). Telephone advice for out of hours calls in general practice. *British Journal of General Practice, 40*, 19–21.

Mechaber, J., McNerney, H., & Chorney, E. (1974). Analysis of the triage system in a neighborhood health center. *Journal of Nursing Administration, 4*, 29–32.

Moorhead, G. V. & Koehler, G. (1986). *Emergency Medical Dispatcher Guidelines.* Sacramento, CA: Emergency Medical Services Authority.

Morse, S. (1990). Poison information: A phone call away. *Journal of Emergency Nursing, 16*, 9–11.

Murphy, D. (1975). Nursing by telephone. *American Journal of Nursing, 75*, 1137–1139.

National Association of Emergency Medical Services Physicians. (1987). Emergency medical dispatching. *Prehospital and Disaster Medicine, 4* (2), 163–166.

Nelson, E. W., Van Cleve, S., Swartz, M. K., Kessen, W., & McCarthy, P. L. (1991). Improving the use of early follow-up care after emergency department visits. *American Journal of Diseases of Children, 145*, 440–444.

Nickerson, H. J., Biechler, L., & Witte, L. F. (1975). How dependable is diagnosis and management of earache by telephone? *Clinical Pediatrics, 14*, 920–923.

Nicklin, W. M. (1986). Postdischarge concerns of cardiac patients as presented via a telephone callback system. *Heart and Lung, 15*, 268–272.

Oberkaid, F., Bell, J., & Duke, V. (1983). Pediatric telephone consultation: A neglected area of health service delivery. *Australian Pediatric Journal, 20*, 113–114.

Pachter, L. M., Ludwig, S., & Groves, A. (1991). Night people: Utilization of a pediatric emergency department during the late night. *Pediatric Emergency Care, 7*(1), 12–14.

Perkins, A. H., Copel, M., & Fairbanks, K. R. (1986). National nutrition month hotline. *Journal of the American Diatetic Association, 86*, 365–367.

Pierce, J. M., & Kellerman, A. L. (1990). "Bounces": An analysis of short term return visits to a public hospital emergency department. *Annals of Emergency Medicine, 19*, 752–757.

Pitts, J. & Whitby, M. (1990) Out-of-hours workload of a suburban general practice: deprivation or expectation. *British Medical Journal, 300*, 1113–1115.

Plumlee, K. (1985). Nurse telephone service blends hospitals' marketing and mission. *Health Progress, 10*, 68.

Purvis, A. (1991, July 22). Reach out and cure someone. *Time*, p. 54.

Rabinow, J. (1989, February). Where you stand in the eyes of the law. *Nursing 89*, 34–40.

Ranan, W., & Blodgett, A. (1983, January). Using telephone therapy for "unreachable" clients. *The Journal of Contemporary Social Work*, 39–43.

Rauen, K. (1985). The telephone as stethoscope. *Maternal-Child Nursing, 10*, 122–124.

Reagan, M. D. (1987). Physicians as gatekeepers. *New England Journal of Medicine, 317*, 1731–1733.

Rezazadeh, M. & Evans, N. E. (1988). Remote vital-signs monitor using a dial up telephone line. *Medical and Biological Engineering and Computing, 26*, 557–561.

Russo, R. M., Gururaj, V. J., & Allen, J. E. (1974). Ambulatory care triage. *American Family Physician, 9*, 125–130.

Seller, R. (1986). *Differential diagnosis of common complaints*. Philadelphia: W. B. Saunders.

Sergi-Swinehart, P. (1985). Hospice home care: How to get patients home and help them stay there. *Seminars in Oncology, 1*, 461–465.

Shah, C. P., Elan, T. J., & Bona, H. W. (1980). An expanded emergency service: The role of telephone services in the emergency department. *Annals of Emergency Medicine, 9*, 617–623.

Shaughnessy, S. (1978). A telephone screening system that works. *Group Practice, 27*, 24–25.

Shesser, R., Smith, M., Adams, S., Walls, R., & Paxton, M. (1986). The effectiveness of an organized emergency department follow-up system. *Annals of Emergency Medicine, 15*, 911–915.

Siegal, L. P., & Krieble, T. (1988). "In touch" telephone message system for teenagers. *Delaware Medical Journal, 60*, 708.

Silverstone, B., & Hyman, H. K. (1976). *You and your aging parent*. New York: Pantheon.

Simon, J. L., Johnson, C. A., & Liese, B. S. (1988). A family practice "breastfeeding hotline": description and preliminary results. *Family Medicine, 20*, 224–226.

Simon, H., Reisman, A., Javad, S., & Sachs, D. (1979). An index of accessibility for ambulatory health services. *Medical Care, 17*, 894–898.

Singh, G., Barton, D., & Bodiwala, G. G. (1991). Accident and emergency department's response to patients' inquiries by telephone. *Journal of the Royal Society of Medicine, 84*(6), 345–346.

Spencer, D. C., & Daugird, A. J. (1990). The nature and content of telephone prescribing habits in a community practice. *Family Medicine, 22*, 205–209.

Strasser, P. H., Levy, J., Lamb, G. A., & Rosekrans, J. (1979). Controlled clinical trial of pediatric telephone protocols. *Pediatrics, 64*, 553–557.

Sturtz, G. S., & Brown, R. T. (1969). Concerning A. G. Bell's invention. *Clinical Pediatrics, 8*, 378–380.

Taniguchi, R. T. (1980). Community drug information services by telephone. *Contemporary Pharmacy Practice, 3*, 82–84.

Tanner, C. A., Padrick, K. P., Westfall, U. E., & Putzier, D. J. (1987). Diagnostic reasoning strategies of nurses and nursing students. *Nursing Research, 36*, 358–363.

Tekavcic-Grad, O., & Farberow, N. L. (1989). A cross-cultural comparison of ideal and undesirable qualities of crisis line workers. *Crisis, 10*(2), 152–163.

Tennenhouse, D. J. (1987). Abandoning your patients—a constant legal peril. *California Nursing Review, 11*, 33–34.

Tripp, S. (1971). Telephone techniques in pediatric practice. *American Journal of Nursing, 71*, 1722–1724.

Valenzuela, T. D., Criss, E. A., Spaite, D., Meislin, H. W., Wright, A. L., & Clark, L. (1990). Cost effectiveness analysis of paramedic emergency medical services in treatment of prehospital cardiopulmonary arrest. *Annals of Emergency Medicine, 19*, 1407–1411.

Van Every, S. L., & Curwen, L. H. (1985). Combating heart attacks on the home front. *Nursing 85, 15*, 55–57.

Walfish, S. (1983). Crisis telephone counselor's views of clinical interaction situations. *Community Mental Health Journal, 19*, 219–226.

Williams, L. (1985, April 14). Lawyer says doctor shopped while patient was dying. *San Francisco Examiner*, p. A2.

Winter, J. P., Hornfeldt, C. S., Weiland, M. J., & Ling, L. J. (1988). Analysis of initial requests for information of non-exposure related topics at a regional poison center. *Veterinary and Human Toxicology, 30(2)*, 108–109.

Woodward, C. T., Stevenson, J. G., & Poremba, A. (1990). Assessing the quality of pharmacist answers to telephone drug information questions. *American Journal of Hospital Pharmacy, 47*, 798–799.

Yeatman, G. W. (1981). Twenty-four hour telephone triage: An expedient to ambulatory child care. *Military Medicine, 146*, 249–253.

Zborowski, M. (1952). Cultural components in response to pain. *Journal of Social Issues, 8*, 16–30.

Zylke, J. W. (1990). Physicians need better line on how, when to respond to patients via telephone. *Journal of the American Medical Association, 264*, 1797–1798.

AUDIO ACTIVITIES

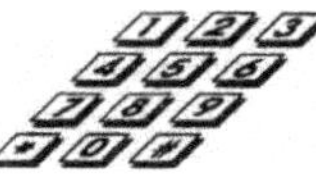

OBJECTIVES:

Upon completion of these exercises, participants will be able to:

1. Use a case study methodology to analyze telephone triage calls
2. Differentiate and select roles appropriate to each case study
3. Differentiate and select strategies appropriate to each case study
4. Identify practitioner flaws
5. Suggest additional or alternative management strategies
6. Identify major guideline(s) illustrated by each case study

METHOD:

This 60-minute CD contains 10 case study vignettes-each about 3-7 minutes long. Each case study is a reenactment of an actual or fictitious telephone triage call that illustrates either effective or ineffective telephone triage management. Using the following case study approach, analyze and critique each call. It will take approximately 20-30 minutes to complete each exercise and to compare your answers with the key. The total time to complete the entire audiotape activity is approximately 4-5 hours.

You will need four items to complete these exercises:

1. a watch with a sweep hand,
2. the scoresheet and case study questions,
3. the information sheets found at the end of the exercises (see tabbed pages), and
4. the ***Telephone Triage Audio CD,*** which will be mailed to you separately after you purchase the book.

Review the scoresheet, questions, and the information sheets now. You will also be provided with a protocol to refer to during the call.

CASE STUDY APPROACH

Each exercise consists of the scoresheet, case study approach questions, a protocol, and an answer key. Listen to each case study and use the case study scoresheet and your intuition to score the call.

Keep track of the time. First collect data and get an intuitive sense of the call. Use the scoresheet to evaluate the nurses' performance before answering case study approach questions 2–10. Remember that all categories of skill and data collection may not apply to each call. In these cases write NA-1 and count as 1 point when adding up the scores. A passing score is 25. Failure to demonstrate a minimum of helpfulness, ask open-ended questions (except for medical crisis calls), or determine age results in an automatic failure.

It may be necessary to listen more than once. Make notes as appropriate on the scoresheet. Then use the data from the information sheet at the end of the exercises (see tabbed pages) and your notes to answer the case study approach questions 2–10.

Score and analyze your results by referring to the answer key that follows the tabbed pages and listening to the follow-up comments on the audiotape. Please remember that you are free to go at your own pace, to stop or replay the tape as often as you like, and to score the case studies in any order you wish. Please note that there may be more than one correct answer.

ADDITIONAL TEACHING AND LEARNING STRATEGIES

The audiotape can be used with individuals or groups in the following ways:

1. Individual learning study
   —play the tape and complete each exercise at your own pace
2. Teaching strategies
   —play the tape straight through and then lead a group discussion
   —interrupt the tape at strategic points and conduct a group discussion or have participants role play what they might do in the given situation.

The first case study is designed as a "warm-up" to illustrate an example of effective telephone triage. You do not need to score it, but after listening to the tape, read the answer key and listen to the follow-up comments to get an idea of how to do subsequent exercises.

Case Study Scoresheet:

ROLE	SCORE	COMMENT/EXAMPLES
*Helping		
Teaching/Coaching		
Diagnostic		
Monitoring of Intervention		
Crisis Intervention		
INTERVIEW SKILLS	SCORE	COMMENT/EXAMPLES
*Asks open-ended questions		
Concrete data collection/directions		
Uses confrontation appropriately		
Speaks directly to client		
Uses lay language		
Restates problem		
States working diagnosis		
States disclaimer		
Elicits hidden agenda		
Elicits verbal contract		
Uses time frames		
Uses protocol		
DATA COLLECTION SKILLS	SCORE	COMMENT/EXAMPLES
*Age		
Symptoms		
Characteristics		
Course/ADL		
History of complaint		
Onset of symptoms		
Location of symptoms		
Altering factors		
Pregnant, breastfeeding status		
Allergies		
Medications		
Previous chronic illness		
Emotional status		
Recent injury, illness, ingestion		
Pertinent negatives		
TOTAL SCORE		

CASE STUDY APPROACH QUESTIONS:

Use data from the your notes and the information sheet (see tabbed pages) to answer the following questions.

(1. Collect data using the scoresheet.)

2. Determine the type, level, and length of the call. Was the call length adequate?

___

3. What is the desired outcome?

___

___

4. What are the major client and practitioner weaknesses and strengths?

___

___

5. What, if at all, was the nature of any call management problem(s)?

___

___

6. What practitioners' role(s) are illustrated?

___

___

7. What are the interpersonal dynamics of this call?

___

___

8. What, if any, additional or alternative strategies (interpersonal or technical) could be used to manage the call?

___

___

9. What would be the most effective strategy?

___

___

10. What important guideline(s) did this practitioner follow?

___

___

NOTE: MAKE 9 COPIES EACH OF THE SCORESHEET AND QUESTIONS TO USE WHILE YOU COMPLETE EACH EXERCISE.

SAMPLE EXERCISE

Refer to Figure A.0 while listening to the sample case study.

FIGURE A.0 Prototype: Burns (Thermal—First, Second, Third Degree)

SPECIFIC QUESTIONS	DISPOSITION/ADVICE
EMERGENT/URGENT SYMPTOMS	**ED/MD IN 0–2 HOURS**
THIRD DEGREE • Absence of pain-Loss of skin? • Third degree in excess of 10% body surface? • Third degree in excess of 3% body surface–child? • Third degree of face, hands, feet, or groin? • SECOND DEGREE in excess of 20%–child, 30%–adult? • White, dark, charred appearances? • *Degree, Percentage, Location, Complications, Age?*	• **Immed. cool (not ice) water × 10 min** • Wrap in clean wet sheet or saran wrap • Transport to ED
SEMI-URGENT SYMPTOMS	**MD/APPT IN 2–24 HOURS**
SECOND DEGREE • Red, mottled color, blisters, extreme pain? • Facial, neck, genitals, hands, feet? • Deep sunburn? • Uncomplicated second degree of 10-20%–child? • "Moderate Burn" + High Risk Factor (SAVED)? • AGE - 0-5 yrs., 60 + yrs. = Thin skin, low immunity? FIRST DEGREE (Poss. fatal if 2/3 surface involved)? • *Degree, Percentage, Location, Complications, Age?* • *Infectious process requiring antibiotics?* • *Painful conditions requiring prescription drugs?* • *Failure to improve after 48 hours on Antibiotic?*	• **Immed. cool (not ice) water × 10 min** • Wrap in clean wet sheet or saran wrap
ROUTINE SYMPTOMS	**MD/APPT IN 24 HOURS - 2 WEEK**
FIRST DEGREE: • Red, mild swelling, moderate pain, no blisters? • Sunburn?	• **Immed. cool (not ice) water × 10 min** • *Remain at home and begin treatment* • *Call back if symptoms become markedly worse or fail to improve with treatment within 48 hours*
CROSS REFERENCE	**BASIC TEACHING**
INHALATION BURNS ELECTRICAL BURNS	RULE OF NINES–ADULT–Head/Neck–9, Post. Trunk–1 Ant. Trunk–18, Arm–9, Perineum–1, Legs–18 CHILD–Head–18, Post. Trunk 18, Ant. Trunk 18, Arm–9, Leg–14 • COMPLICATIONS: Airway problems, pain/anxiety or fluid loss leading to shock, swelling, infection • SA TECH: Measure using hand = 1%

SCORESHEET: Sample Exercise Answer Key
Crisis Intervention—Burn or possible child abuse

ROLE	SCORE	COMMENT/EXAMPLES
*Helping	1	
Teaching/Coaching	1	
Diagnostic	1	
Monitoring of Intervention	1	Client to perform follow-up call
Crisis Intervention	1	Obtained address, phone, and age
INTERVIEW SKILLS	**SCORE**	**COMMENT/EXAMPLES**
*Asks open-ended questions	1	
Concrete data collection/directions	1	
Uses confrontation appropriately	1	
Speaks directly to client	NA-1	pre-verbal client
Uses lay language	1	"genitals" translated
Restates problem	1	
States working diagnosis	1	
States disclaimer	NA-1	Not appropriate—hi-level call
Elicits hidden agenda	1	explored possible child abuse
Elicits verbal contract	1	
Uses time frames	1	
Uses protocol	1	Modified protocol–i. e. pain med, ED in 1 hour
DATA COLLECTION SKILLS	**SCORE**	**COMMENT/EXAMPLES**
*Age	1	
Symptoms	1	
Characteristics	1	
Course/ADL	1	Blisters getting worse
History of complaint	1	Elicited possible child abuse history
Onset of symptoms	1	
Location of symptoms	1	1/2 R arm and whole R leg
Altering factors	1	Cool water makes it better
Pregnant, breastfeeding status	NA-1	
Allergies	1	None known, ruled out allergy before advising Tylenol
Medications	1	
Previous chronic illness	1	Elicited health history
Emotional status	1	Panic stricken mother, crying child
Recent injury, illness, ingestion	1	Ruled out possible child abuse
Pertinent negatives	1	No burns to genitals
TOTAL SCORE	32	

QUESTIONS:

2. *Type of call*—crisis intervention
   Level of call—high-level
   Length of call—approximately 6 minutes (appropriate)
3. *Desired outcome*—prevent further injury from burn
4. *Weaknesses:*
   Client— pre-verbal infant, second-party call, panic stricken mother, recent immigrant, Spanish speaking, questionable reliability, no transportation
   Practitioner— none
   Strengths:
   Client— assertive, resourceful, treatment on-hand
   Practitioner— expertise/charisma, sufficient data collection, sufficient time, consulted with colleague, resourceful
5. *Nature of call management problem*—effectively managed the problem of contracting/compliance
6. *Practitioner role(s)*—all roles including monitoring via follow-up call
7. *Interpersonal dynamics*—authoritative, collaborative, empowering
8. *Additional or alternative strategies*—none needed
9. *Most effective strategy*—implement first-aid
10. *Guideline(s) followed*—
    always obtain age, remain with caller, err on the side of caution, make corrections for own fallibility

LISTEN TO THE FOLLOW-UP COMMENTS FOR THE SAMPLE CASE STUDY NOW.

EXERCISE 1 Refer to Figure A.1 while listening to case study 1.

FIGURE A.1 Poison Control Form

PCC Log Book #:
Computer Case #:

Phone line: 800 476 8058 911 5338 3182

Substance 1: ________ Amt 1: ____ Size: ____ Units: ____

PCode 1: [ ] SF Code 1: [ ]

Substance 2: ________ Amt 2: ____ Size: ____ Units: ____

PCode 2: [ ] SF Code 2: [ ]

Units:
1 Bite 10 Swallow/Sip
2 Grains 11 Tbls
3 Grams 12 Tsp
4 lick/taste 13 Tabs/Caps
5 μgrams 14 Vial/Ampute
6 mgrams 15 Whiff
7 mliters 16 Unknown
8 Oz. 17 Other
9 Splash/Spill

Total # Subs:
1 or ________

PATIENT DATA

Name: ________
Phone: ( ) ________
Address: ________ ZIP: ________
Age: ___Yr Mo UNI Unkn Infant UC2 Unkn 2-5 Y UC6 Unkn 6-12 Y UAL Unkn Adolesc UAD Unkn Adult UAG Unkn Age
Sex: M F Weight: ________ Pds Kgs Unk
Route(s): _Ingestion _Ocular _Bite/Sting _Unkn _Inhal/Nasal _Dermal _Parenteral _Other ________
Time since exposure: ________ Min. Hr. Day or Chronic
PMHx: (mark all that apply) Pregnant?: T F Unk
_Alcoholism _Drug Abuse _Pulm-Asthma/COPD
_Allergy-Drug _Hepatic Dis. _Pulm-Other
_Allergy-Other _Medications _Renal Dis.
_Cardiac/CHF _Ment. Handicap _Seizure Dis.
_Down's Synd. _Psych./Schizoph _Other

CALLER DATA

Name: ________
Relation: Moth Fath Self Oth
Title: MD RN Pharm Oth
Hospital: ________
ZIP: ________ Phone:( ) ________
Address: ________
City: ________ State: ________
County: ________

Site of Caller:		Site of Exposure:
____	Residence	____
____	Workplace	____
____	Health Care Facility	____
____	School	____
____	Other	____
____	Unknown Site	____

Notes:

Call type:	Victim:	Exposure Type:
1 Exposure 3 Poison Info. 2 Drug Info. 4 Med./Other	1 Human 2 Animal	1 Acute 2 Chronic 3 Unknown

Reason for Exposure:
1 Acc Gen 5 Acc Unkn 9 Int Unkn
2 Acc Occup 6 Int Suicide 10 Adv Rxn Drug
3 Acc Environ 7 Int Misuse 11 Adv Rxn Food
4 Acc Misuse 8 Int Abuse 12 Adv Rxn Oth
13 Unk.

Initial Sx:
1 Asymptomatic
2 Symp., Related
3 Symp., Unrelated
4 Symp., Unkn if Related
5 Unkn if Symptomatic
6 Late Symptom Develop.

Symptoms:
_CNS-Coma _Gi-Minor
_CNS-Sz _Gi-Major
_CNS-Major _Met. Acid.
_CNS-Minor _Renal Fail.
_CV-Hypotens. _Rhapdo.
_CV-Hypertens. _Resp.-Major
_CV-Minor _Resp-Minor
_CV-Ser. EKG _Skin/Eye-Major
_Hyperthermia _Skin/Eye-Minor
_Other

Care Provided:
1 No therapy nec.
2 Observation only
3 Patient refused
IF THERAPY PROVIDED, LEAVE BLANK OR ENTER "0"

PCC #2? True False

Decontamination:
_Ipecac _Lavage _Fresh Air
_Act. Charcoal _Dilute _Other decon.
_Cathartic _Irrigate/Wash _Other ematic

Other Therapies:
_Acidification _Deferoxamine _NAC, IV
_Alkalinization _EDTA _NAC, PO
_Anticonvulsants _Ethanol _Naloxone
_Antihistamines _Exchg. Transf. _Oxygen
_Antivenin _Fab Fragmnts _2-Pam
_Atropine _Forced diuresis _Penicillamine
_BAL _Glucose _Perit dialys
_CPR _Hemodialysis _Physosogmine
_Char Hemoper. _Hyperbar Oxy _Pyndoxine
_Cyanide Kit _Methylene blue _Resin Hemoperf.
_Other

Patient Flow:
1 Managed on site (non HCF)
2 Patient already in/enroute to HCF
3 Treated and released
4 Admitted for medical care
5 Admitted for psych care/eval
6 Lost to follow-up/left AMA
7 Patient was referred by PCC to HCF
8 Treated and released
9 Admitted for medical care
10 Admitted for psych care/eval
11 Refused ref/didn't arr HCF
12 Lost to follow-up/left AMA
13 Other
14 Unknown

# of F/U: ____

Outcome:
1 No effect
2 Minor effect
3 Moderate effect
4 Major effect
5 Unkn. nontoxic
6 Unkn. pot toxic
7 Unrelated effect
8 Death

Teaching Case?: (free area #1) Y N

HCF #2? ________ (name)

HazMat? True False

Foreign Language? (free area #2) Y N

Signed: ________ Reviewed: ________
Complete?: True False
Entered in Computer: ________

EXERCISE 2 Refer to Figure A.2 while listening to case study 2.

FIGURE A.2 Poison Control Form

PCC Log Book #:
Computer Case #:

Phone line: 800 476 8058 911 5338 3182

Substance 1: ____ Amt 1: ___ Size: ___ Units: ___

PCode 1: [| | | | | |] SF Code 1: [| |]

Substance 2: ____ Amt 2: ___ Size: ___ Units: ___

PCode 2: [| | | | | |] SF Code 2: [| |]

Units:
1 Bite 10 Swallow/Sip
2 Grains 11 Tbls
3 Grams 12 Tsp
4 lick/taste 13 Tabs/Caps
5 μgrams 14 Vial/Ampute
6 mgrams 15 Whiff
7 mliters 16 Unknown
8 Oz. 17 Other
9 Splash/Spill

Total # Subs: 1 or ____

PATIENT DATA

Name: ____
Phone: ( ) ____
Address: ____ ZIP: ____
Age: __Yr Mo UNI Unkn Infant UAL Unkn Adolesc UC2 Unkn 2-5 Y UAD Unkn Adult UC6 Unkn 6-12 Y UAG Unkn Age
Sex: M F Weight: ____ Pds Kgs Unk
Route(s): _Ingestion _Ocular _Bite/Sting _Unkn _Inhal/Nasal _Dermal _Parenteral _Other ____
Time since exposure: ____ Min. Hr. Day or Chronic
PMHx: (mark all that apply) Pregnant?: T F Unk
_Alcoholism _Drug Abuse _Pulm-Asthma/COPD
_Allergy-Drug _Hepatic Dis. _Pulm-Other
_Allergy-Other _Medications _Renal Dis.
_Cardiac/CHF _Ment. Handicap _Seizure Dis.
_Down's Synd. _Psych./Schizoph _Other

CALLER DATA

Name: ____
Relation: Moth Fath Self Oth
Title: MD RN Pharm Oth
Hospital: ____
ZIP: ____ Phone:( ) ____
Address: ____
City: ____ State: ____
County: ____

Site of Caller:		Site of Exposure:
____	Residence	____
____	Workplace	____
____	Health Care Facility	____
____	School	____
____	Other	____
____	Unknown Site	____

Notes:

Call type:	Victim:	Exposure Type:
1 Exposure 3 Poison Info. 2 Drug Info. 4 Med./Other	1 Human 2 Animal	1 Acute 2 Chronic 3 Unknown

Reason for Exposure:
1 Acc Gen 5 Acc Unkn 9 Int Unkn
2 Acc Occup 6 Int Suicide 10 Adv Rxn Drug
3 Acc Environ 7 Int Misuse 11 Adv Rxn Food
4 Acc Misuse 8 Int Abuse 12 Adv Rxn Oth
13 Unk.

Initial Sx:
1 Asymptomatic
2 Symp., Related
3 Symp., Unrelated
4 Symp., Unkn if Related
5 Unkn if Symptomatic
6 Late Symptom Develop.

Symptoms:
_CNS-Coma _Gi-Minor
_CNS-Sz _Gi-Major
_CNS-Major _Met. Acid.
_CNS-Minor _Renal Fail.
_CV-Hypotens. _Rhapdo.
_CV-Hypertens. _Resp.-Major
_CV-Minor _Resp-Minor
_CV-Ser. EKG _Skin/Eye-Major
_Hyperthermia _Skin/Eye-Minor
_Other

Care Provided:
1 No therapy nec.
2 Observation only
3 Patient refused
IF THERAPY PROVIDED. LEAVE BLANK OR ENTER "0"

PCC #2? True False

Decontamination:
_Ipecac _Lavage _Fresh Air
_Act. Charcoal _Dilute _Other decon.
_Cathartic _Irrigate/Wash _Other ematic

Other Therapies:
_Acidification _Deferoxamine _NAC, IV
_Alkalinization _EDTA _NAC,PO
_Anticonvulsants _Ethanol _Naloxone
_Antihistamines _Exchg.Transf. _Oxygen
_Antivenin _Fab Fragmnts _2-Pam
_Atropine _Forced diuresis _Penicillamine
_BAL _Glucose _Perit dialys
_CPR _Hemodialysis _Physosogmine
_Char Hemoper. _Hyperbar Oxy _Pyndoxine
_Cyanide Kit _Methylene blue _Resin Hemoperf.
_Other

Patient Flow:
1 Managed on site (non HCF)
2 Patient already in/enroute to HCF
3 Treated and relased
4 Admitted for medical care
5 Admitted for psych care/eval
6 Lost to follow-up/left AMA
7 Patient was referred by PCC to HCF
8 Treated and relased
9 Admitted for medical care
10 Admitted for psych care/eval
11 Refused ref/didn't arr HCF
12 Lost to follow-up/left AMA
13 Other
14 Unknown

# of F/U: ____

Outcome:
1 No effect
2 Minor effect
3 Moderate effect
4 Major effect
5 Unkn. nontoxic
6 Unkn. pot toxic
7 Unrelated effect
8 Death

Teaching Case?: (free area #1) Y N

HCF #2? ____ (name)

HazMat? True False

Foreign Language? (free area #2) Y N

Signed: ____ Reviewed: ____

Complete?: True False

Entered in Computer: ____

EXERCISE 3 Refer to Figure A.3 while listening to case study 3.

FIGURE A.3 Pre-Arrival Instruction (Crash Card)

DISPATCH LIFE SUPPORT™

B ARREST – CHILD

For use through Exclusive License only Pat. Pend. ©8/90 Medical Priority

1 PATIENT TO PHONE	2 CHECK AIRWAY	3 CHECK BREATHING
Listen carefully. I'll tell you how to help your child. **Get him/her as close to the phone as possible.** I'm going to tell you how to do CPR. **Don't hang up. Go do it now.**	Listen carefully. **Lay him/her flat on his/her back on the floor.** Remove any **pillows.** Now place your **hand** under the **neck** and **shoulders** and **tilt** the **head** back. Then **look** in the **mouth. Go do it now** and come right back to the phone.	I want you to see if s/he is **breathing.** Put your **ear** next to his/her **mouth.** See if you can **feel** or **hear** any breathing, or if you can **see** the **chest rise. Go do it now** and come right back to the phone. ***(If I'm not here, stay on the line.)***
WHERE is the child now?	**Is there VOMIT in the mouth?**	**Can you FEEL or HEAR any breathing?**
→2	NO→3 YES→13	NO/UNCRTN→4 YES→16
4 START M-TO-M	**5 GIVE BREATHS**	**6 CHECK PULSE**
I'm going to tell you how to give Mouth-to-Mouth. Place your **hand** under the **neck** and **shoulders** and **tilt** the **head** back. **Pinch** the **nose** closed. Completely **cover** his/her **mouth** with your **mouth.**	Blow **2 soft breaths** of air into the lungs just like you are blowing up a balloon. **Watch** for the **chest** to **rise** with each breath. When you have done this come right back to the phone. **Don't hang up. Go do it now.** ***(If I'm not here, stay on the line.)***	I want you to **check** his/her **pulse. Place** your index and middle **fingers** over his/her left nipple. **Feel carefully for a pulse.** Don't press too hard. Feel for **5 seconds. Go do it now** and come right back to the phone. ***(If I'm not here, stay on the line.)***
	Can you FEEL the air going in? Did you SEE the chest rising?	**Can you FEEL a PULSE?**
→5	NO→14 YES→6	NO→7 YES→17
7 RECHECK PULSE	**8 CPR LANDMARKS**	**9 COMPRESSIONS**
I want you to **check** for a **pulse** again on his/her upper arm. Use your index and middle **fingers** to feel on the **inside** of his/her **upper arm** for a pulse. Feel carefully for **5 seconds. Go do it now** and come right back to the phone.	Listen carefully. I'll tell you what to do next. Put the **heel** of **one hand** on the **breast-bone** in the **center** of his/her **chest,** right between the **nipples.**	Push down with your hand **1½ inches** with only the **heel** of one hand touching the chest. Do it **5 times,** just like you are **"pumping"** his/her chest **twice** a second. When you have done this come right back to the phone. **Don't hang up. Go do it now.**
Do you FEEL a PULSE now?		
NO→8 YES→17	→9	→10

PRE-ARRIVAL INSTRUCTIONS

EXERCISE 4 Refer to Figure A.4 while listening to case study 4.

FIGURE A.4 Master Format

SPECIFIC DATA	DISPOSITION/ADVICE
EMERGENT/URGENT SYMPTOMS	**ED/MD IN 0–2 HOURS**
SEMI-URGENT SYMPTOMS	**MD/APPT IN 2–24 HOURS**
• "SAVED"? • *Any infectious process requiring antibiotics?* • *Painful conditions requiring prescription drugs?* • *Failure to improve after 48 hours on antibiotic?*	
ROUTINE SYMPTOMS	**MD/APPT IN 24 HOURS–2 WEEK**
• *Self-limiting symptoms existing over 1 week but not becoming markedly worse?*	• *Remain at home and begin treatment* • *Call back if symptoms become markedly worse or fail to improve with treatment within 48 hours*
CROSS-REFERENCE	**BASIC TEACHING**

EXERCISE 5 Refer to Figure A.5 while listening to case study 5.

FIGURE A.5 Master Format

SPECIFIC DATA	DISPOSITION/ADVICE
EMERGENT/URGENT SYMPTOMS	**ED/MD IN 0–2 HOURS**
SEMI-URGENT SYMPTOMS	**MD/APPT IN 2–24 HOURS**
• "SAVED"? • *Any infectious process requiring antibiotics?* • *Painful conditions requiring prescription drugs?* • *Failure to improve after 48 hours on antibiotic?*	
ROUTINE SYMPTOMS	**MD/APPT IN 24 HOURS–2 WEEK**
• *Self-limiting symptoms existing over 1 week but not becoming markedly worse?*	• *Remain at home and begin treatment* • *Call back if symptoms become markedly worse or fail to improve with treatment within 48 hours*
CROSS-REFERENCE	**BASIC TEACHING**

EXERCISE 6 Refer to Figure A.6 while listening to case study 6.

FIGURE A.6 Abdominal Pain Protocol

SUBJECT: Surgery Advice Protocols	NUMBER: 2	PAGE 1 OF
TITLE: Abdominal Pain	EFFECTIVE DATE: 10/75	
PERSONNEL APPLICABLE TO:	REVISION DATE: 8/80, 4/81, 6/90	

ABDOMINAL PAIN

1. Inquire from patient:
   a. Where is it?
   b. How long have you had it?
   c. Have you had recent surgery? If so, what and where and when?
   d. How severe is it?
   e. Have you vomited? If so, what?
   f. Do you have fever?
   g. Do you have headache or muscle aches?
   h. Do you have frequent or painful urination?
   i. Do you have diarrhea, bloody or black stools?
   j. Do you have gall stones, ulcers or chronic intestinal disease?
   k. Do you have yellow eyes or skin?
   l. For women: When was your last period? Do you have any vaginal bleeding or discharge?
2. If patient has had:
   a. Surgery recently (within one month)
   b. Is being followed for a specific problem by a surgeon, refer message to patient's surgeon, surgeon on-call, or clinic surgeon.
3. If patient complains of:
   a. Severe pain of recent onset.
   b. Vomiting of blood or coffee ground emesis.
   c. Bloody or tarry stools.
   d. High fever (over 101).
   e. Yellow eyes or skin or dark urine.
   f. Localized abdominal tenderness.
   g. Heavy vaginal bleeding.

   DIRECT PATIENT TO THE EMERGENCY DEPARTMENT.
4. If patient complains of:
   a. Pelvic pain as in menstrual cramps, abnormal bleeding (less than heavy) vaginal discharge.

   TRANSFER TO GYNECOLOGY ADVICE NURSE
5. All others transfer to Medical Advice Nurse.

EXERCISE 7 Refer to Figure A.7 while listening to case study 7.

FIGURE A.7 Master Format

SPECIFIC DATA	DISPOSITION/ADVICE
EMERGENT/URGENT SYMPTOMS	**ED/MD IN 0–2 HOURS**
SEMI-URGENT SYMPTOMS	**MD/APPT IN 2–24 HOURS**
• "SAVED"? • *Any infectious process requiring antibiotics?* • *Painful conditions requiring prescription drugs?* • *Failure to improve after 48 hours on antibiotic?*	
ROUTINE SYMPTOMS	**MD/APPT IN 24 HOURS–2 WEEK**
• *Self-limiting symptoms existing over 1 week but not becoming markedly worse?*	• *Remain at home and begin treatment* • *Call back if symptoms become markedly worse or fail to improve with treatment within 48 hours*
CROSS-REFERENCE	**BASIC TEACHING**

EXERCISE 8 Refer to Figure A.8 while listening to case study 8.

FIGURE A.8 AIDS Guidelines

DATA COLLECTION

Elicit the following information *as appropriate:*

Age
Sexual orientation
Education and literacy level
Language barriers
Any symptoms of illness?
Risk factors (IV drugs, alcohol, drug experience, unprotected sex, blood transfusions)
Sexual experience (in detail)
Perception of risk (denial, panic, knowledge deficit, confusion)
Emotional status
Resources (living at home, on street, college)

INTERVIEW APPROACHES

Expect shyness, anxiety, denial, anger
Avoid being judgmental
Elicit feedback regarding client's knowledge
Give concrete directives
Reassure anxious clients ("worried well"):

Remedy knowledge deficits about 3 items—

- HIV must be present in partner
- There must be an adequate amount of fluid
- Fluid must enter into bloodstream

TREAT THE WHOLE CLIENT

Intellectually—remedy knowledge deficits by educating regarding risk factors
Emotionally—address emotional needs as appropriate; for clients not ready to confront issue—offer opportunity to call back
Referral—resources (books, groups, hot lines)

EXERCISE 9 Refer to Figure A.9 while listening to case study 9. Also, please use suicide intervention scoresheet on page 325.

FIGURE A.9 SUICIDE INTERVENTION PROTOCOL

INTERVENTION TASKS:

Engage person in conversation that focuses on feelings
Identify if client is suicidal
Inquire about reasons for and against suicide at this point in time
Assess the degree of risk for suicide at this point in time
Prevent the immediate risk by agreeing to a plan with the person

PREVENTION PLAN:

Specificity—formulated a detailed plan of action
Limited objectives—intervene until immediate danger or threat has passed
Mutuality—collaborate with the client about plan of action
Commitment—elicit a "no suicide" agreement
Crisis contact—confirm the back-up plan if first plan cannot be carried out
Follow-up—Set time and date for another meeting between you and the client or whatever follow-up resources agreed upon.

(Above guidelines adapted from *The California Helper's Handbook,* 1991, pp. vi, vii.)

LETHALITY ASSESSMENT:

Predictors:	***Indicators:***
LACK OF RESOURCES	Alcohol/drugs
PLAN	2nd party call
PRIOR ATTEMPTS	Symptoms
	Stress
	Sex
	Age
	Medical problems
	Life-style
	Season/day/place

EXERCISE 9 SUICIDE INTERVENTION SCORESHEET

ROLE	SCORE	COMMENT/EXAMPLES
*Helping		
Teaching/Coaching		
Diagnostic		
Monitoring of Intervention		
Crisis Intervention		
INTERVENTION TASKS	SCORE	COMMENT/EXAMPLES
Engaged/focused on feelings		
Identified if client is suicidal		
Inquired about suicidal ambivalence		
Assessed degree of risk		
Prevented immediate risk through plan		
PREVENTION PLAN	SCORE	COMMENT/EXAMPLES
Specificity—formulated detailed plan of action		
Limited objectives—addressed immediate danger		
Mutuality—collaborated effectively		
Commitment—elicited agreement to plan		
Crisis contact—confirmed back-up plan		
Follow-up—confirmed follow-up plan		
Used protocol		
LETHALITY ASSESSMENT	SCORE	COMMENT/EXAMPLES
PREDICTORS		
LACK OF RESOURCES		
PLAN/METHOD		
PRIOR ATTEMPTS		
INDICATORS		
Alcohol/drugs		
2nd party call		
Symptoms		
Stress		
Sex		
Age		
Medical problems:		
Lifestyle		
Season/day/place		
SCORE		

INFORMATION SHEET

Use this information to answer questions 2–10. Each section relates to the numbers of the exercise questions. **Select the answer or answers that are most correct** from the section below.

CALL CLASSIFICATION

QUESTION 2. Determine the type, level, and length of call. Was the call length adequate?

TYPE
- Informational/referral
- Triage/advice
- Counsel/reassurance
- Crisis intervention

LEVEL
- Low-level—Informational only, routine advice only
- Mid-level—Appointment needed
- High-level—Crisis

CALL LENGTH

Informational/referral:	3–7 minutes minimum
Triage/advice:	5–7 minutes minimum (English-speaking client) 7–12 minutes minimum (communications with some elderly, non-English speaking, new immigrants)
Counsel/reassurance:	5–7 minutes minimum
Crisis intervention:	1–3 minute maximum for intervention/coaching (Medical) plus time remaining on line with caller **3–30 minutes^{+} for suicidal call

DESIRED OUTCOME

QUESTION 3. What is the desired outcome?

- Prevention of death
- Prevention of further injury or complications
- Prevention of loss of limb, organ
- Facilitate access to care or referral
- Remedy knowledge deficit
- Problem facilitation/ownership

MAJOR WEAKNESSES AND STRENGTHS

QUESTION 4. What are major client and practitioner weaknesses and strengths?

CLIENT WEAKNESSES
- Age (very young, very old, inarticulate teen)
- Panic, denial
- Language barrier
- Second-party call
- Unreliability
- Distance from help

CLIENT STRENGTHS
- Sophistication
- Treatment/medication on-hand
- Can self-transport
- Other adults present

PRACTITIONER WEAKNESSES
- Lack of rapport
- Failure to follow protocols (pre-arrival instructions) appropriately
- Inadequate data collection
- Inadequate "talk time"
- Stereotyping clients or problems
- Failure to talk directly with client
- Self-diagnoses and second guessing
- Failure to elicit hidden agenda
- Overreacting, underreacting, and fatigue
- Denial

PRACTITIONER STRENGTHS
- Expertise/charisma
- Allows sufficient time
- Elicits hidden agendas
- Talks directly with client
- Consults with colleagues in questionable cases
- Alert to client self-diagnosis
- Remains alert to denial
- Uses protocol appropriately

NATURE OF PROBLEM

QUESTION 5. What, if at all, was the nature of any call management problem(s)?

Deficit of:
- Interpersonal skill
- Assessment skill
- Diagnostic skill
- Intervention skills—Contracting/compliance
- Educational skills for self-evaluation

ROLES

QUESTION 6. What practitioners' role(s) are illustrated?

Helping— creates a healing relationship, "presencing" (ie. being present), maximizes clients' control, and provides comfort through voice (charisma).

Coaching/Teaching—	uses timing, elicits interpretations of illness, and provides rationales for home treatment; identifies "client readiness", seizes opportunities to facilitate clients in learning to change behaviors and attitudes.
Diagnostic—	detects significant changes in the client's condition, anticipates problems, and formulates treatment strategies.
Monitoring of Interventions—	minimizes the risks and complications of interventions.
Crisis Intervention—	able to instantly grasp and effectively manage rapidly changing situations.

INTERPERSONAL DYNAMICS

QUESTION 7. What are the interpersonal dynamics of this call?

+ Anticipates problems and prepares clients
+ Collaborative approach
+ Authoritative approach
+ Empowering attitude

– Authoritarian attitude
– Client passivity, dependency
– Power struggle/interpersonal conflict

MANAGEMENT STRATEGIES

QUESTION 8. What, if any, additional or alternative strategies could be used to manage the call?

QUESTION 9. What would be the most effective strategy?

DATA COLLECTION
- Allows sufficient time
- Uses open-ended questions
- Uses lay language
- Follows protocol directive appropriately
- Anticipate problems, prepares client
- Elicits significant data (SAVED, SCHOLAR, PAMPER, ADL)
- Elicits pertinent negatives
- Facilitates client self-assessment
- Uses time frames

DIAGNOSIS
- Formulates/states working diagnosis

INTERVENTION/INFORMATION AND REFERRAL BROKERING

Microteaching
Self-care and self-help referral
Facilitates contracting/compliance
Elicits hidden agendas
Facilitates ED access through interface

EVALUATION

Educates client in self-evaluation
Gives follow-up instructions

MEDICAL CRISIS INTERVENTION STRATEGIES

Strategies primarily intended for emergency medical dispatch use, but applicable to ED nurse with appropriate modifications.

Stylistic

Calm, authoritative manner
Engenders trust
Remains with caller

Data collection/diagnosis

Four Commandments
Determines the address from which the call is made
Uses standardized pre-arrival instructions
Determines proximity of phone to caller

Intervention/self-evaluation

Implements first-aid measures
Anticipates predictable panic
Coaching/repetitive persistence
Determines proximity of caller to ED

SUICIDAL CRISIS INTERVENTION STRATEGIES

Stylistic

Buys time while establishing trust
Authentic
Resourceful
Active listening skills
Remains with the caller

Assessment/diagnosis suicidal calls

Confronts the issue
Determines lethality
History of prior suicide attempts
Second-party calls
Age, sex
Alcohol or drug use
Lack of resources

Recent stress
Physical symptoms of depression
Medical status
Life-style
Season/day/place

Diagnosis/intervention

Formulates working diagnosis of lethality
Fosters client ownership of the problem
Reinforces coping strategies

GUIDELINES

QUESTION 10. What important guideline(s) did this practitioner follow?

—Always obtain the age
—Always err on the side of caution
—Speak directly to the client whenever possible
—When the caller says they have an emergency, the burden of proof is not theirs
—For all medication calls, obtain pregnancy and breastfeeding status, list of any allergies, and list of any medications currently using
—The more vague the symptom, the greater the need for data collection
—Remain with the caller when possible
—Make corrections for fallibility
—Speed does not equal competence
—Consider distance and traffic flow

Acknowledgements:

Figures A.0, A.4, A.5, and A.7 courtesy of Wheeler and Associates
Figures A.1 and A.2 courtesy of San Francisco Bay Area Regional Poison Control Center, San Francisco, CA
Figure A.3 reprinted with permission of Jeff Clawson, M.D.
Figure A.6 reprinted with permission of Kaiser Permanente, South San Francisco, CA
Figure A.9 adapted from The California Helper's Handbook, *1991, pp. vi, vii*
Case study 3 is adapted with permission of Jeff Clawson (Clawson & Dernocoeur, 1988, p. 262)
Case study 9 formulated in collaboration with Marin Suicide Prevention Center, Marin County, CA.

SCORESHEET: Exercise 1 Answer Key
Crisis Intervention—Iron overdose

ROLE	SCORE	COMMENT/EXAMPLES
*Helping	1	
Teaching/Coaching	1	
Diagnostic	1	
Monitoring of Intervention	NA-1	
Crisis Intervention	1	
INTERVIEW SKILLS	**SCORE**	**COMMENT/EXAMPLES**
*Asks open-ended questions	1	
Concrete data collection/directions	1	
Uses confrontation appropriately	1	
Speaks directly to client	NA-1	pre-verbal client
Uses lay language	1	
Restates problem	1	
States working diagnosis	1	
States disclaimer	NA-1	
Elicits hidden agenda	NA-1	
Elicits verbal contract	1	Ipecac, transport
Uses time frames	1	15 minutes, 1 hr from ED
Uses protocol	1	
DATA COLLECTION SKILLS	**SCORE**	**COMMENT/EXAMPLES**
*Age	1	1 1/2 years
Symptoms	1	conscious, breathing
Characteristics	NA-1	
Course/ADL	0	
History of complaint	0	
Onset of symptoms	NA-1	
Location of symptoms	NA-1	
Altering factors	NA-1	
Pregnant, breastfeeding status	NA-1	
Allergies	NA-1	
Medications	0	
Previous chronic illness	0	
Emotional status	1	
Recent injury, illness, ingestion	1	
Pertinent negatives	1	sitting, playing
TOTAL SCORE	28	

QUESTIONS:

2. *Type of call*—crisis intervention
   Level of call—high-level
   Length of call—approximately 3 minutes (appropriate)
3. *Desired outcome*—prevent further injury, complications (progression or worsening of overdose)
4. *Weaknesses:*
   Client— questionable reliability, pre-verbal client, second-party call, **distance from help (65 miles)**
   Practitioner— may have called ahead to ED to inform of client arrival to facilitate care

   Strengths:
   Client— sophisticated client, with partner to help, can self-transport, antidote available
   Practitioner— expertise, articulate, rapport
5. *Nature of call management problem*—no major deficits
6. *Practitioner role(s)*—all roles except monitoring
7. *Interpersonal dynamics*—authoritative, collaborative, empowering
8. *Additional or alternative strategies*—elicit additional details about ADL, health history, anticipating problems in administering ipecac (uncooperative child), prepared parent with strategies ahead of time
9. *Most effective strategy*—(see Crisis Intervention Strategies in information sheet), implement first-aid measures
10. *Guideline(s) followed*—always obtain age, err on the side of caution, consider distance and traffic flow

LISTEN TO THE FOLLOW-UP COMMENTS FOR CASE STUDY 1 NOW.

SCORESHEET: Exercise 2 Answer Key
Crisis Intervention—Multiple bee stings on head

ROLE	SCORE	COMMENT/EXAMPLES
*Helping	1	
Teaching/Coaching	1	
Diagnostic	1	
Monitoring of Intervention	1	
Crisis Intervention	1	Potential for crisis
INTERVIEW SKILLS	SCORE	COMMENT/EXAMPLES
*Asks open-ended questions	1	
Concrete data collection/directions	1	
Uses confrontation appropriately	0	Seems irritated: intimidated caller
Speaks directly to client	0	
Uses lay language	1	
Restates problem	1	
States working diagnosis	NA-1	
States disclaimer	NA-1	
Elicits hidden agenda	NA-1	
Elicits verbal contract	1	
Uses time frames	1	
Uses protocol	1	
DATA COLLECTION SKILLS	SCORE	COMMENT/EXAMPLES
*Age	1	31, 27
Symptoms	1	
Characteristics	1	Elicited very few details
Course/ADL	1	Elicited few details
History of complaint	NA-1	
Onset of symptoms	1	"5 minutes ago"
Location of symptoms	1	repeated sting head/arms
Altering factors	0	
Pregnant, breastfeeding status	NA-1	
Allergies	1	none known
Medications	0	
Previous chronic illness	0	
Emotional status	1	
Recent injury, illness, ingestion	1	
Pertinent negatives	1	denies allergies, negative health history
TOTAL SCORE	27	

QUESTIONS:

2. *Type of call*—triage advice (potentially crisis intervention)
   Level of call—mid-level
   Length of call—approximately 5 minutes
3. *Desired outcome*—prevent further injury (due to allergic response)
4. *Weaknesses:*
   - Client— distance from help, second-party caller, questionable reliability
   - Practitioner— initial lack of rapport, failure to talk directly with client, fatigue (?)

   Strengths
   - Client— sophistication, three adults, self-transport, medication on-hand
   - Practitioner— expertise
5. *Nature of call management problem*—initial lack of interpersonal skill
6. *Practitioner role(s)*—all (monitoring performed by follow-up call later)
7. *Interpersonal dynamics*—initial interpersonal conflict, authoritarian attitude, client passivity, power struggle
8. *Additional or alternative strategies*—adopt a more collaborative approach initially, **talk with clients directly,** elicit more data
9. *Most effective strategy*—talk directly to clients
10. *Guideline(s) followed*—always obtain age, speak directly to client when possible, err on the side of caution, consider distance and traffic flow

LISTEN TO THE FOLLOW-UP COMMENTS FOR CASE STUDY 2 NOW.

SCORESHEET: EXERCISE 3 Answer Key
Crisis Intervention—Child near drowning

ROLE	SCORE	COMMENT/EXAMPLES
*Helping	1	
Teaching/Coaching	1	
Diagnostic	1	
Monitoring of Interventions	1	
Crisis Intervention	1	
INTERVIEW SKILLS	SCORE	COMMENT/EXAMPLES
*Asks open-ended questions	1	
Concrete data collection/directions	1	Pinch nose, give 4 breaths
Uses confrontation appropriately	1	
Speaks directly to client	NA-1	
Uses lay language	1	
Restates problem	NA-1	
States working diagnosis	NA-1	
States disclaimer	NA-1	
Elicits hidden agenda	NA-1	
Elicits verbal contract	1	Effectively enlisted caller cooperation
Uses time frames	1	Determined length of time in pool
Uses protocol	1	
DATA COLLECTION SKILLS	SCORE	COMMENT/EXAMPLES
*Age	1	2-year-old
Symptoms	1	
Characteristics	1	Color is purple
Course/ADL	1	Worsening condition
History of complaint	1	Fell into pool, time unknown
Onset of symptoms	NA-1	
Location of symptoms	NA-1	
Altering factors	NA-1	
Pregnant, breastfeeding status	NA-1	
Allergies	NA-1	
Medications	NA-1	
Previous chronic illness	NA-1	
Emotional status	1	Panic stricken mother
Recent injury, illness, ingestion	1	Unobserved accident
Pertinent negatives	NA-1	
TOTAL SCORE	32	

QUESTIONS:

2. *Type of call*—crisis intervention
   Level of call—high-level
   Length of call—under 3 minutes (appropriate)
3. *Desired outcome*—prevent death
4. *Weaknesses:*
   Client— panic
   Practitioner— lack of protocol (no formal protocols in 1976)
   Strengths
   Client— cooperative, two other adults present to assist
   Practitioner— established rapport, resourceful use of CPR instruction
5. *Nature of call management problem*—no deficits, effective intervention, (contracting/compliance)
6. *Practitioner role(s)*—all roles
7. *Interpersonal dynamics*—authoritative, collaborative approach
8. *Additional or alternative strategies*—standardized pre-arrival instructions
9. *Most effective strategy*—use formal protocol, pre-arrival instructions
10. *Guideline(s) followed*—always obtain age, remain with the caller

LISTEN TO THE FOLLOW-UP COMMENTS FOR CASE STUDY 3 NOW.

SCORESHEET: EXERCISE 4 Answer Key Hidden Agenda—Teen overdose

ROLE	SCORE	COMMENT/EXAMPLES
*Helping	1	Only in most basic sense—appt. given
Teaching/Coaching	0	
Diagnostic	0	
Monitoring of Intervention	0	
Crisis Intervention	0	
INTERVIEW SKILLS	**SCORE**	**COMMENT/EXAMPLES**
*Asks open-ended questions	1	Elicited very little detail
Concrete data collection/directions	1	
Uses confrontation appropriately	0	
Speaks directly to client	0	Major flaw—should talk to client directly
Uses lay language	1	
Restates problem	0	Never gave working diagnosis
States working diagnosis	0	
States disclaimer	0	Gave appointment
Elicits hidden agenda	0	
Elicits verbal contract	0	
Uses time frames	1	
Uses protocol	1	Used Master protocol
DATA COLLECTION SKILLS	**SCORE**	**COMMENT/EXAMPLES**
*Age	1	
Symptoms	1	Minimal data collection
Characteristics	1	
Course/ADL	1	
History of complaint	0	No past history of similar symptom elicited
Onset of symptoms	1	Started at midnight
Location of symptoms	NA-1	
Altering factors	1	7-Up not helping
Pregnant, breastfeeding status	0	Possible hidden agenda (?), teen pregnancy (?)
Allergies	0	
Medications	0	Possible hidden agenda (?), recreational drugs, alcohol (?)
Previous chronic illness	0	
Emotional status	1	Worried parent
Recent injury, illness, ingestion	0	Possible hidden agenda (overdose)
Pertinent negatives	0	
TOTAL SCORE	14	

QUESTIONS:

2. *Type of call*—perceived as advice/triage but actually crisis intervention
   Level of call—high-level (nurse failed to recognize)
   Length of call—1–2 minutes (very inadequate)
3. *Desired outcome*—prevention of loss of organ (liver) or death
4. *Weaknesses:*
   - Client— teenager, second-party caller
   - Practitioner— inadequate data collection/talk time, failed to talk directly with client, believed client self-diagnosis, failed to elicit hidden agenda

   Strengths
   - Client— assertive mother
   - Practitioner— used protocol
5. *Nature of call management problem*—assessment deficit
6. *Practitioner role(s)*—helped at minimal level only
7. *Interpersonal dynamics*—authoritatarian attitude
8. *Additional or alternative strategies*—sufficient talk time, data collection, talk with client directly
9. *Most effective strategy*—talk with client directly
10. *Guideline(s) followed*—always obtain age, err on the side of caution

LISTEN TO THE FOLLOW-UP COMMENTS FOR CASE STUDY 4 NOW.

EXERCISE 5 Answer Key

SCORESHEET: Stereotyping Symptoms—Difficulty sleeping

ROLE	SCORE	COMMENT/EXAMPLES
*Helping	1	Basic level only
Teaching/Coaching	1	Based on stereotyped symptom
Diagnostic	0	
Monitoring of Intervention	0	
Crisis Intervention	0	
INTERVIEW SKILLS	**SCORE**	**COMMENT/EXAMPLES**
*Asks open-ended questions	1	
Concrete data collection/directions	0	
Uses confrontation appropriately	0	
Speaks directly to client	NA-1	
Uses lay language	1	
Restates problem	0	
States working diagnosis	1	Faulty diagnosis, stereotyped
States disclaimer	0	
Elicits hidden agenda	0	
Elicits verbal contract	0	
Uses time frames	0	
Uses protocol	0	Did not follow directives of Master protocol
DATA COLLECTION SKILLS	**SCORE**	**COMMENT/EXAMPLES**
*Age	1	7-month-old
Symptoms	1	Difficulty sleeping
Characteristics	0	
Course/ADL	0	
History of complaint	0	Did not elicit past history of sleeping difficulties
Onset of symptoms	0	
Location of symptoms	NA-1	
Altering factors	0	
Pregnant, breastfeeding status	NA-1	
Allergies	NA-1	
Medications	1	On Augmentin × 4 days
Previous chronic illness	0	
Emotional status	1	Anxious mother
Recent injury, illness, ingestion	1	
Pertinent negatives	1	
TOTAL SCORE	15	

QUESTIONS:

2. *Type of call*—triage/advice
   Level of call—mid-level
   Length of call—less than 2 minutes (very inadequate)
3. *Desired outcome*—prevention of complications
4. *Weaknesses:*
   - Client— denial (?), second-party caller, very young client
   - Practitioner— inadequate talk time, data collection, stereotyping problem, underreacting, failed to follow Master protocol: "failure to improve on antibiotic"

   Strengths:
   - Client— None
   - Practitioner— None
5. *Nature of call management problem*—assessment deficit
6. *Practitioner role(s)*—minimal helping
7. *Interpersonal dynamics*—authoritarian attitude, client passivity
8. *Additional or alternative strategies*—sufficient talk time, data collection, follow protocol directives
9. *Most effective strategy*—sufficient data
10. *Guideline(s) followed*—always obtain age

LISTEN TO THE FOLLOW-UP COMMENTS FOR CASE STUDY 5 NOW.

SCORESHEET: EXERCISE 6 Answer Key
Stereotyping Symptoms—Abdominal pain

ROLE	SCORE	COMMENT/EXAMPLES
*Helping	1	
Teaching/Coaching	0	
Diagnostic	0	
Monitoring of Intervention	0	
Crisis Intervention	0	
INTERVIEW SKILLS	SCORE	COMMENT/EXAMPLES
*Asks open-ended questions	1	Elicited minimal detail
Concrete data collection/directions	1	Minimal
Uses confrontation appropriately	0	
Speaks directly to client	1	
Uses lay language	1	
Restates problem	0	
States working diagnosis	1	Wrong working diagnosis
States disclaimer	0	
Elicits hidden agenda	0	
Elicits verbal contract	1	
Uses time frames	1	
Uses protocol	0	Failed to follow abdominal pain protocol
DATA COLLECTION SKILLS	SCORE	COMMENT/EXAMPLES
*Age	1	
Symptoms	1	
Characteristics	1	
Course/ADL	1	
History of complaint	0	Did not elicit past history of abdominal pains
Onset of symptoms	1	
Location of symptoms	0	No specifics
Altering factors	0	Did not elicit details of patient attempts at treatment
Pregnant, breastfeeding status	0	Not elicited, unlikely at age 48, but possible
Allergies	0	
Medications	0	
Previous chronic illness	0	
Emotional status	1	Anxious, in pain
Recent injury, illness, ingestion	1	Recent surgery increases risk
Pertinent negatives	0	
TOTAL SCORE	15	

QUESTIONS:

2. *Type of call*—perceived as Triage/advice, actually Crisis level
   Level of call—high-level
   Length of call—about 1–2 minutes (very inadequate)
3. *Desired outcome*—prevent complications (of surgery)
4. *Weaknesses:*
   - Client— none
   - Practitioner— inadequate talk time, inadequate data collection, stereotyping symptoms, failed to follow abdominal pain protocol

   Strengths:
   - Client— assertive (went to ED within the hour without calling nurse again)
   - Practitioner— none
5. *Nature of call management problem*—assessment deficit
6. *Practitioner role(s)*—minimal helping
7. *Interpersonal dynamics*—authoritarian
8. *Additional or alternative strategies*—adequate data collection/talk time, open-ended questioning
9. *Most effective strategy*—adequate data collection
10. *Guideline(s) followed*—always obtain age

LISTEN TO THE FOLLOW-UP COMMENTS FOR CASE STUDY 6 NOW.

SCORESHEET: EXERCISE 7 Answer Key
Stereotyping Symptoms—Vague symptoms

ROLE	SCORE	COMMENT/EXAMPLES
*Helping	1	
Teaching/Coaching	0	
Diagnostic	0	
Monitoring of Intervention	0	
Crisis Intervention	0	
INTERVIEW SKILLS	SCORE	COMMENT/EXAMPLES
*Asks open-ended questions	1	
Concrete data collection/directions	0	
Uses confrontation appropriately	0	
Speaks directly to client	1	
Uses lay language	0	
Restates problem	0	
States working diagnosis	0	
States disclaimer	0	
Elicits hidden agenda	0	
Elicits verbal contract	0	
Uses time frames	0	
Uses protocol	0	Failed to follow protocol directives
DATA COLLECTION SKILLS	SCORE	COMMENT/EXAMPLES
*Age	1	
Symptoms	1	
Characteristics	1	
Course/ADL	1	
History of complaint	0	Failed to elicit history of symptoms in past
Onset of symptoms	1	
Location of symptoms	1	"aches all over"
Altering factors	0	
Pregnant, breastfeeding status	0	
Allergies	0	
Medications	0	
Previous chronic illness	0	
Emotional status	0	
Recent injury, illness, ingestion	0	
Pertinent negatives	0	
TOTAL SCORE	9	

QUESTIONS:

2. *Type of call*—Triage/advice
   Level of call—perceived as mid-level, should have been treated as high-level
   Length of call—less than one minute (very inadequate)
3. *Desired outcome*—prevent further complications
4. *Weaknesses:*
   Client— none
   Practitioner— inadequate data collection and talk time, stereotyping, failed to follow protocol directives: SAVED, signs of infectious process

   Strengths:
   Client— can self-transport
   Practitioner— none
5. *Nature of call management problem*—ineffective assessment skill
6. *Practitioner role(s)*—helping at minimal level
7. *Interpersonal dynamics*—authoritarian approach
8. *Additional or alternative strategies*—adequate time, data collection, elicit significant data, formulate a working diagnosis
9. *Most effective strategy*—follow protocol directives appropriately
10. *Guideline(s) followed*—always obtain age

LISTEN TO THE FOLLOW-UP COMMENTS FOR CASE STUDY 7 NOW.

SCORESHEET: EXERCISE 8 Answer Key Informational/Counseling Call—Teenager with possible AIDS exposure

ROLE	SCORE	COMMENT/EXAMPLES
*Helping	1	
Teaching/Coaching	1	
Diagnostic	1	Assessed risk factors effectively
Monitoring of Intervention	NA-1	
Crisis Intervention	NA-1	
INTERVIEW SKILLS	**SCORE**	**COMMENT/EXAMPLES**
*Asks open-ended questions	1	
Concrete data collection/directions	1	
Uses confrontation appropriately	1	
Speaks directly to client	1	
Uses lay language	1	
Restates problem	1	
States working diagnosis	1	
States disclaimer	NA-1	
Elicits hidden agenda	1	
Elicits verbal contract	1	
Uses time frames	1	
Uses protocol	1	Followed AIDS guidelines
DATA COLLECTION SKILLS	**SCORE**	**COMMENT/EXAMPLES**
*Age	1	
Symptoms	NA-1	
Characteristics	NA-1	
Course/ADL	1	
History of complaint	1	Sexual history
Onset of symptoms	1	Determined when exposure occurred
Location of symptoms	NA-1	
Altering factors	NA-1	
Pregnant, breastfeeding status	1	
Allergies	NA-1	
Medications	1	Elicited recreational drug history
Previous chronic illness	1	Elicted STD history
Emotional status	1	Panic, denial
Recent injury, illness, ingestion	1	Recent exposure to STD possibly AIDS
Pertinent negatives	NA-1	
TOTAL SCORE	32	

QUESTIONS:

2. *Type of call*—informational/referral/counseling
   Level of call—low-level
   Length of call—7–8 minutes (excellent call length)
3. *Desired outcome*—prevent further high-risk behavior, STD, facilitate access to care, facilitate problem ownership, remedy knowledge deficits
4. *Weaknesses:*
   - Client— young age, inarticulate teen, denial, panic, questionable reliability
   - Practitioner— none

   Strengths:
   - Client— demonstrates assertiveness by calling
   - Practitioner— expertise, charisma, sufficient talk time/data collection, remained alert to client denial, used protocol
5. *Nature of call management problem*—none, but had potential for deficit of intervention skill, compliance
6. *Practitioner role(s)*—all except monitoring and crisis intervention
7. *Interpersonal dynamics*—collaborative, anticipatory, authoritarian
8. *Additional or alternative strategies*—none needed, they were all used
9. *Most effective strategy*—microteaching, contracting/compliance
10. *Guideline(s) followed*—always obtain age, err on the side of caution, remain with the caller

LISTEN TO THE FOLLOW-UP COMMENTS FOR CASE STUDY 8 NOW.

FIGURE A.9 EXERCISE 9 ANSWER KEY

ROLE	SCORE	COMMENT/EXAMPLES
*Helping	1	Warmth, empathy
Teaching/Coaching	1	
Diagnostic	1	Used lethality scale appropriately
Monitoring of Intervention	1	Set up alternative plan
Crisis Intervention	1	
INTERVENTION TASKS	SCORE	COMMENT/EXAMPLES
Engaged/focused on feelings	1	
Identified if client is suicidal	1	
Inquired about suicidal ambivalence	1	
Assessed degree of risk	1	
Prevented immediate risk through plan	1	
PREVENTION PLAN	SCORE	COMMENT/EXAMPLES
Specificity—formulated detailed plan of action	1	
Limited objectives—addressed immediate danger	1	
Mutuality—collaborated effectively	1	
Commitment—elicited agreement to plan	1	
Crisis contact—confirmed back-up plan	1	
Follow-up—confirmed follow-up plan	1	
Used protocol	1	
LETHALITY ASSESSMENT	SCORE	COMMENT/EXAMPLES
PREDICTORS		
LACK OF RESOURCES	1	Church, family
PLAN/METHOD	1	Partial plan, no bullets
PRIOR ATTEMPTS	0	
INDICATORS		
Alcohol/drugs	1	Currently sober; Hx of alcoholism
2nd party call	1	Daughter-in-law called initially
Symptoms	1	Depression symptoms
Stress	1	Recent retirement
Sex	1	Male
Age	1	High-risk group
Medical problems:	1	Back pain
Lifestyle	1	Widower
Season/day/place	1	First Christmas alone
SCORE	28	

QUESTIONS:

2. *Type of call*—crisis intervention
   Level of call—high-level
   Length of call—appropriate
3. *Desired outcome*—prevention of death
4. *Weaknesses:*
   - Client— age, possible unreliability
   - Practitioner— none

   Strengths:
   - Client— other adults present
   - Practitioner— charisma, expertise
5. *Nature of call management problem*—none
6. *Practitioner role(s)*—Helping, Diagnostic, Crisis intervention
7. *Interpersonal dynamics*—collaborative, empowering, anticipating
8. *Additional or alternative strategies*—all crisis intervention strategies listed
9. *Most effective strategy (Crisis Intervention)*—remain with the caller
10. *Guideline(s) followed*—remain with the caller

LISTEN TO THE FOLLOW-UP COMMENTS FOR CASE STUDY 9 NOW.

INDEX

www.ingramcontent.com/pod-product-compliance
Lightning Source LLC
Chambersburg PA
CBHW080902220326
41598CB00034B/5445

* 9 7 8 0 9 8 3 0 7 6 9 3 3 *